Atlas of Thyroid Cytopathology

Syed Z. Ali, MD, FRCPath, FIAC
Professor of Pathology and
Radiology
Director of Cytopathology
The Johns Hopkins Hospital
Baltimore, Maryland

Ritu Nayar, MD
Professor of Pathology
Director of Cytopathology
Northwestern University, Feinberg School of
Medicine
Northwestern Memorial Hospital
Chicago, Illinois

Jeffrey F. Krane, MD, PhD
Associate Professor of Pathology
Associate Director, Cytology Division
Chief, Head and Neck Pathology Service
Brigham and Women's Hospital
Harvard Medical School
Boston, Massachusetts

William H. Westra, MD
Professor of Pathology, Oncology and
Otolaryngology-Head & Neck Surgery
Associate Director of Surgical Pathology
The Johns Hopkins Hospital
Baltimore, Maryland

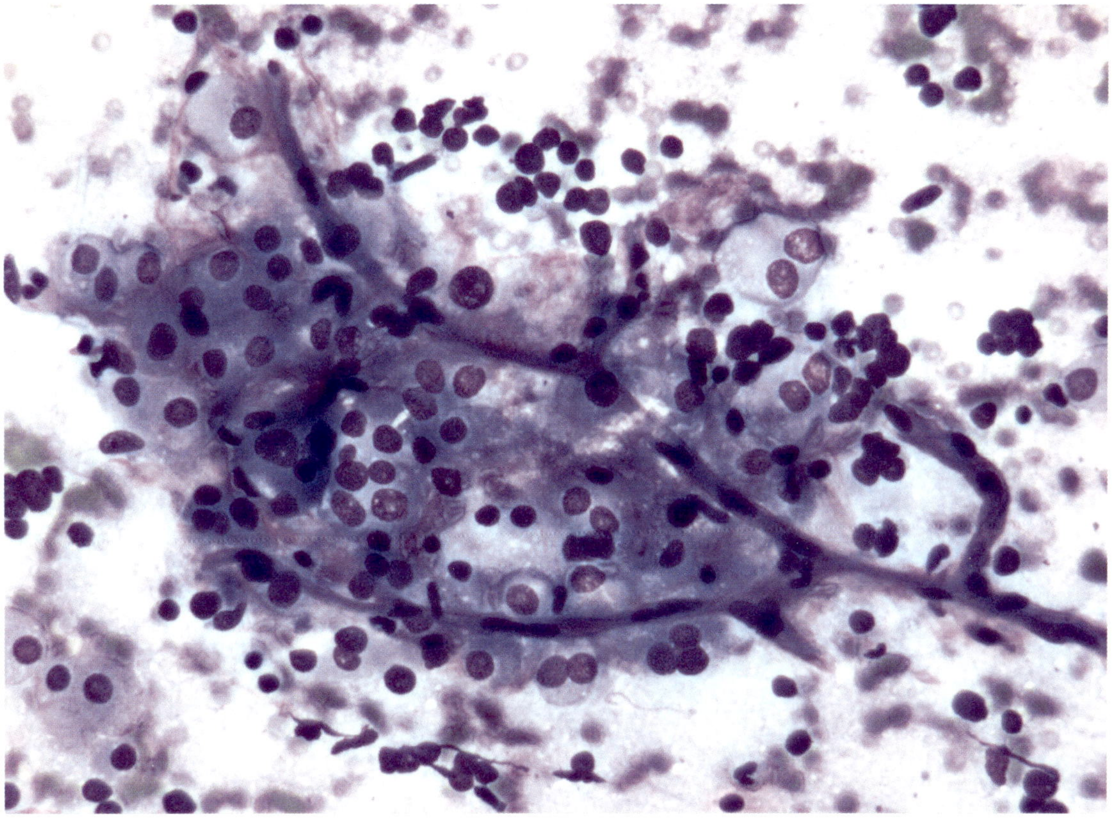

Atlas of Thyroid Cytopathology

With Histopathologic Correlations

demosMEDICAL
New York

Visit our website at www.demosmedpub.com

ISBN: 9781933864952
e-book ISBN: 9781935281498

Acquisitions Editor: Rich Winters
Compositor: diacriTech

Library of Congress Cataloging-in-Publication Data
Ali, Syed Z., author.
Atlas of thyroid cytopathology with histopathologic correlations / by Syed Z. Ali, Ritu Nayar, Jeffrey F. Krane, William H. Westra.
p. ; cm.
Includes bibliographical references and index.
ISBN 978-1-933864-95-2 — ISBN 978-1-935281-49-8 (e-book)
I. Nayar, Ritu, author. II. Krane, Jeffrey F., author. III. Westra, William H., author. IV. Title.
[DNLM: 1. Thyroid Diseases—diagnosis—Atlases. 2. Thyroid Diseases—pathology—Atlases. 3. Cytodiagnosis—Atlases. WK 17]
RC655
616.4'4—dc23

2013025694

Printed in the United States of America by Bradford & Bigelow.
13 14 15 16 17 / 5 4 3 2 1

Contents

Contributors

Zubair W. Baloch, MD, PhD
Professor of Pathology & Laboratory Medicine
Department of Pathology & Laboratory Medicine
Hospital of the University of Pennsylvania
Philadelphia, Pennsylvania

Ulrike M. Hamper, MD, MBA
Professor of Radiology and Pathology
Director of Diagnostic Ultrasound
Department of Radiology and Radiological Science
The Johns Hopkins Hospital
Baltimore, Maryland

Armanda Tatsas, MD
Assistant Professor of Pathology
Division of Cytopathology
The Johns Hopkins Hospital
Baltimore, Maryland

Foreword

With this atlas of thyroid cytopathology and histopathology, Drs. Ali, Nayar, Krane, and Westra have provided a valuable tool for cytologists learning (and continuing to learn) fine needle aspiration (FNA) cytology of the thyroid. The authors beautifully illustrate the wide variety of lesions that can be encountered, from the commonplace benign follicular nodule to the rarest of thyroid neoplasms.

This atlas follows a logical outline, adhering to the categories of The Bethesda System for Reporting Thyroid Cytopathology, widely used in the United States and elsewhere for reporting the results of thyroid aspiration biopsies. This makes the content immediately easy to follow, as the authors weave a path from benign nodules to cases that are atypical or suspicious, ending with unequivocally malignant neoplasms.

The authors include a wide variety of sample preparation methods—smears, liquid-based preparations, and cell blocks—as well as the commonly used stains—Papanicolaou, Romanowsky, and hematoxylin & eosin—providing the reader with the greatest flexibility in recognizing cytomorphologic patterns. Relevant immunocytochemical stains are included for good measure.

Ultimately, however, it is the juxtaposition of histopathologic and cytologic images that makes this book so valuable. In many cases, the caption headings of the cytologic images reflect a retrospective diagnosis based on histologic follow-up. The text is careful to point out, for example, that it is rarely possible to make a definitive diagnosis of a poorly differentiated carcinoma of the thyroid on a fine needle aspiration sample. The same applies to adenomatoid nodules, follicular adenoma, follicular carcinoma, and a variety of other less common entities. Histologic correlation is an excellent teacher, but limitations to cytologic classification remain, and the reader must learn to report cytologic findings using cytologic, not histologic terminology.

This book, with its beautiful images illustrating thyroid cytologic-histologic correlation, provides the ammunition a cytologist needs to master thyroid FNA interpretation.

Edmund S. Cibas, MD
Boston, Massachusetts

Preface

This atlas is published at an exciting time for the diagnosis of thyroid disease by cytopathology. Thyroid fine needle aspiration in conjunction with ultrasonographic imaging has transformed the management of clinically frequent thyroid nodules. More recently, and with significant contributions by the authors of this atlas, The Bethesda System for Reporting Thyroid Cytopathology (TBSRTC), has provided unifying terminology in the United States and elsewhere for the reporting of thyroid aspirates. Among the strengths of TBSRTC framework are the associations of defined risks of malignancy and expected management approaches with each of the six major diagnostic categories.

At the same time, we must acknowledge that there remain significant challenges and limitations in the recognition of thyroid cancer sonographically, cytologically, and histologically. Cytomorphologic evaluation on fine needle aspiration remains to date the initial diagnostic modality of choice for a patient with a thyroid nodule and hence we all have witnessed an "epidemic" of thyroid aspirations in our practices. Surgical follow-up of indeterminate cytologic diagnoses most frequently yields benign histologic outcomes revealing the need for improved triage of patients for surgery. Additionally, the ability to diagnose smaller, incidental thyroid cancers in this typically indolent disease poses important dilemmas about which nodules to image and sample cytologically and in determining who needs surgery, what the extent of surgery should be, and for whom additional treatment, such as radioiodine therapy, is appropriate. Accordingly, there is tremendous interest and excitement regarding the potential role of molecular testing both for resolving diagnostic uncertainty and for refining clinical management. As yet, however, consensus regarding appropriate and cost effective use of this promising tool remains a goal rather than a reality.

Solutions to these difficult questions will require interdisciplinary cooperation amongst endocrinologists, surgeons, radiologists, cytopathologists, and surgical pathologists. This atlas embraces the importance of an interdisciplinary approach and is intended to capture our current state of knowledge for diagnosing thyroid nodules by ultrasound imaging, fine needle aspiration cytology, and gross and histologic evaluation of surgical pathology specimens. It is our sincere hope and belief that the quantity and quality of the images included herein will provide the reader with valuable and practical insights into the current state of the art in this rapidly evolving field and will further enrich the knowledge and learning acquired since the publication of TBSRTC.

Syed Z. Ali
Ritu Nayar
Jeffrey F. Krane
William H. Westra

1

Thyroid Fine Needle Aspiration Biopsy: General Considerations

Zubair W. Baloch

Thyroid nodules are common and have been affecting human kind since ancient times. They can be seen in artworks and artifacts of many cultures. Though, in the current era iodine supplementation has greatly reduced the number of thyroid enlargements, epidemiologic studies have shown the prevalence of palpable thyroid nodules to be approximately 5% in women and 1% in men living in iodine-sufficient parts of the world. In contrast, high resolution ultrasound (US) can detect thyroid nodules in 15% to 67% of the population with higher frequencies in women and the elderly [1–3]. The main purpose of thyroid nodule evaluation is to exclude thyroid cancer which is seen in 5% to 10% of cases requiring surgical intervention. It has been shown that the prevalence of thyroid nodularity and thyroid cancer is related to age, gender, radiation exposure history, family history of thyroid carcinoma in first degree relative, and other factors such as rapid growth and hoarseness [1,4–6]. The follicular cell derived—well-differentiated thyroid cancer, that is, papillary and follicular carcinoma, comprises the vast majority (90%) of all thyroid cancers. According to the recent figures 44,760 new cases of differentiated thyroid cancer were diagnosed in 2010 which resulted in death in 1,690 patients. It is projected that these numbers may be increasing in the future. Furthermore, 2 out of 3 cases are found in people with an age range of 22 to 55 years [7,8].

EVALUATION OF THYROID NODULES

Clinical Evaluation

Thyroid nodule is a discrete lesion within the thyroid gland which appears distinct from the surrounding thyroid parenchyma either by palpation or on ultrasound examination. Most sizeable thyroid nodules are palpable except the ones situated in the posterior aspect of the thyroid lobes. Ultrasound evaluation of the thyroid gland can detect many nonpalpable thyroid nodules of all sizes and shapes; often termed as "incidentalomas." It has been shown that the risk of malignancy is similar between palpable and incidentally discovered thyroid nodules [1,9]. Initially, it was thought that a solitary thyroid nodule is more prone to harbor malignancy as compared to those seen in the setting of multinodular goiter; however, several authors have proven by studying large case cohorts that risk of malignancy is the same in solitary vs. multiple nodules [10,11]. According to the American Thyroid Association the initial evaluation of all patients with thyroid nodules should include serum thyrotropin (TSH) level determination followed by radionuclide imaging if it is suppressed to exclude a hyperfunctioning (AKA hot) nodule [1]. It is prudent that the cytopathologists should be made aware of or obtain this data since the functional status of the thyroid or that of the biopsied nodule affects the cell morphology seen in cytologic specimens. For example evidence of chronic lymphocytic thyroiditis and oncocytic metaplasia in hypothyroid and presence of random nuclear enlargement and atypia in hyperthyroid patients and hyperfunctioning (toxic) nodule(s) [12,13]. The other laboratory tests performed as part of a pre-fine-needle aspiration (FNA) panel include serum thyroglobulin and calcitonin measurements; these are not practiced routinely in the United States.

Ultrasound Evaluation

It is recommended that thyroid ultrasound be performed in all patients found to have solitary or multiple thyroid nodules to define the anatomical detail, structure, and the exact extent and location of true nodule(s) [14–17]. Many clinicians who employ thyroid ultrasound also use it as an adjunct to their physical examination. Multiple nodules palpated in Hashimoto thyroiditis may not correlate with the nodule reported on ultrasound thus avoiding biopsy of multiple nodules. The ultrasound features that are suspicious for malignancy include micro-calcifications, marked hypo-echogenicity, an irregular or micro-lobulated margin, a longitudinal dimension larger than the cross sectional dimension, intrinsic vascularity, and direct tumor invasion of adjacent tissue. Neck ultrasound in patients with suspicious thyroid nodules can be helpful in detection of abnormal vs. benign lymph nodes to assess the extent of disease for proper surgical management [15,18,19]. Though ultrasound is more sensitive than clinical and laboratory evaluation of a patient with nodular enlargement of the thyroid it is a poor predictor of malignancy. For example, hypoechoic thyroid nodules are more likely to be malignant; however, most benign nodules are also hypoechoic [14,15].

At present besides its few aforementioned uses ultrasound is commonly employed to guide the FNA biopsy needle to obtain adequate diagnostic material from a thyroid nodule.

Fine-Needle Aspiration Biopsy

Fine-needle aspiration biopsy (FNAB) of the thyroid has now been established as reliable and safe and has become an integral part in the management of thyroid nodules. Based on the examination of a few groups of cells it can effectively triage cases which require clinical or surgical follow-up.

Procedure

Thyroid FNAB can be performed manually by palpation or employing ultrasound guidance. It is recommended that FNAB is performed by a clinician, radiologist, or pathologist who is proficient/experienced in thyroid FNAB [20]. The use of ultrasound guidance ensures that the sample is obtained from the nodule in question and allows directing the needle into the solid portions of a complex solid and cystic nodule, thus improving the diagnostic yield [14,20]. The specimen should be obtained by using either a 25 or 27-gauge needle which can be either attached or not (non-aspiration technique) to a syringe; however, the former method is the most favored one. The correlation between the gauge of the needle and the cellularity of the specimen has been discussed in the literature [21]. A higher rate of specimen adequacy has been reported with a thinner gauge needle. Various studies have compared FNAB of thyroid by employing aspiration and non-aspiration (capillary action) techniques. Some authors have shown no difference between the two sampling techniques while others have reported a higher rate of adequacy with non-aspiration technique. In any event this is highly dependent upon the preference and experience of the operator with either technique [21–24]. Multiple passes in a thyroid nodule may not prove to be useful in acquiring adequate cellularity as thyroid nodules are inherently vascular and lead to increased bleeding resulting in diluted specimen [22,25].

Specimen

It is well understood that the precise and management based cytologic diagnosis is highly dependent upon an adequate specimen with well-preserved cellular details. Therefore, regardless of the cytologic preparation, that is, smears, cytospins, monolayer preps, and cell block, an adequate and well-preserved thyroid FNAB specimen is important for rendering cytologic interpretation [26–29]. Many experts have proposed various criteria for cell adequacy in thyroid FNAB specimens [30–33]; it is well understood that these criteria of adequacy apply to solid nodules, solid and cystic nodules and not to cystic nodules with no solid component on ultrasound evaluation. The most commonly used criterion for specimen adequacy is: six to eight groups of follicular cells with 10 to 20 cells per group on two different slides. Adequate cellularity of a thyroid FNAB specimen reflects adequate and representative sampling of the nodule; granted, this is highly operator dependent [33]. In my experience an adequate and representative thyroid FNAB specimen is acquired by using ultrasound-guidance and making sure that the biopsy needle samples multiple rather than one portion of the nodule.

On-Site Evaluation

The on-site evaluation of thyroid FNAB specimens with performance of rapid stains leads to adequate specimens and lessens nondiagnostic rates; however, this may not be possible in all clinical settings. The clinical utility of the on-site assessment of thyroid FNA is similar to the interpretation of frozen sections in surgical pathology. A number of questions can be answered by on-site evaluation, which include adequacy of specimen, classification of lesion, primary vs. metastatic, and if additional studies are needed (flow cytometry, serum calcitonin measurements to rule out medullary carcinoma and molecular studies) [25,34,35].

The number of on-site smears should be kept low, 2 to 3 smears/pass; they can be air dried for Romanowsky stain or fixed in 95% alcohol or spray fixed for Papanicolaou stain. The Romanowsky staining method is one of the best available methods for immediate evaluation of FNA specimens; however, some authors have proposed the rapid Papanicolaou staining method. Papanicolaou stain is vital to the diagnosis of thyroid lesion. It effectively highlights the nuclear details and alterations (grooves and inclusions), which are crucial for the diagnosis of papillary thyroid carcinoma. It also is helpful in the diagnosis of Hürthle cell and C-cell lesions. If one is not providing on-site assessment then an FNAB specimen can be placed into an appropriate medium for monolayer preparation (ThinPrep®, SurePath®, etc.) or other concentration techniques and preparations [25].

It is well established now that molecular testing can serve to further refine the cytologic interpretation. Therefore, a portion or an entire thyroid FNAB pass maybe processed for molecular diagnosis. This is highly dependent upon the molecular test(s). In case of BRAF mutational analysis DNA can be extracted from the FNAB material in routinely air-dried smears or left-over needle rinse, however, mutational analysis for multiple genes will require a dedicated FNAB pass stored at –80°C [36].

Core Needle Biopsy

Although, FNAB is the most commonly employed method for obtaining diagnostic material from a thyroid nodule, in some cases it may not yield sufficient diagnostic material even with multiple passes and repeat procedures. It has been shown that core biopsy (18–20 gauge needle) can increase the diagnostic yield by 10% as compared to FNA. The core biopsy does provide a large amount of histologic material to be examined for evaluation of cytologic as well as architectural features; however, the success of this procedure is highly dependent upon the operator being well versed in this procedure as there is also an increased risk of complications such as hematoma formation [25, 37, 38].

DIAGNOSTIC CLASSIFICATION

Thyroid FNA specimens are usually classified by employing a tiered system. Several classification schemes have been proposed by various authors based on personal/institutional experiences. In 2007, the National Cancer Institute hosted a two day state of the art scientific meeting regarding thyroid fine needle aspiration. The participants included endocrinologists, radiologists, surgeons, and pathologists. This meeting led to various position statements on the selection of patients for thyroid biopsy, handling of thyroid FNA specimens, and their cytopathologic diagnosis. At this conference many participants agreed to a six-tiered scheme for classifying thyroid FNA's (Table 1.1). Each diagnostic category was assigned a risk

Table 1.1 — The Bethesda System for Reporting Thyroid Cytopathology: Implied Risk of Malignancy and Recommended Clinical Management [39,40,41]

Diagnostic Category	Risk of Malignancy (%)	Usual Management
Nondiagnostic or unsatisfactory		Repeat FNA with ultrasound guidance
Benign	0%–3%	Clinical follow-up
Atypia of undetermined significance or follicular lesion of undetermined significance	~5%–15%	Repeat FNA
Follicular neoplasm or suspicious for a follicular neoplasm	15%–30%	Surgical lobectomy
Suspicious for malignancy	60%–75%	Near-total thyroidectomy or surgical lobectomy
Malignant	97%–99%	Near-total thyroidectomy

of malignancy based on literature review along with recommendations for management. It is also recommended that for some of the diagnostic categories, some degree of sub categorization can be informative and is often appropriate. Additional descriptive comments (beyond such sub categorization) are optional and left to the discretion of the cytopathologist [39,42]).

The brief description of the diagnostic categories in the Bethesda Classification is as follows:

I. **Nondiagnostic or Unsatisfactory:**

a. This diagnostic category applies to specimens which are nondiagnostic due to limited cellularity, no follicular cells and adequate specimens which are uniterpretable due to poor fixation and preservation, that is, obliteration of cellular details.

b. In some cases of solid nodules it may be prudent to process and examine the entire specimen.

c. It is recommended that solid nodules with repeat nondiagnostic FNA results should be excised because malignancy is eventually diagnosed in about 9% of such cases.

II. **Benign:**

a. The reported rate of malignancy for this diagnostic category is 0% to 3%

b. The diagnostic terms in this category include, but are not limited to, nodular goiter, hyperplastic/adenomatoid nodule in goiter, chronic lymphocytic thyroiditis and sub-acute thyroiditis.

c. A thyroid nodule with a benign diagnosis should be followed periodically by US examination; a repeat FNA may be considered if the nodule increases in size (as per American Thyroid Association (ATA) guidelines the increase should be in 20% in two dimensions of the nodule; and that of solid component in case of cystic nodules).

III. **Atypia of undetermined significance/Follicular lesion of undetermined significance (AUS/FLUS):**

a. The literature review of the large cases series published after Bethedsa classification scheme shows that this represents a heterogeneous diagnostic category (a true Gray Zone). The reported malignancy risk for cases diagnosed as such in these studies ranges from 6% to 48% [43–45].

b. It is recommended that the number of cases diagnosed as such should be kept to a minimum; 7% of the total diagnoses. The question arises what can serve as a guide for keeping the AUS/FLUS diagnosis in an acceptable range. One obvious answer is to use the AUS/FLUS:malignant diagnoses ratio similar to ASCUS:SIL ratio in cervical cytology, however, this needs to be proven by independent studies from multiple institutions.

c. It is optional to describe the reason(s) for AUS/FLUS diagnosis. Some authors have shown that subclassifying this diagnosis further stratifies the risk of malignancy for this diagnostic catergory.

d. It has been shown that repeat FNA is effective in arriving at definite management based diagnosis in thyroid nodules initially diagnosed as indeterminate. Therefore, repeat FNA should be recommended in cases diagnosed as AUS/FLUS. It is clearly evident that repeat fine needle aspiration (RFNA) has a definite role in the management of patients with thyroid nodules diagnosed as FLUS/AUS.

IV. **Follicular/follicular neoplasm with oncocytic features (AKA Hürthle cell) neoplasm or suspicious for follicular or follicular neoplasm with oncocytic features (AKA Hürthle cell) neoplasm:**

a. These diagnostic terms encompasses both benign and malignant tumors; that is, follicular adenoma and carcinoma and oncocytic follicular adenoma and carcinoma. The cytologic diagnosis of "neoplasm" reflects the limitations of thyroid cytology, since the diagnosis of follicular carcinoma is only based on the demonstration of capsular and/or vascular invasion. Several authors have shown that, at most, only 20% to 30% of cases diagnosed as "follicular neoplasm" are diagnosed as malignant on histological examination and the rest are either follicular adenomas or cellular adenomatoid nodules, that is, benign.

b. Several studies have shown that half or more of the malignant cases diagnosed as follicular neoplasm or suspicious for follicular neoplasm (FON/SFN) are found to be follicular variant of papillary thyroid carcinoma (FVPC) on surgical excision. It is well-known that the surgical pathology diagnosis of FVPC (the so called "Gold Standard") can be problematic even for experts due to multifocal rather than diffuse distribution of nuclear features of papillary carcinoma. Thus, the sampling of the areas lacking diagnostic nuclear features is the main reason for the under-diagnosis of these cases as SFN/FON.

V. **Suspicious for malignancy:**

a. This term includes suspicious for: papillary carcinoma (malignancy risk 60%–75%), medullary carcinoma, other malignancies, lymphoma (flow cytometry can be recommended with repeat FNA), metastatic carcinoma/secondary tumor and carcinoma (includes poorly differentiated and anaplastic carcinoma).

VI. **Malignant:**

a. The thyroid FNA cases diagnosed as such carry a 97% to 100% risk of malignancy. The malignant tumors of the thyroid diagnosed on FNA include: papillary carcinoma and variants, medullary carcinoma, poorly differentiated carcinoma, anaplastic carcinoma, metastatic carcinoma (with immunohistochemistry), and lymphoma (combined with flow cytometry).

Bethesda Thyroid FNA Classification Across Atlantic

The United Kingdom Royal College of Pathologists has recommended a tiered diagnostic classification scheme based on the similar needs which led to the formulation of Bethesda Thyroid FNA Classification. Basically, this scheme has adopted all the diagnostic categories with altered names to incorporate the "British Thy terminology" designations. This has also led the European cytopathologists to consider the need for a standard scheme for reporting thyroid FNA specimens similar to Bethesda terminology. Therefore, it is not bold to forecast that in the near future Bethesda terminology or ones similar to it will be adapted to meet the needs of diagnosing thyroid nodules in different parts of the world [46,47].

Reflex Molecular Testing of Thyroid FNAB Specimens

Similar to other organ systems new perspectives for reclassification and diagnosis of thyroid tumors especially papillary and follicular carcinoma have emerged based on identification of somatic mutations. At present there is a dearth of information regarding molecular analyses of thyroid FNA specimens for BRAF gene mutation, RET/PTC translocation, PAX8-PPRA-gamma, and RAS-gene mutations. As mentioned previously thyroid FNA cannot differentiate between follicular adenoma and carcinoma and in this a majority of FNA samples obtained from follicular variant of papillary carcinoma are classified as follicular neoplasm or suspicious for papillary thyroid carcinoma due to paucity of the diagnostic features. Based on the molecular data available several authors have used one or all of the above-mentioned markers to diagnose papillary and follicular thyroid carcinoma in FNA specimens. These studies have shown much promise with high positive predictive value of malignancy. This role of molecular markers as an adjunct to the cytopathologic diagnosis of thyroid nodules is growing at a speedy rate. Therefore, "reflex" molecular testing of thyroid FNA specimens diagnosed as AUS/FLUS, FON/SFN, and suspicious for papillary carcinoma is considered as standard practice by many laboratories [48–51].

REFERENCES

1. Cooper DS, Doherty GM, Haugen BR, et al. Revised American thyroid association management guidelines for patients with thyroid nodules and differentiated thyroid cancer. *Thyroid.* 2009;19:1167–1214.
2. Baloch ZW, LiVolsi VA. Fine-needle aspiration of thyroid nodules: past, present, and future. *Endocr Pract.* 2004;10: 234–241.
3. Henrichsen TL, Reading CC. Thyroid ultrasonography. Part 2: nodules. *Radiol Clin North Am.* 2011;49:417–424, v.
4. Mazzaferri EL, de los Santos ET, Rofagha-Keyhani S. Solitary thyroid nodule: diagnosis and management. *Med Clin North Am.* 1988;72:1177–1211.

5. Mazzaferri EL. Solitary thyroid nodule. 2. Selective approach to management. *Postgrad Med.* 1981;70:107–109, 112, 116.
6. Gonzalez-Gonzalez A, Mate-Valdezate A, Parra-Arroyo A, Tenias-Burillo JM. New guidelines for the management of thyroid nodules and differentiated thyroid cancer. *Minerva Endocrinologica.* 2011;36:7–12.
7. Yu GP, Li JC, Branovan D, McCormick S, Schantz SP. Thyroid cancer incidence and survival in the national cancer institute surveillance, epidemiology, and end results race/ethnicity groups. *Thyroid.* 2010;20:465–473.
8. Wartofsky L. Increasing world incidence of thyroid cancer: increased detection or higher radiation exposure? *Hormones (Athens).* 2010;9:103–108.
9. Moon HJ, Son E, Kim EK, Yoon JH, Kwak JY. The diagnostic values of ultrasound and ultrasound-guided fine needle aspiration in subcentimeter-sized thyroid nodules. *Ann Surg Oncol.* 2012;19:52–59.
10. Barroeta JE, Wang H, Shiina N, Gupta PK, Livolsi VA, Baloch ZW. Is fine-needle aspiration (FNA) of multiple thyroid nodules justified? *Endocr Pathol.* 2006;17:61–65.
11. Frates MC, Benson CB, Doubilet PM, et al. Prevalence and distribution of carcinoma in patients with solitary and multiple thyroid nodules on sonography. *J Clin Endocrinol Metab.* 2006;91:3411–3417.
12. Khayyata S, Barroeta JE, LiVolsi VA, Baloch ZW. Papillary hyperplastic nodule: pitfall in the cytopathologic diagnosis of papillary thyroid carcinoma. *Endocr Pract.* 2008;14:863–868.
13. Baloch Z, LiVolsi VA. Diagnostic dilemmas in thyroid pathology: follicualr variant of papillary thyroid carcinoma and classic papillary thyroid carcinoma arising in lymphocytic thyroiditis. *Pathol Case Rev.* 2003;8:47–56.
14. Moon WJ, Baek JH, Jung SL, et al. Ultrasonography and the ultrasound-based management of thyroid nodules: consensus statement and recommendations. *Korean J Radiol.* 2011;12:1–14.
15. Shapiro RS. Management of thyroid nodules detected at sonography: society of radiologists in ultrasound consensus conference statement. *Thyroid.* 2006;16:209–210.
16. Frates MC, Benson CB, Charboneau JW, et al. Management of thyroid nodules detected at US: Society of Radiologists in Ultrasound consensus conference statement. *Ultrasound Q.* 2006;22:231–238; discussion 239–240
17. Frates MC, Benson CB, Charboneau JW, et al. Management of thyroid nodules detected at US: Society of Radiologists in Ultrasound consensus conference statement. *Radiology.* 2005;237:794–800.
18. Rago T, Di Coscio G, Basolo F, et al. Combined clinical, thyroid ultrasound and cytological features help to predict thyroid malignancy in follicular and Hürthle cell thyroid lesions: results from a series of 505 consecutive patients. *Clin Endocrinol.* 2007;66:13–20.
19. Marqusee E, Benson CB, Frates MC, et al. Usefulness of ultrasonography in the management of nodular thyroid disease. *Ann Intern Med.* 2000;133:696–700.
20. Gharib H, Papini E, Valcavi R, et al. American Association of Clinical Endocrinologists and Associazione Medici Endocrinologi medical guidelines for clinical practice for the diagnosis and management of thyroid nodules. *Endocr Pract.* 2006;12:63–102.
21. Cappelli C, Pirola I, Gandossi E, De Martino E, Agosti B, Castellano M. Fine-needle aspiration cytology of thyroid nodule: does the needle matter? *South Med J.* 2009;102(5):498–501.
22. Carpi A, Di Coscio G, Iervasi G, et al. Thyroid fine needle aspiration: how to improve clinicians' confidence and performance with the technique. *Cancer Lett.* 2008;264:163–171.
23. Carpi A, Ferrari E, Sagripanti A, et al. Aspiration needle biopsy refines preoperative diagnosis of thyroid nodules defined at fine needle aspiration as microfollicular nodule. *Biomed Pharmacother.* 1996;50:325–328.
24. Carpi A, Ferrari E, Toni MG, Sagripanti A, Nicolini A, Di Coscio G. Needle aspiration techniques in preoperative selection of patients with thyroid nodules: a long-term study. *J Clin Oncol.* 1996;14:1704–1712.
25. Pitman MB, Abele J, Ali SZ, et al. Techniques for thyroid FNA: a synopsis of the National Cancer Institute Thyroid Fine-Needle Aspiration State of the Science Conference. *Diagn Cytopathol.* 2008;36:407–424.
26. Baloch ZW, LiVolsi VA. Fine-needle aspiration of the thyroid: today and tomorrow. *Best Pract Res.* 2008;22:929–939.
27. Baloch ZW, Tam D, Langer J, Mandel S, LiVolsi VA, Gupta PK. Ultrasound-guided fine-needle aspiration biopsy of the thyroid: role of on-site assessment and multiple cytologic preparations. *Diagn Cytopathol.* 2000;23:425–429.
28. Tulecke MA, Wang HH. ThinPrep for cytologic evaluation of follicular thyroid lesions: correlation with histologic findings. *Diagn Cytopathol.* 2004;30:7–13.
29. Malle D, Valeri RM, Pazaitou-Panajiotou K, Kiziridou A, Vainas I, Destouni C. Use of a thin-layer technique in thyroid fine needle aspiration. *Acta Cytol.* 2006;50:23–27.
30. Kini SR, Miller JM, Hamburger JI. Cytopathology of thyroid nodules. *Henry Ford Hosp Med J.* 1982;30:17–24.

31. Oertel YC, Burman K, Boyle L, et al. Integrating fine-needle aspiration into a daily practice involving thyroid disorders: the Washington Hospital Center approach. *Diagn Cytopathol.* 2002;27:120–122.
32. Hamburger JI. Fine needle biopsy diagnosis of thyroid nodules. Perspective. *Thyroidology.* 1988 Apr;(1):21–34
33. Goellner JR, Gharib H, Grant CS, Johnson DA. Fine needle aspiration cytology of the thyroid. *Acta Cytol.* 1987;31:587–590.
34. Redman R, Zalaznick H, Mazzaferri EL, Massoll NA. The impact of assessing specimen adequacy and number of needle passes for fine-needle aspiration biopsy of thyroid nodules. *Thyroid.* 2006;16:55–60.
35. Ghofrani M, Beckman D, Rimm DL. The value of onsite adequacy assessment of thyroid fine-needle aspirations is a function of operator experience. *Cancer.* 2006;108:110–113.
36. Ferraz C, Eszlinger M, Paschke R. Current state and future perspective of molecular diagnosis of fine-needle aspiration biopsy of thyroid nodules. *J Clin Endocrinol Metab.* 2011;96:2016–2026.
37. Park KT, Ahn SH, Mo JH, et al. Role of core needle biopsy and ultrasonographic finding in management of indeterminate thyroid nodules. *Head Neck.* 2011;33:160–165.
38. Zhang S, Ivanovic M, Nemcek AA Jr, Defrias DV, Lucas E, Nayar R. Thin core needle biopsy crush preparations in conjunction with fine-needle aspiration for the evaluation of thyroid nodules: a complementary approach. *Cancer.* 2008;114:512–518.
39. Cibas ES, Ali SZ. The Bethesda system for reporting thyroid cytopathology. *Thyroid.* 2009;19:1159–1165.
40. Ali SZ. Thyroid cytopathology: Bethesda and beyond. *Acta Cytol.* 2011;55:4–12.
41. Baloch ZW, Cibas ES, Clark DP, et al. The National Cancer Institute Thyroid fine needle aspiration state of the science conference: a summation. *Cytojournal.* 2008;5:6
42. Baloch ZW, LiVolsi VA, Asa SL, et al. Diagnostic terminology and morphologic criteria for cytologic diagnosis of thyroid lesions: a synopsis of the National Cancer Institute Thyroid Fine-Needle Aspiration State of the Science Conference. *Diagn Cytopathol.* 2008;36:425–437.
43. Faquin WC, Baloch ZW. Fine-needle aspiration of follicular patterned lesions of the thyroid: Diagnosis, management, and follow-up according to National Cancer Institute (NCI) recommendations. *Diagn Cytopathol.* 2010;38:731–739.
44. Layfield LJ, Morton MJ, Cramer HM, Hirschowitz S. Implications of the proposed thyroid fine-needle aspiration category of "follicular lesion of undetermined significance": A five-year multi-institutional analysis. *Diagn Cytopathol.* 2009;37(10):710–714.
45. Nayar R, Ivanovic M. The indeterminate thyroid fine-needle aspiration: experience from an academic center using terminology similar to that proposed in the 2007 National Cancer Institute Thyroid Fine Needle Aspiration State of the Science Conference. *Cancer Cytopathol.* 2009;117(3):195–202.
46. Cross PA, Poller D. The Bethesda thyroid terminology and progress towards international agreement on thyroid FNA cytology reporting. *Cytopathology.* 2010;21:71–74.
47. Kocjan G, Chandra A, Cross PA, et al. The interobserver reproducibility of thyroid fine-needle aspiration using the UK Royal College of Pathologists' classification system. *Am J Clin Pathol.* 2011;135:852–859.
48. Nikiforov YE, Steward DL, Robinson-Smith TM, et al. Molecular testing for mutations in improving the fine-needle aspiration diagnosis of thyroid nodules. *J Clin Endocrinol Metab.* 2009;94:2092–2098.
49. Cantara S, Capezzone M, Marchisotta S, et al. Impact of proto-oncogene mutation detection in cytological specimens from thyroid nodules improves the diagnostic accuracy of cytology. *J Clin Endocrinol Metab.* 2010;95:1365–1369.
50. Wang CC, Friedman L, Kennedy GC, et al. A large multicenter correlation study of thyroid nodule cytopathology and histopathology. *Thyroid.* 2011;21:243–251.
51. Xing M, Tufano RP, Tufaro AP, et al. Detection of BRAF mutation on fine needle aspiration biopsy specimens: a new diagnostic tool for papillary thyroid cancer. *J Clin Endocrinol Metab.* 2004;89:2867–2872.

2

Radiologic Characteristics of Thyroid Disease

Ulrike M. Hamper

High-resolution ultrasonography (7.5–15MHz) with gray-scale and Color Doppler Ultrasound (CDUS) is ideally suited for the evaluation of normal thyroid anatomy and pathologic conditions. This technique has become increasingly utilized for the diagnosis of nodular and diffuse thyroid disease. In this chapter we will review the sonographic characteristics of the normal gland, and present examples of diffuse and nodular thyroid disease, normal and abnormal lymph nodes (LNs), and examples of fine needle aspiration biopsies (FNABs).

NORMAL THYROID GLAND

The thyroid parenchyma demonstrates a homogeneous, medium to high-level echogenicity, which makes detection of focal cystic, or hypoechoic nodules relatively obvious. The esophagus is seen laterally and posterior to the left lobe of the gland, not to be mistaken for a focal thyroid nodule. It will demonstrate the target appearance of bowel signature and demonstrates peristalsis during swallowing.

DIFFUSE THYROID DISEASE

The ultrasound (US) appearance of Hashimoto lymphocytic thyroiditis and Graves disease is fairly classical. In addition, US is useful to exclude other pathologies in those patients such as thyroid nodules, thyroid malignancies, and lymphoma. In Graves' disease serial US monitoring has been useful to monitor therapy and assess size and vascularity of the gland.

US Findings in Hashimoto Lymphocytic Thyroiditis

The gland may be normal in size or enlarged with either a hypoechoic or heterogeneous echotexture, demonstrating lobular margins and echogenic fibrous strands. Microlobulations giving a microlobular pattern can be seen. In the active stage the thyroid gland may be hypervascular on Color Doppler Ultrasound (CDUS). In end-stage disease the gland will become atrophic and hypo- or avascular.

US Findings in Graves Disease

The gland is usually diffusely enlarged and hypoechoic without focal nodules. Sometimes the echotexture is more heterogeneous. Hypervascularity on CDUS is characteristic and has been referred to as the "thyroid inferno."

MULTINODULAR GOITER

The gland is usually heterogeneously enlarged and contains multiple nodules of varying size and echotexture. Most nodules are iso- or hypoechoic. Degenerative changes of goitrous nodules may occur and correspond to their sonographic appearance. Nodules may contain anechoic areas caused by colloid or serous fluid. Hemorrhage into a nodule may cause echogenic fluid or fluid-debris levels. Bright echogenic foci with "comet-tail" artifacts in cystic or hypoechoic nodules are most often due to microcrystals and typical for colloid nodules. Calcifications may occur in a central or peripheral location and appear punctate (microcalcifications) or coarse (macrocalcifications). They can be seen with benign or malignant nodules and such nodules should be further evaluated with FNAB. Likewise intracystic solid projection or papillary, particularly when containing flow on CDUS, are more worrisome for malignancy and should be aspirated. The role of US in evaluating a patient with multinodular goiter is to monitor the size of the gland and nodules and to evaluate for dominant or suspicious nodules, which require FNAB.

NORMAL CERVICAL LNs

Normal LNs are oval in shape, demonstrate an echogenic, fatty hilum, have a symmetric hypoechoic cortex and often show a central feeding vessel.

MALIGNANT CERVICAL LNs

Malignant LNs are usually round in shape—"taller than wide," with a loss of the echogenic, fatty hilum. They may be diffusely hypoechoic or demonstrate an asymmetric, lobulated cortex. In addition, they might contain calcifications, irregular vascularity or have a cystic appearance. Sometimes, however, there can be an overlap in appearance with reactive LNs.

BENIGN THYROID NODULES—SONOGRAPHIC FEATURES

These include thyroid cysts or cystic nodules, complex nodules with cystic spaces separated by thin septations in a honeycomb pattern, and cystic or hypoechoic nodules with tiny echogenic foci with "comet-tail" or "ring-down" artifact. These nodules usually do not need FNAB.

WORRISOME/MALIGNANT THYROID NODULES—SONOGRAPHIC FEATURES

Nodules with a hypoechoic echotexture, irregular margins, micro- or macrocalcifications as well as irregular vascular patterns and abnormal LNs have a higher chance of malignancy and should undergo FNAB.

THYROID LESION: "HALO" SIGN

The presence of a thin halo is more suggestive of a benign lesion; however, the thickness cannot reliably distinguish benign from malignant nodules.

THYROID VASCULARITY—PERIPHERAL VERSUS CENTRAL

The presence of peripheral vascularity is more suggestive of a benign nodule, whereas irregular central vascularity is more commonly seen in malignant nodules. However, overlap in the vascular distribution does occur and the vascular pattern cannot reliably differentiate benign from malignant lesions.

THYROID LESION—PERIPHERAL EGGSHELL CALCIFICATIONS

Although this feature usually indicates a higher probability of a benign nodule, it can also be seen in malignant lesions.

PAPILLARY THYROID CARCINOMA—SONOGRAPHIC APPEARANCE

Most lesions (about 90% of cases) demonstrate a hypoechoic appearance with irregular margins and microcalcifications, often without shadowing. On CDUS the majority of lesions demonstrate hypervascularity, often in an irregular pattern. Associated cervical lymphadenopathy, most commonly in the caudal portion of the deep jugular chain is frequently associated. The abnormal LNs may contain punctate microcalcifications or even demonstrate cystic changes due to extensive degeneration.

FOLLICULAR NEOPLASMS: ADENOMA/CARCINOMA

Sonographically, follicular adenomas are typically solid lesions, hyper- iso- or hypoechoic in appearance. They are commonly well marginated, often containing a thin hypoechoic halo. Central linear hypoechoic striations or areas may be present. However, their sonographic appearance is indistinguishable from follicular carcinoma. FNAB also cannot reliably distinguish follicular adenoma from carcinoma and these lesions usually are surgically removed.

MEDULLARY THYROID CARCINOMA

The sonographic appearance of medullary carcinoma can be similar to papillary thyroid carcinoma. The lesions are often solid and slightly hypoechoic, isoechoic, or heterogeneous and tend to be larger lesions. They often contain calcifications, which are coarser and larger than the typical microcalcifications seen in papillary carcinoma. However, (macro- or micro-) calcifications can also be seen in both the primary tumor and LN metastases.

ANAPLASTIC THYROID CARCINOMA—SONOGRAPHIC APPEARANCE

Anaplastic carcinomas are commonly large solid tumors presenting as rapidly enlarging masses extending beyond the thyroid gland and invading adjacent structures such as soft tissues, muscles, and the trachea. Associated lymphadenopathy is frequently seen. These tumors are often inadequately examined by US due to their large size.

THYROID LYMPHOMA

Sonographically the lesions are large and solid, hypoechoic or heterogeneous masses infiltrating the thyroid parenchyma, and sometimes engulfing the trachea.

THYROID METASTASES

The most common primary malignancies metastatic to the thyroid gland are lung cancer, breast cancer, renal cell cancer, and multiple myeloma. Metastases do not have a characteristic US appearance. One can suspect a metastasis if there is a solid nodule on US, which may be PET (Position Emission Tomography) positive in patients with primary extrathyroidal malignancy.

US SCREENING FOR RECURRENCE IN THE NECK LNs

US screening is now routinely performed after thyroidectomy in patients presenting with elevated serum thyroglobulin levels or abnormal nuclear medicine iodine scans.

FNAB

US is ideally suited to guide FNABs of focal thyroid nodules or abnormal cervical LNs. Post biopsy complications such as hematomas are rare, however, can easily be demonstrated and the extent assessed with US.

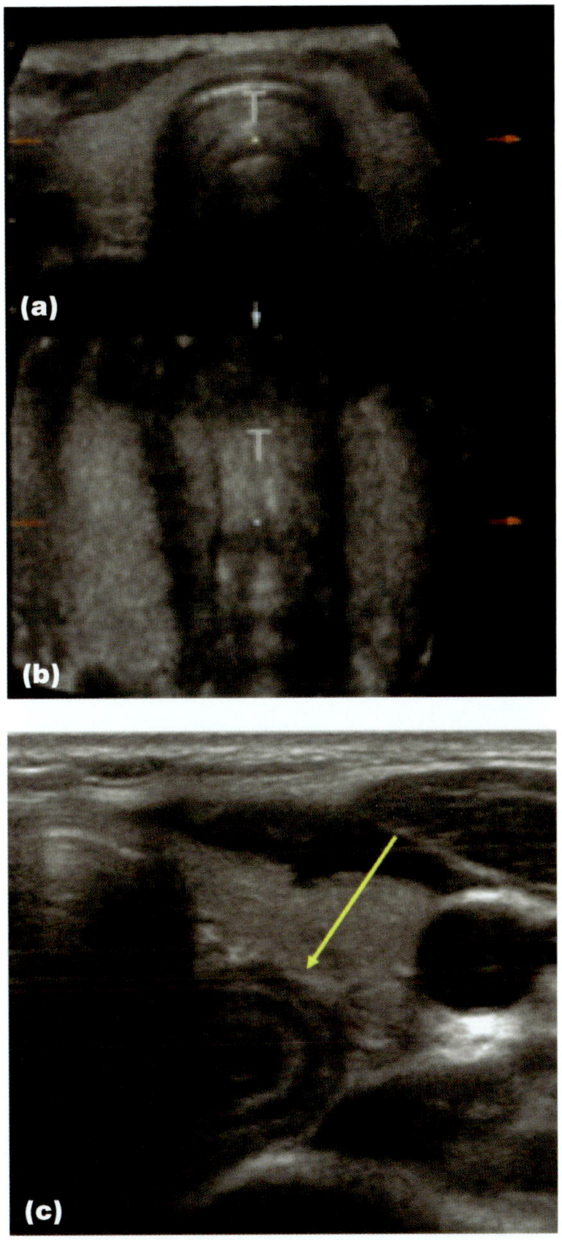

Figure 2.1 — Normal Thyroid Anatomy. Transverse images of both thyroid lobes. (a) The right and left thyroid lobes are symmetric in size and demonstrate a homogeneous echotexture. Normal measurements are 4 to 5 cm in length, 2 cm in anterior-posterior, and 1 to 2 cm in traverse diameter. The isthmus connects the lobes anterior to the trachea (T) and measures ≤5 mm. (b) Three-dimensional reconstruction demonstrates the coronal view of both lobes on either side of the trachea (T). (c) The esophagus is seen in the left para/retrotracheal area (arrow) demonstrating the typical gut signature and peristaltic movement during swallowing.

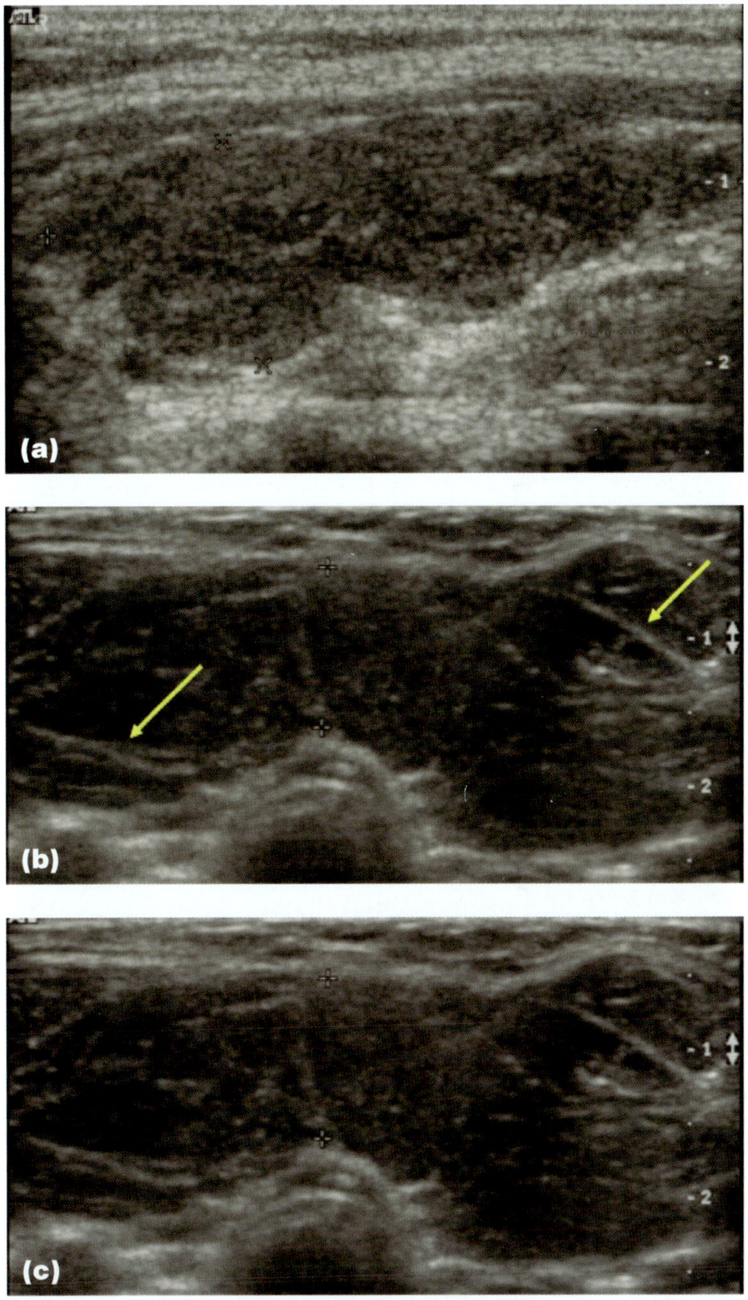

Figure 2.2 — Hashimoto Thyroiditis. (a) Sagittal image of the gland demonstrates an enlarged thyroid with lobular margins and microlobulations (between calipers). (b) Echogenic septae can be seen traversing the gland (arrows). (c) An enlarged isthmus (between calipers) is demonstrated.

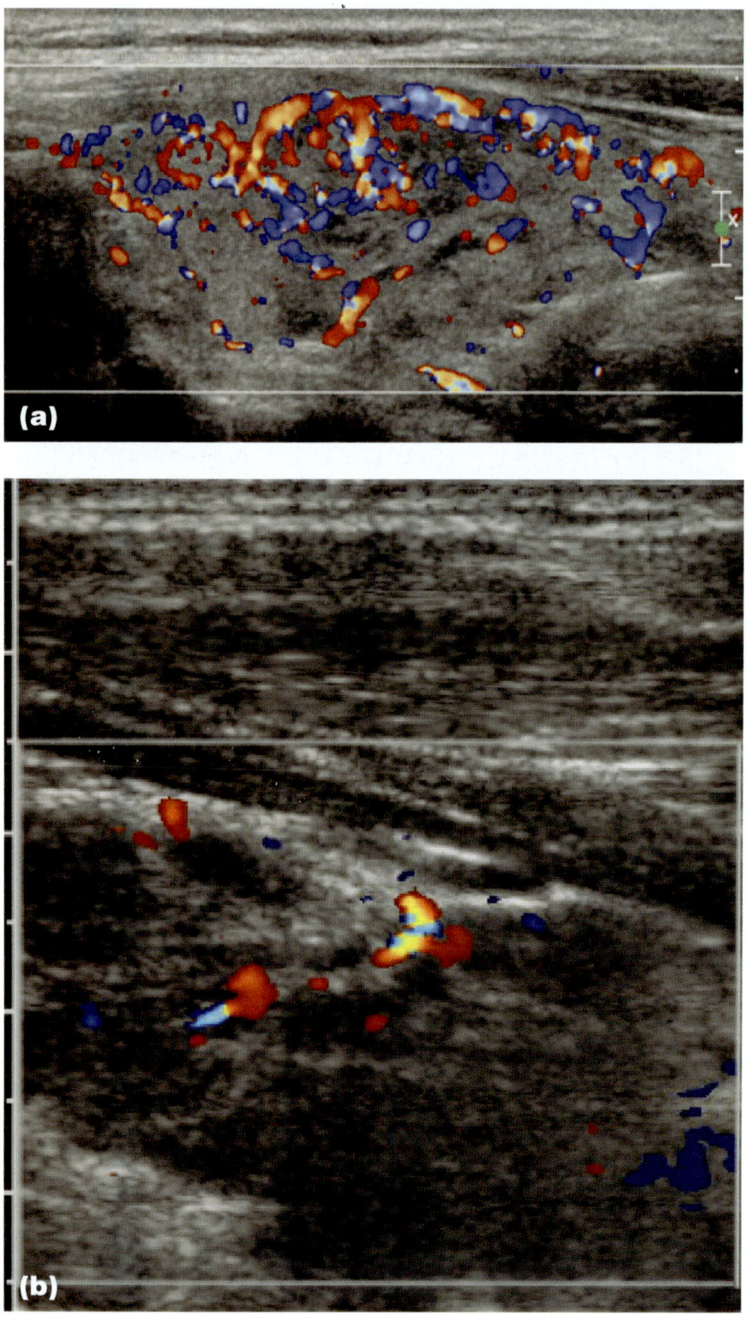

Figure 2.3 — Hashimoto Thyroiditis, Vascularity. The vascularity depends on the stage and activity of the disease. (a) Increased vascularity on CDUS is seen in active disease. (b) Decreased or no vascularity can be seen on CDUS in end-stage disease.

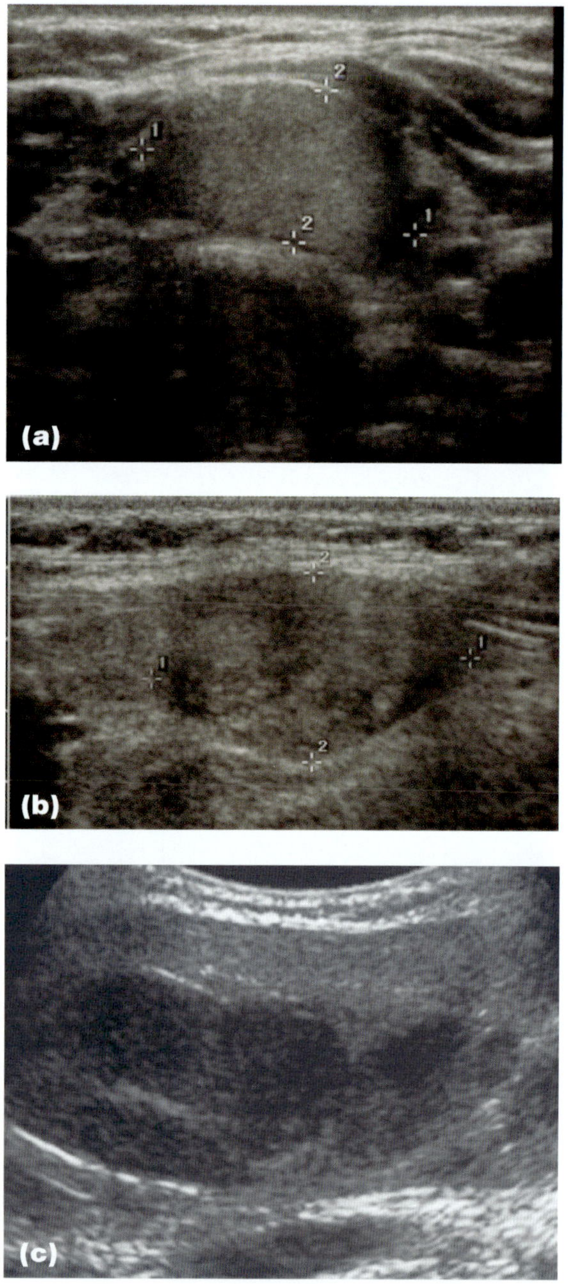

Figure 2.4 — Hashimoto Thyroiditis and Focal Nodules. (a) This gland contains a solid nodule (between calipers) proven to be a benign adenomatoid nodule on FNA. (b) This solid nodule (between calipers) proved to be a papillary carcinoma on FNA. (c) This large hypoechoic nodule was a biopsy proven lymphoma in a background of lymphocytic thyroiditis.

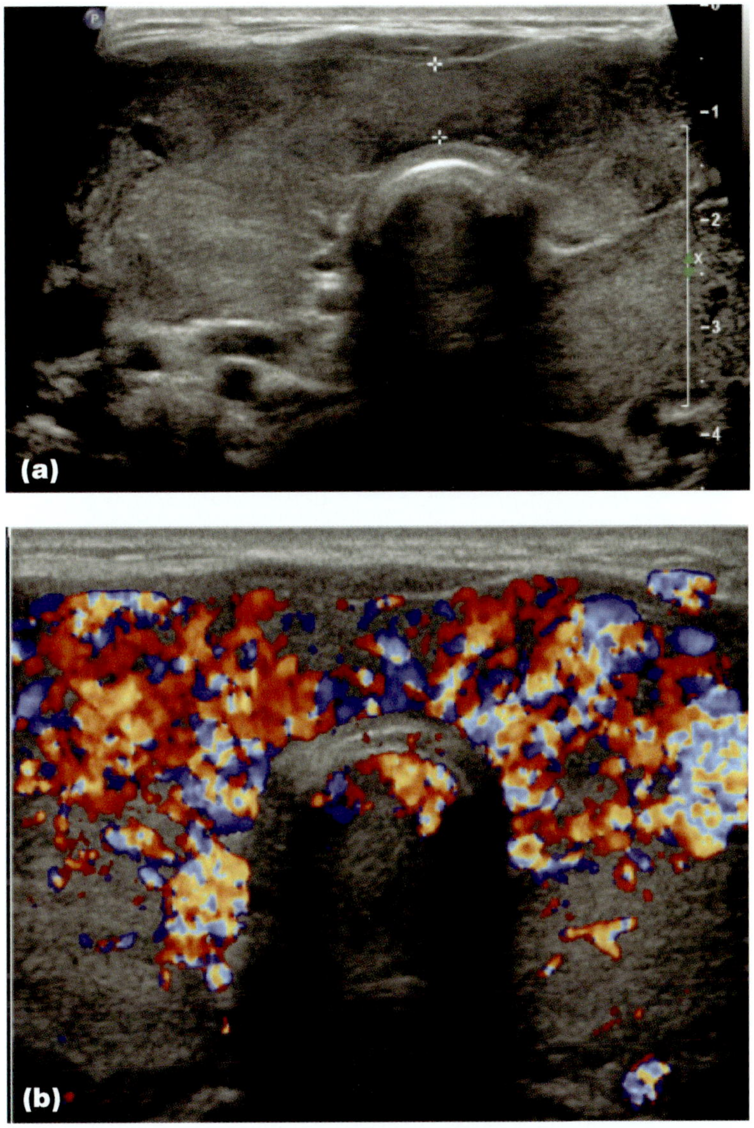

Figure 2.5 — Graves Disease. (a) Transverse grayscale image demonstrates a diffusely enlarged gland with a thick isthmus (between calipers). (b) CDUS demonstrates markedly increased vascularity, giving the appearance of the so called "thyroid inferno."

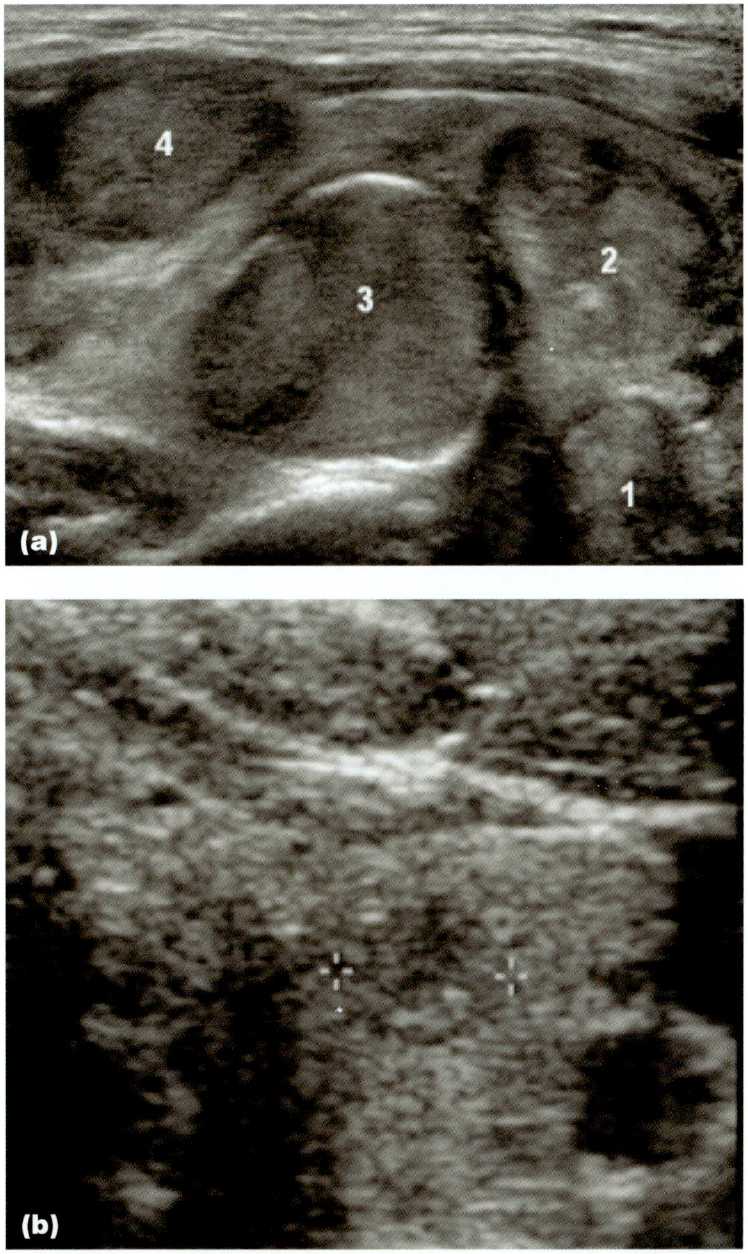

Figure 2.6 — Multinodular Goiter. (a) Sagittal grayscale image demonstrates a diffusely enlarged gland with multiple focal nodules (1–4). (b) A smaller, slightly hypoechoic nodule with microcalcifications (between calipers) proved to be a papillary carcinoma.

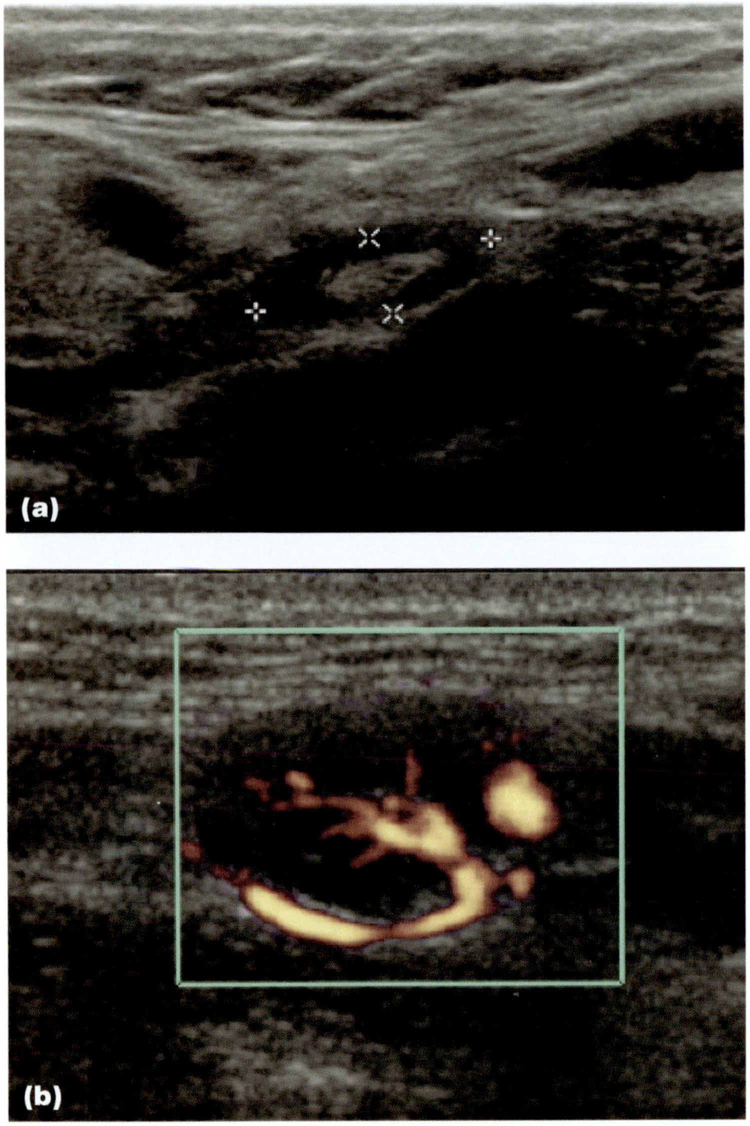

Figure 2.7 — Normal Cervical LN. (a) The node (between calipers) is oval in shape, has a symmetrically hypoechoic cortex and echogenic central hilum. (b) Sometimes a central feeding vessel can be seen.

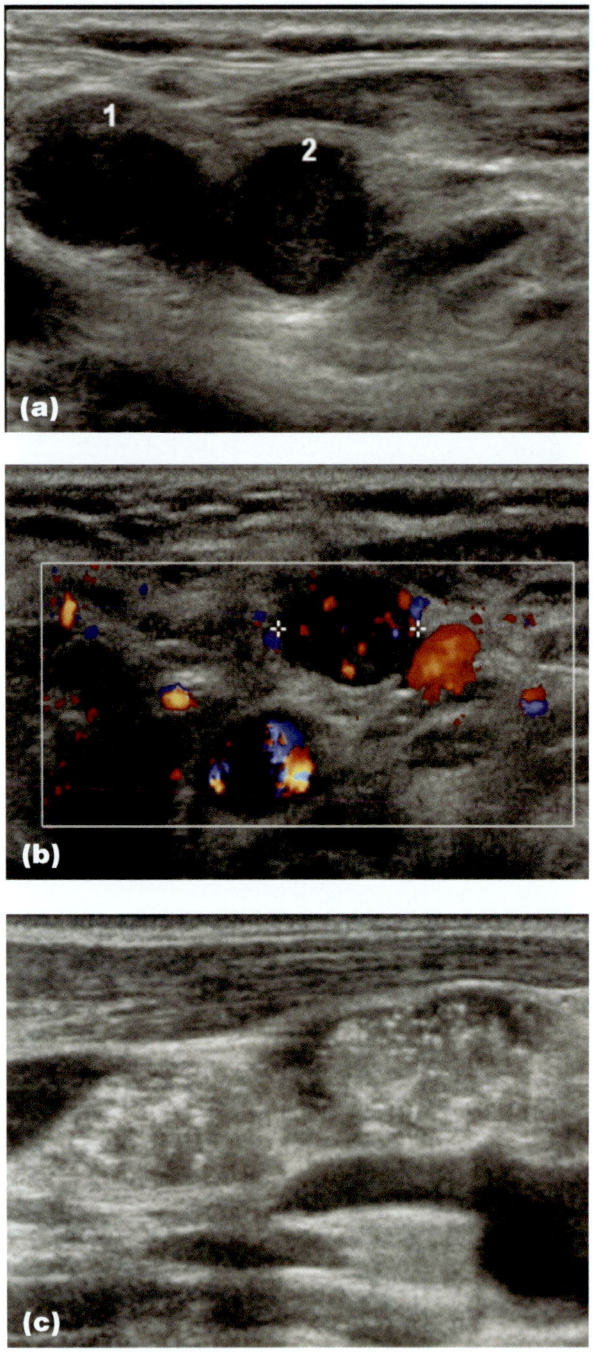

Figure 2.8 — Malignant Cervical LNs from Papillary Thyroid Carcinoma. (a) The nodes (1, 2) are round with loss of the central echogenic hilum and hypoechoic to cystic in appearance. (b) On CDUS irregular vascularity is seen. (c) Enlarged, plump LNs with microcalcifications.

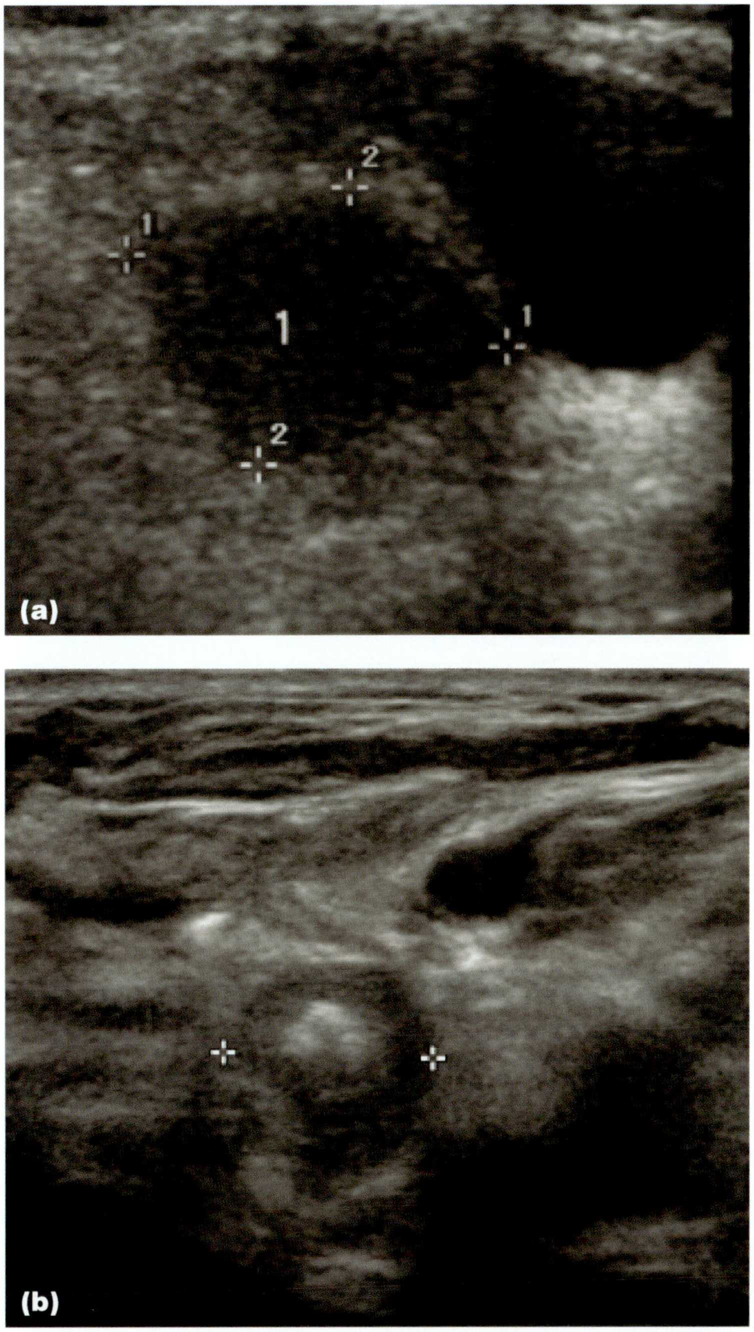

Figure 2.9 — Malignant Cervical LNs from Medullary Thyroid Carcinoma. (a) Hypoechoic node (between calipers) is seen with irregular margins. (b) Hypoechoic, plump LN with loss of fatty hilum and coarser (macro) calcifications (between calipers).

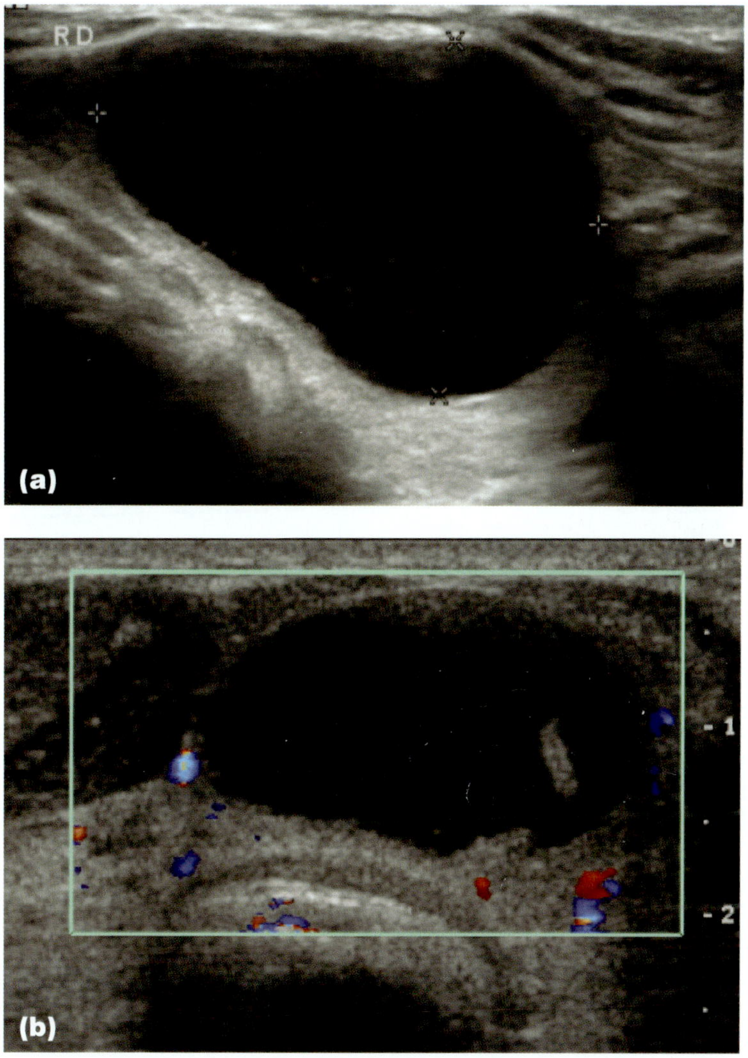

Figure 2.10 — Benign Thyroid Nodules. (a) Thyroid cyst (between calipers) is anechoic in echotexture with a thin wall. (b) On CDUS no wall or internal vascularity is demonstrated.

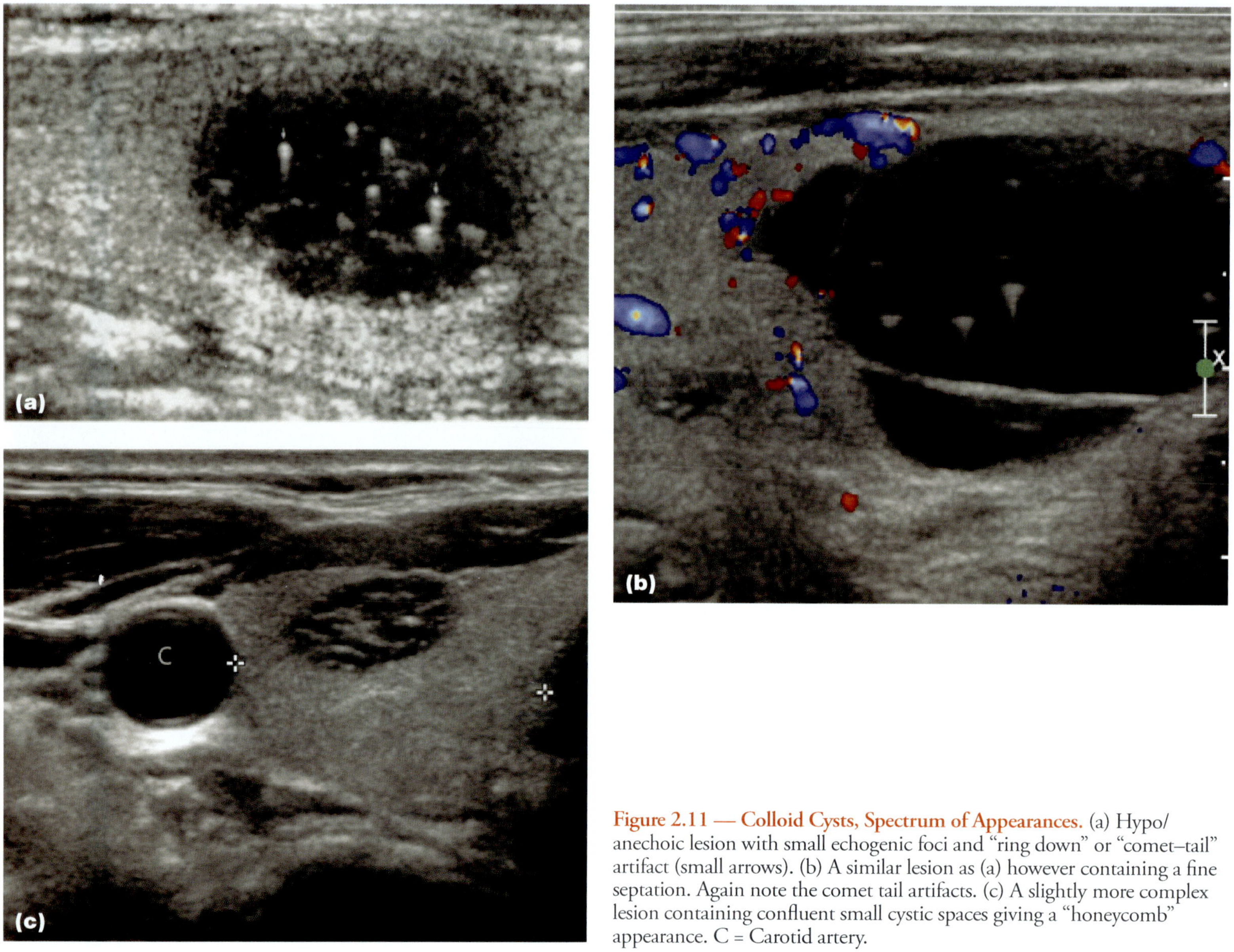

Figure 2.11 — Colloid Cysts, Spectrum of Appearances. (a) Hypo/anechoic lesion with small echogenic foci and "ring down" or "comet–tail" artifact (small arrows). (b) A similar lesion as (a) however containing a fine septation. Again note the comet tail artifacts. (c) A slightly more complex lesion containing confluent small cystic spaces giving a "honeycomb" appearance. C = Carotid artery.

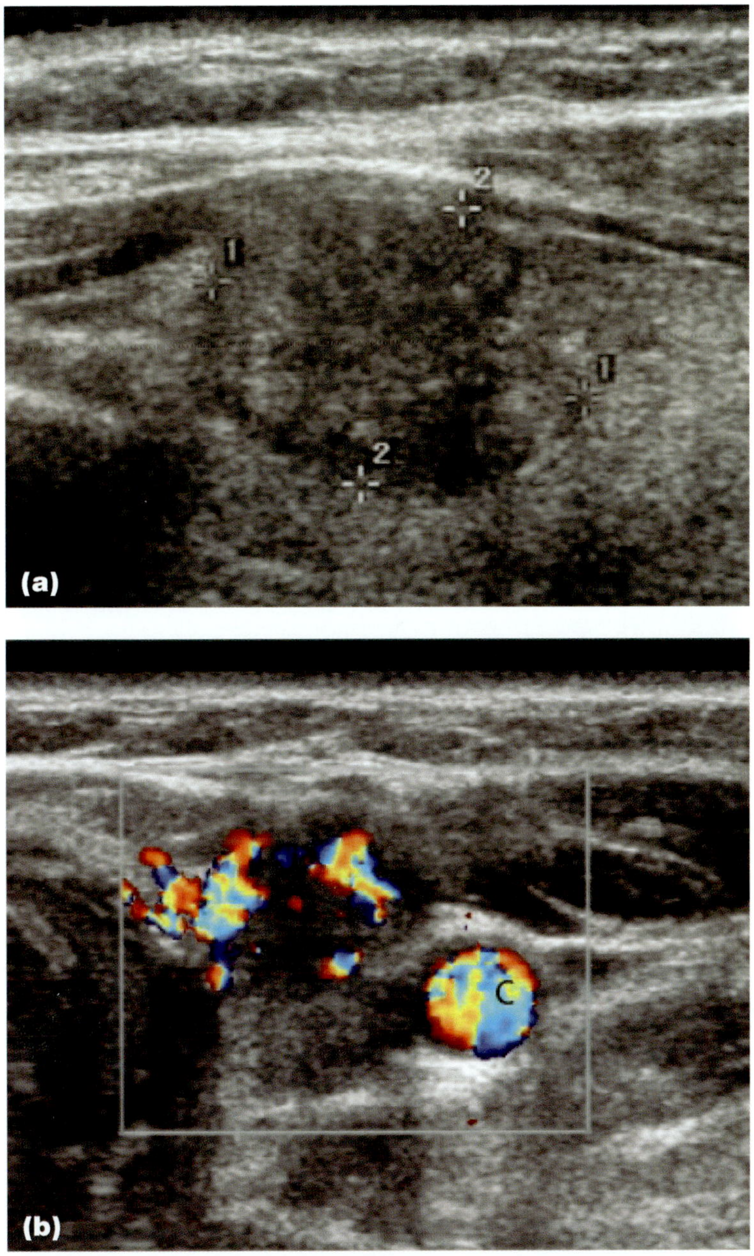

Figure 2.12 — Worrisome/Malignant Nodules. (a) Solid, irregular hypoechoic mass with internal punctate calcifications (between calipers). (b) Abnormal vascularity is seen on CDUS. C = Carotid artery.

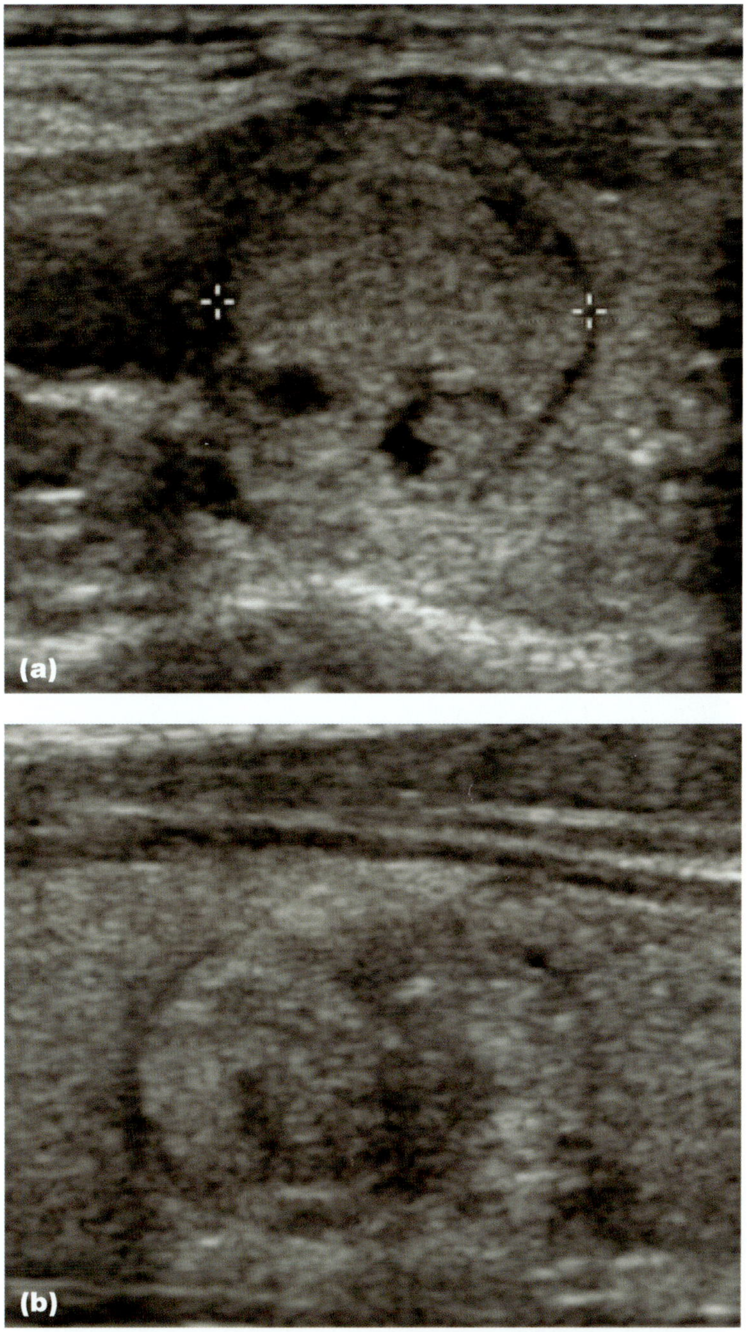

Figure 2.13 — Thyroid Lesion, "Halo Sign." (a) Grayscale image of a lesion with a thin peripheral halo (between calipers) proved to be papillary thyroid carcinoma on FNAB. (b) Solid lesion with a thin halo proved to be a benign adenomatoid nodule on FNAB.

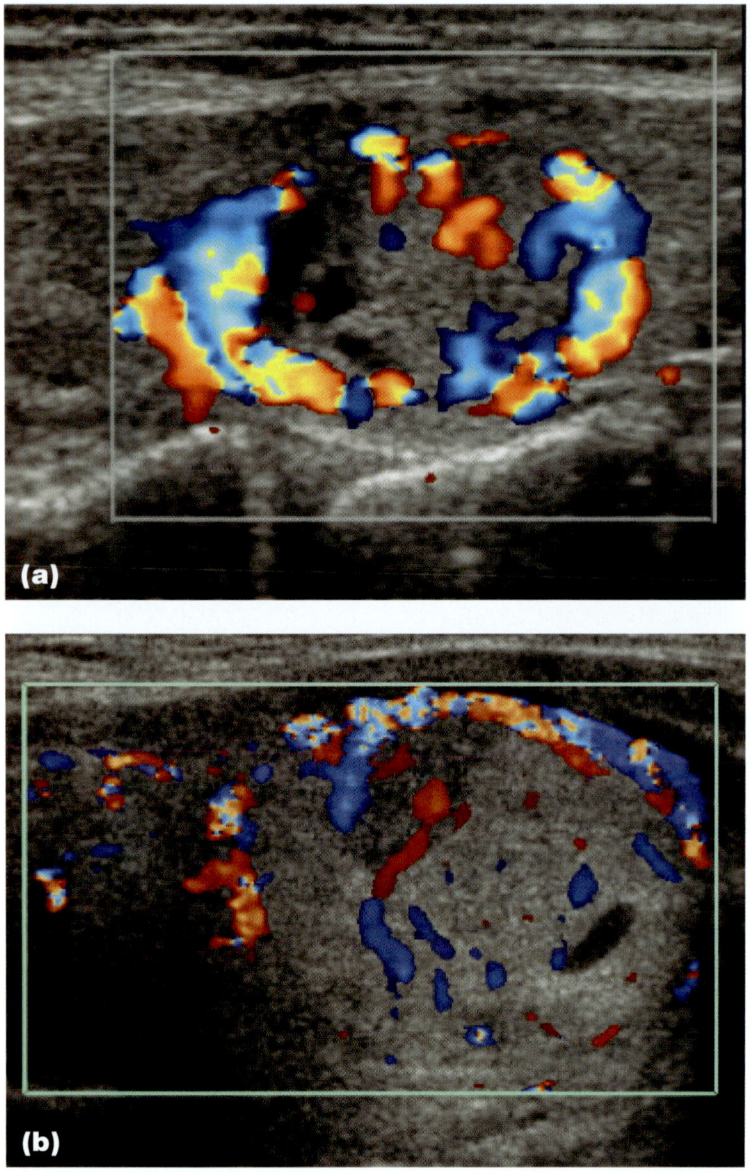

Figure 2.14 — Thyroid Lesions, Vascularity "Central Versus Peripheral." (a) CDUS of a lesion with peripheral and central vascularity showed papillary thyroid carcinoma on FNAB. (b) CDUS of an irregular lesion with central and peripheral vascularity was a biopsy proven benign adenomatoid nodule.

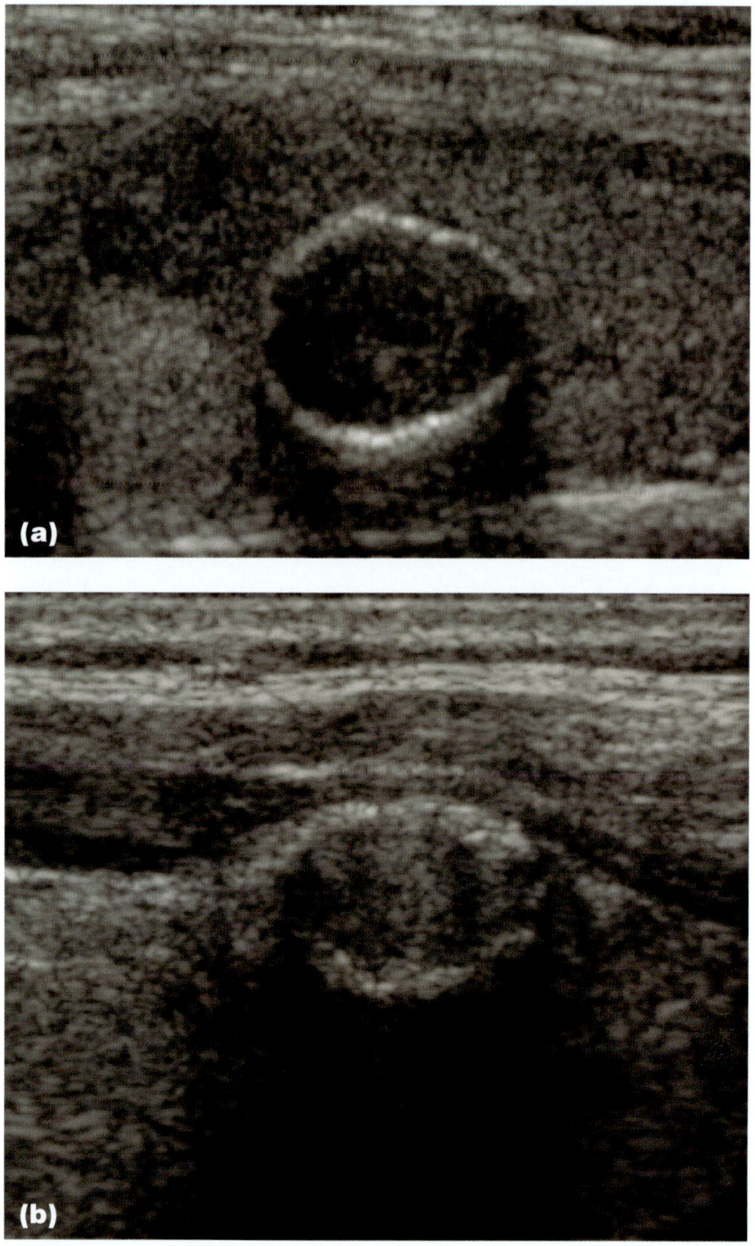

Figure 2.15 — Thyroid Lesions, Peripheral Eggshell Calcifications. (a) Transverse gray scale image demonstrates a lesion with peripheral egg-shell calcifications. On FNAB this lesion was a benign adenomatoid nodule. (b) Grayscale image of another solid lesion with peripheral eggshell calcification, which proved to be a papillary thyroid carcinoma on FNAB.

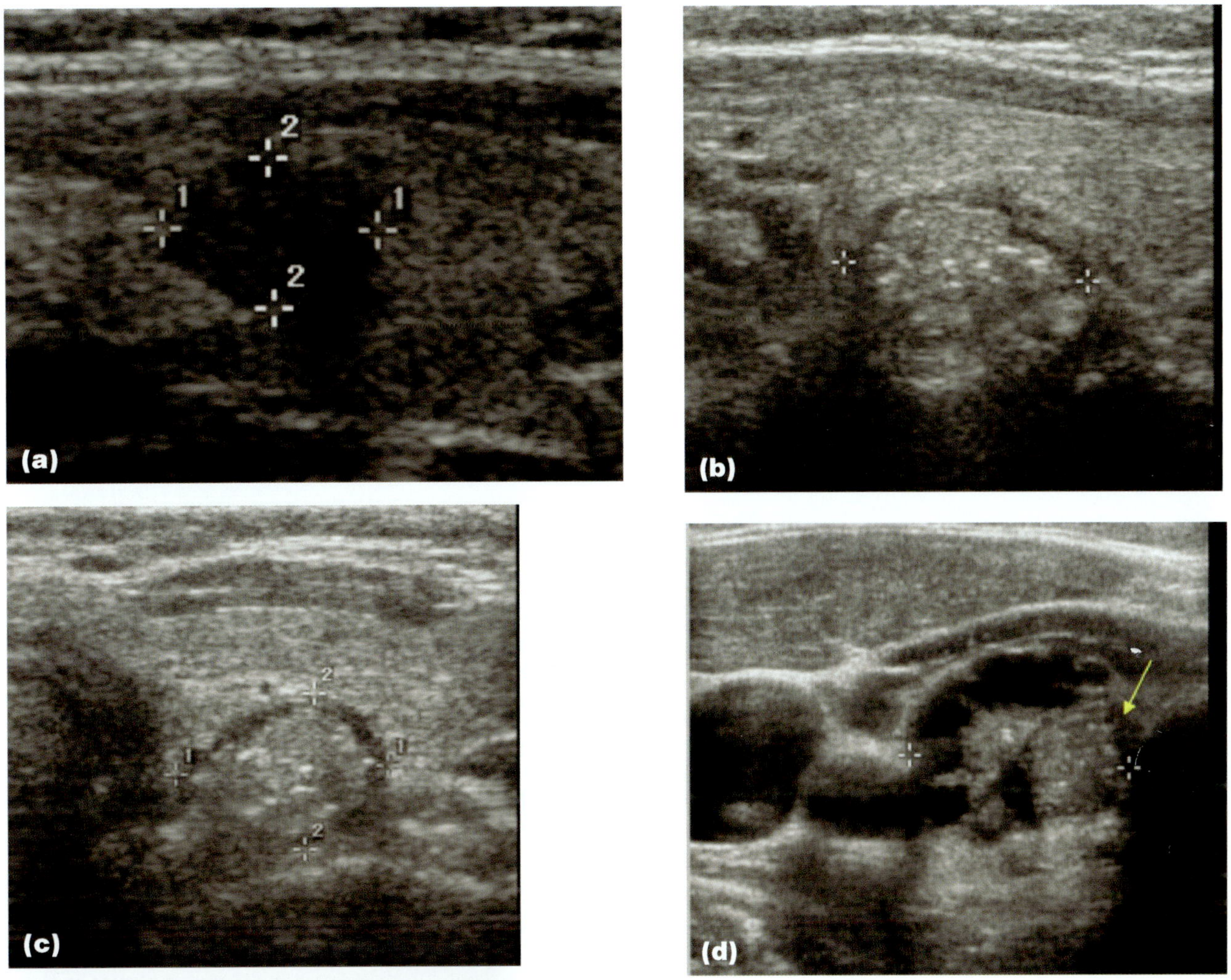

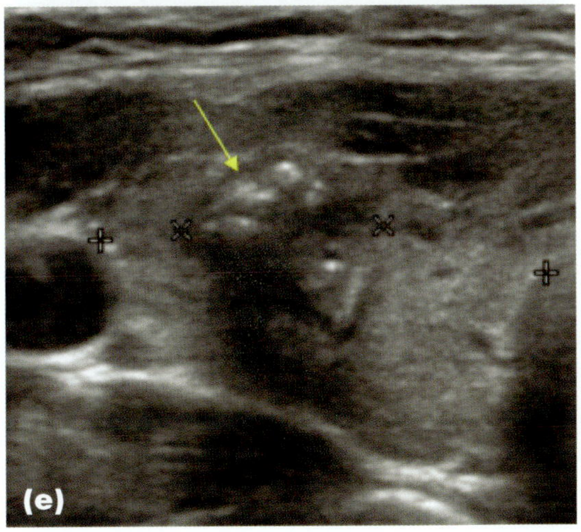

Figure 2.16 — Papillary Thyroid Carcinoma, Spectrum of Sonographic Appearances. (a) Hypoechoic solid nodule without calcifications (between calipers). (b) Solid isoechoic mass (between calipers) with punctate internal calcification. (c) Solid hypoechoic lesion with thick halo and punctate internal calcifications. (d) Partially cystic papillary carcinoma (between calipers) with microcalcifications (arrow). (e) Solid irregular hypoechoic mass with punctate internal calcifications (arrow). (f) LN metastasis (arrow) in the right neck low at level IV nodal station. (g) Heterogeneous mass with irregular margins (between calipers) and (h) LN metastases (1, 2, 3). (i) Small calcified papillary carcinoma (arrow) with (j) large LN metastasis (1,2) and (k) abnormal irregular vascularity.

(*Continued*)

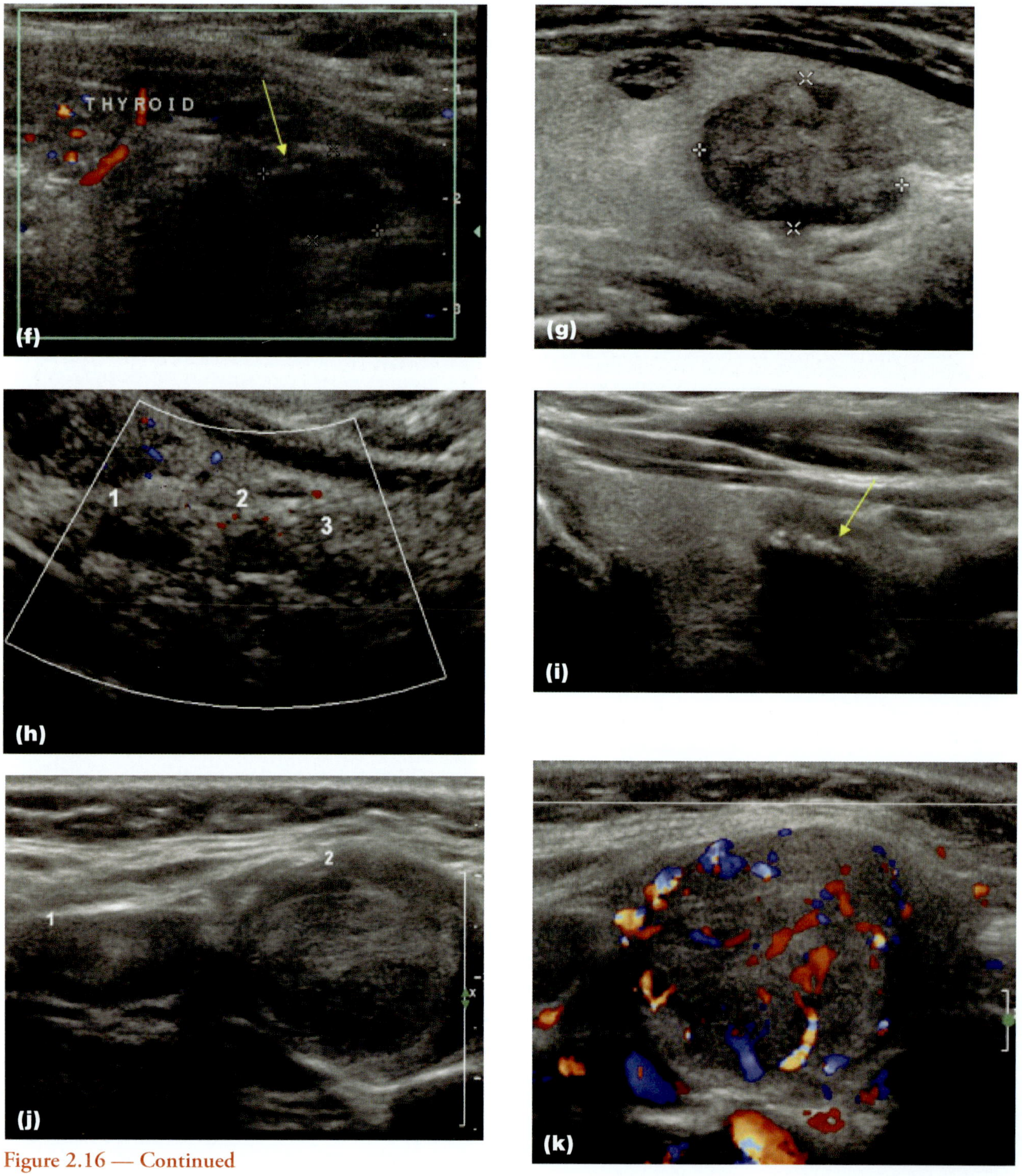

Figure 2.16 — Continued

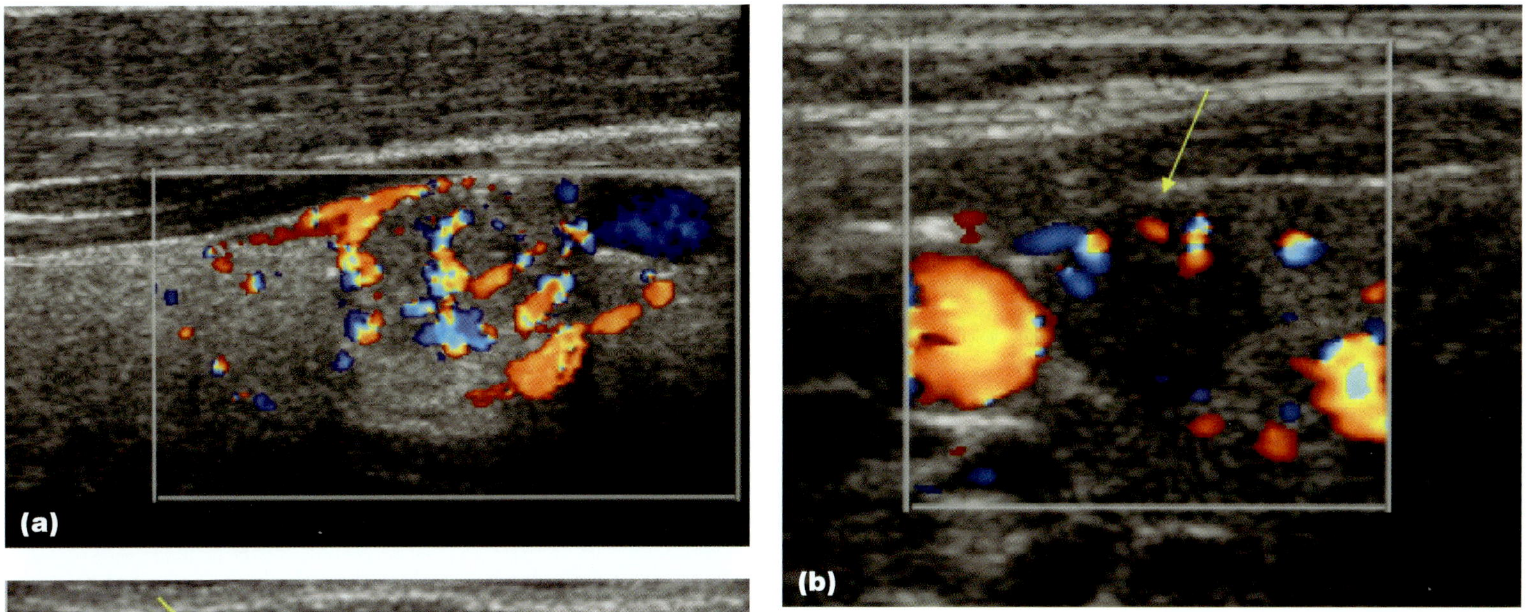

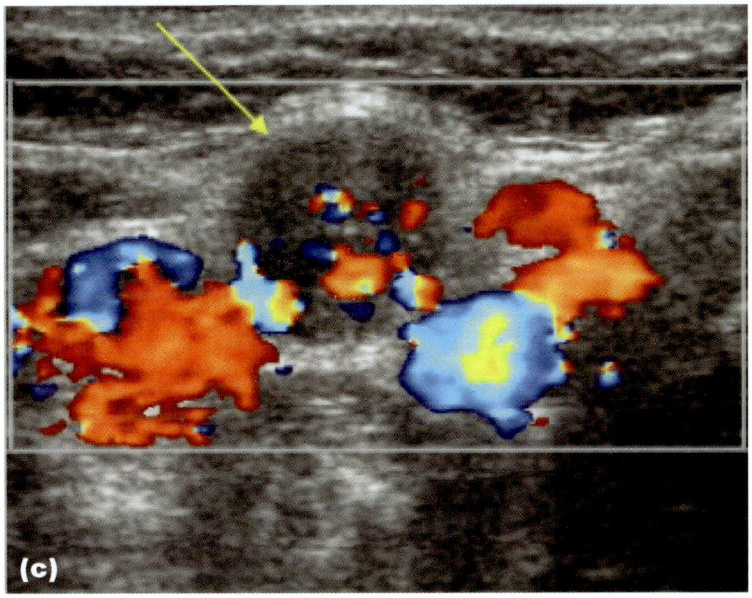

Figure 2.17 — Papillary Thyroid Carcinoma, CDUS Appearance. Blood flow is often, however, not always, increased. (a) Isoechoic mass with diffuse central and peripheral increased vascularity on CDUS. (b) Hypoechoic mass with irregular margins and minimally increased peripheral vascularity on CDUS (arrow). (c) Abnormal LN with internal vascularity (arrow).

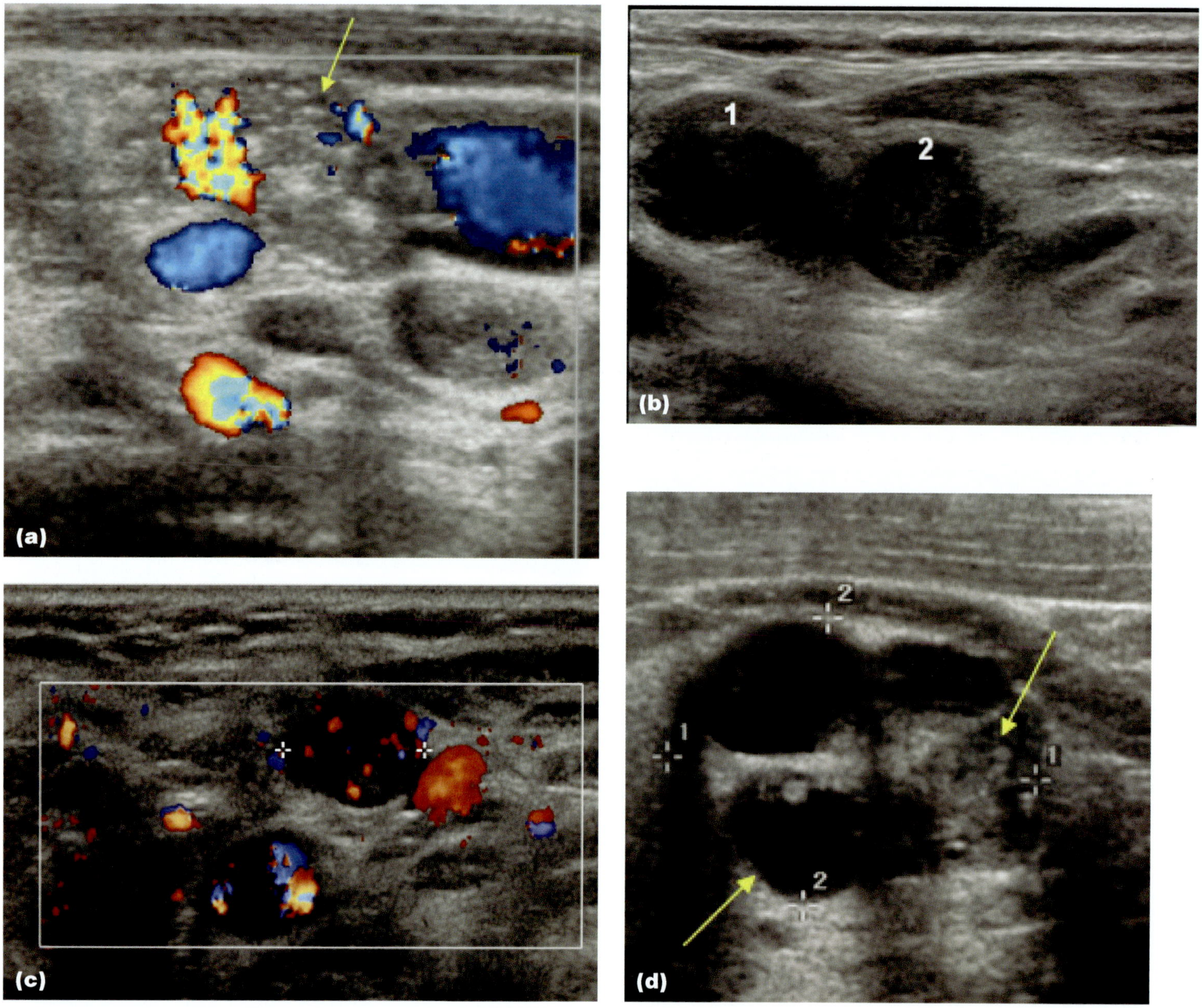

Figure 2.18 — Papillary Thyroid Carcinoma, LN Metastases—Spectrum of Sonographic Appearances. (a) Abnormal cervical LNs with microcalcifications (arrow) and irregular peripheral vascularity. (b) Abnormal cervical LNs (1,2) with cystic areas and (c) irregular vascularity (between calipers). (d) Abnormal cervical LNs with microcalcifications and cystic areas (arrows).

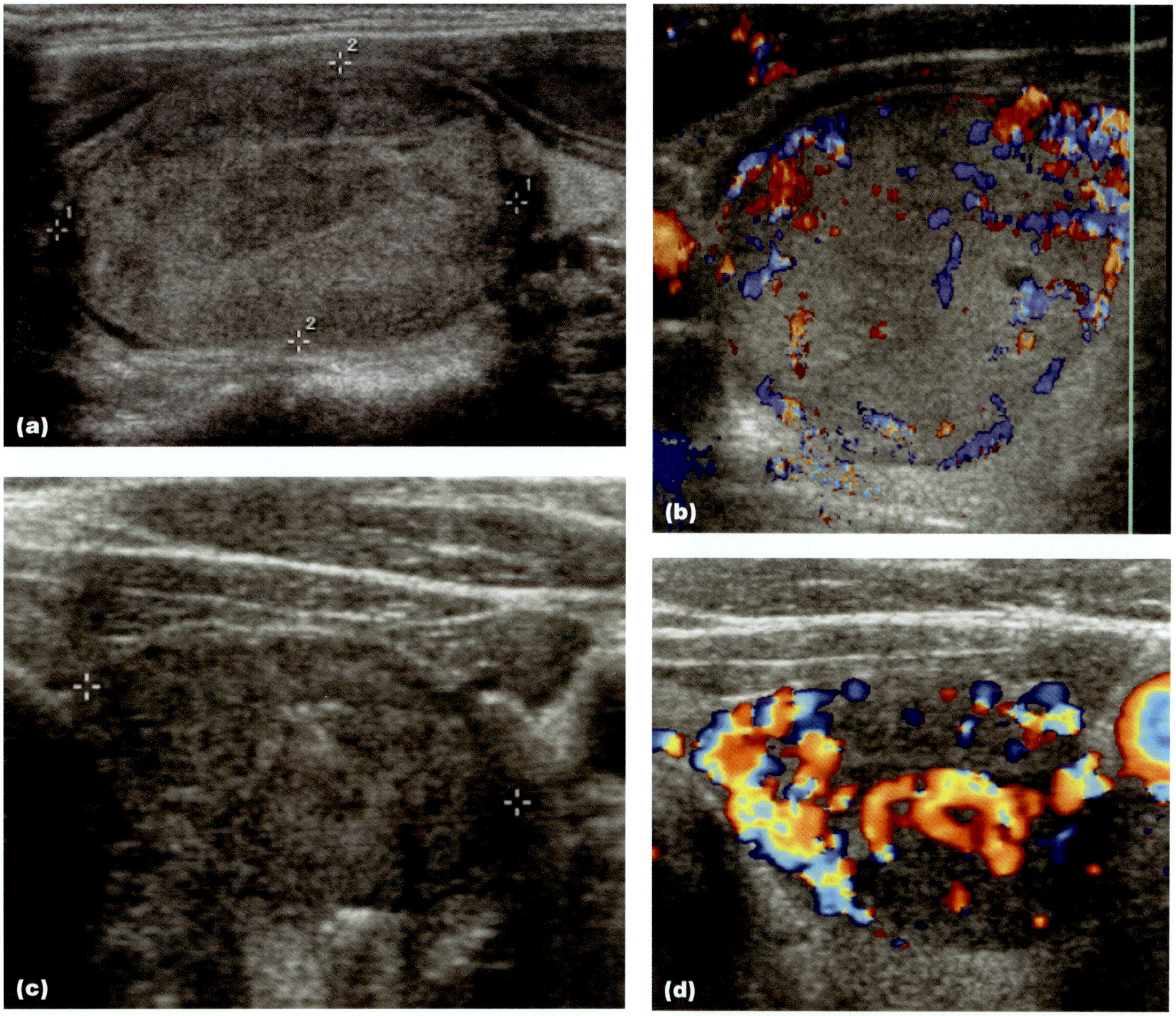

Figure 2.19 — Follicular Neoplasms, Spectrum of Sonographic Appearances. (a) Solid homogeneous mass (between calipers) with thin peripheral halo and linear hypoechoic striations representing a follicular adenoma at surgery. (b) CDUS of the lesion demonstrates irregular central and peripheral vascularity. (c) Solid homogeneous mass (between calipers) with irregular internal vascularity representing a follicular carcinoma with microinvasion at surgery. (d) CDUS of the mass demonstrates irregular central and peripheral vascularity.

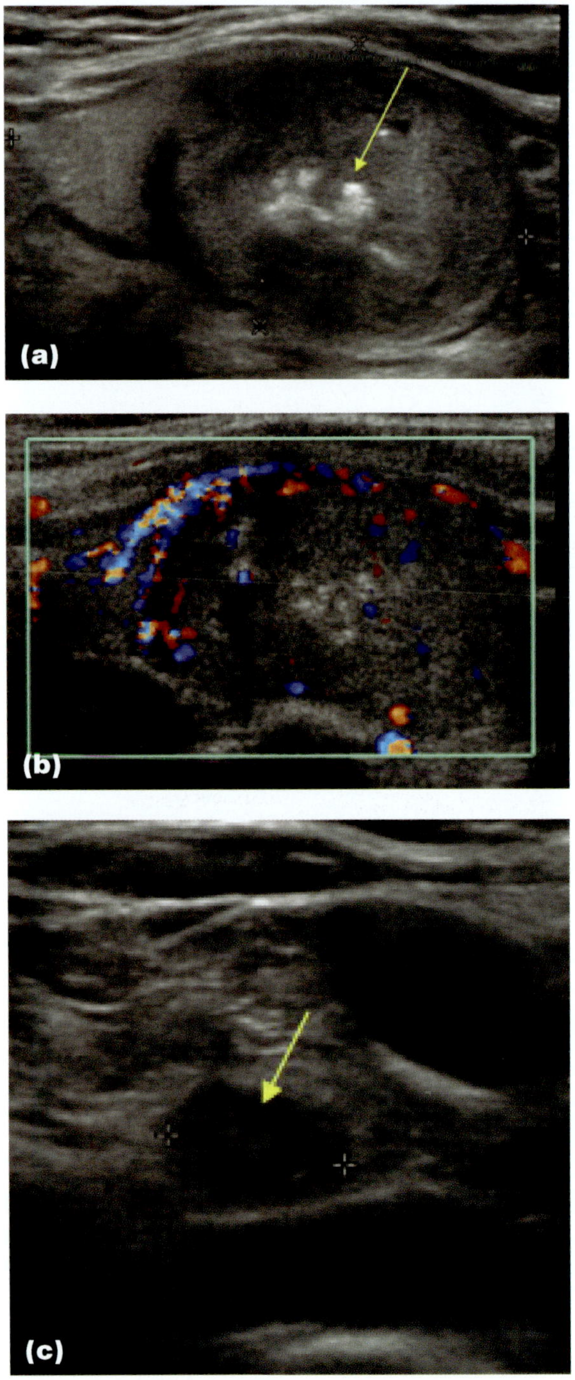

Figure 2.20 — Medullary Thyroid Carcinoma, Spectrum of Sonographic Appearances. (a) Sagittal grayscale image of a large solid, heterogeneous mass in the left thyroid lobe with coarse calcifications (arrow). (b) On CDUS, minimal vascularity is noted. (c) Abnormal cervical LNs with faint calcifications (arrow).

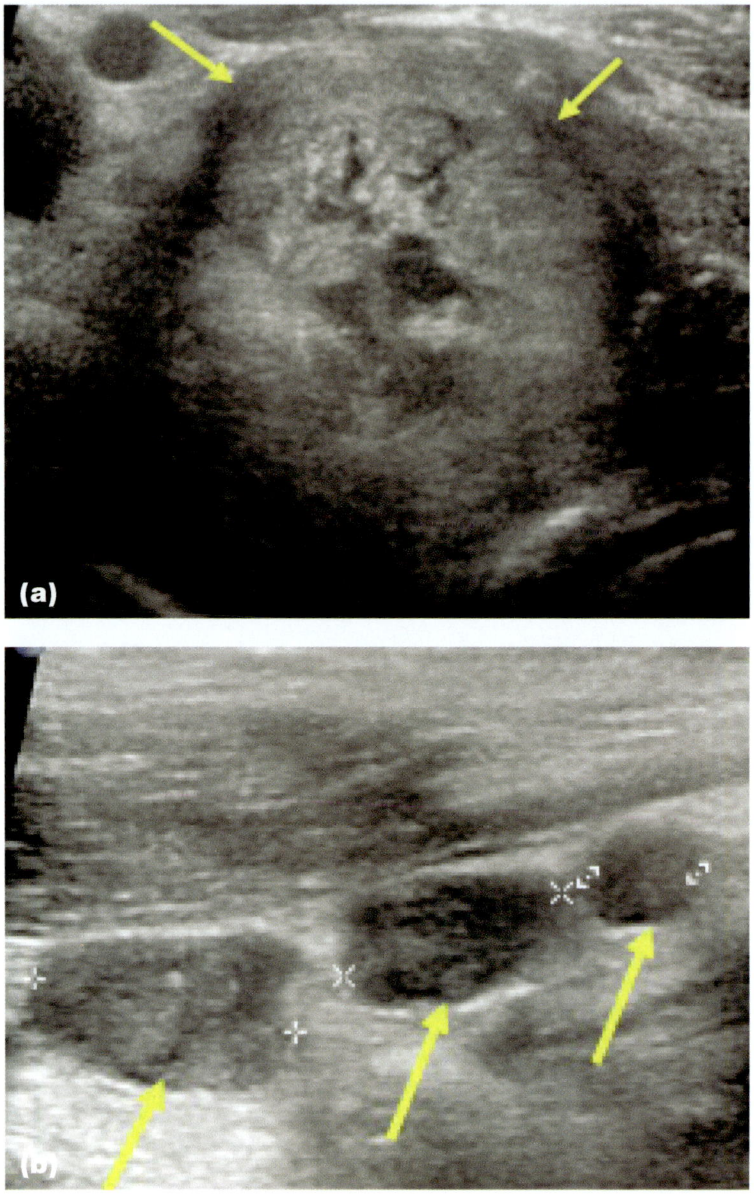

Figure 2.21 — Anaplastic Thyroid Carcinoma, Spectrum of Sonographic Appearances. (a) Large solid ill-defined mass in the left thyroid lobe (arrows) which had invaded adjacent soft tissues and (b) adjacent LNs (arrows).

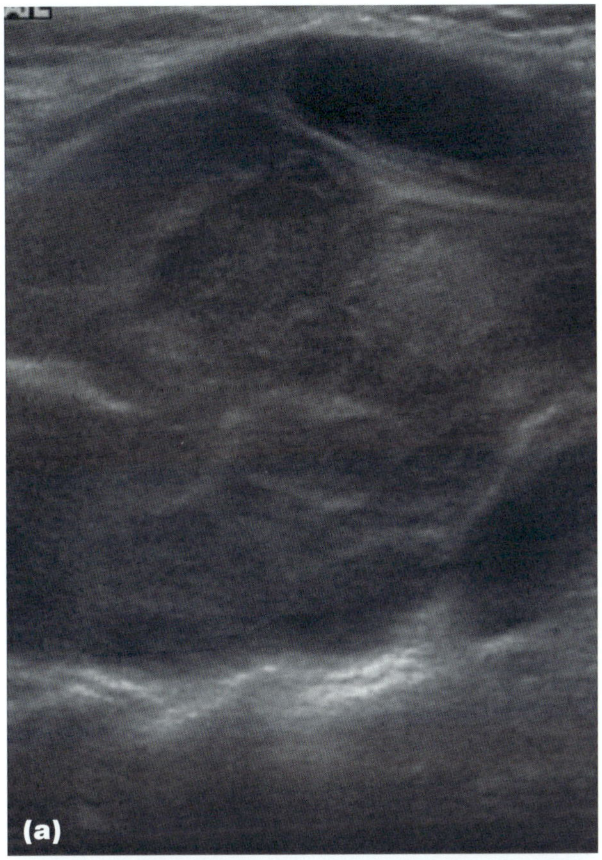

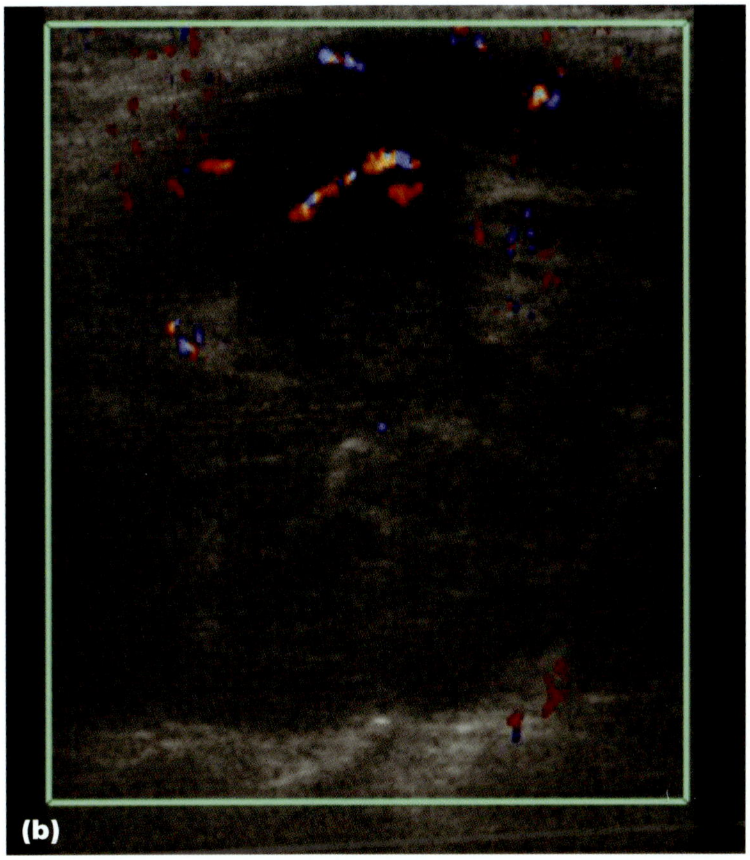

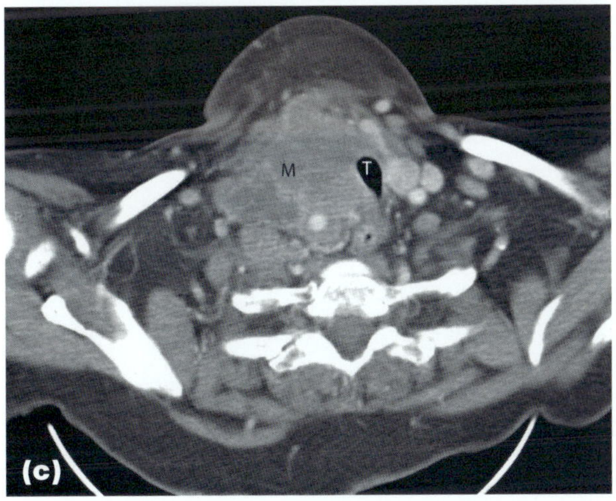

Figure 2.22 — Thyroid Lymphoma, Spectrum of Sonographic Appearances. (a) Large, solid hypoechoic mass replacing the right thyroid lobe. (b) Only minimal internal vascularity is seen on CDUS. (c) Computed Tomography (CT) of the neck shows the large masses (M) engulfing and displacing the trachea (T).

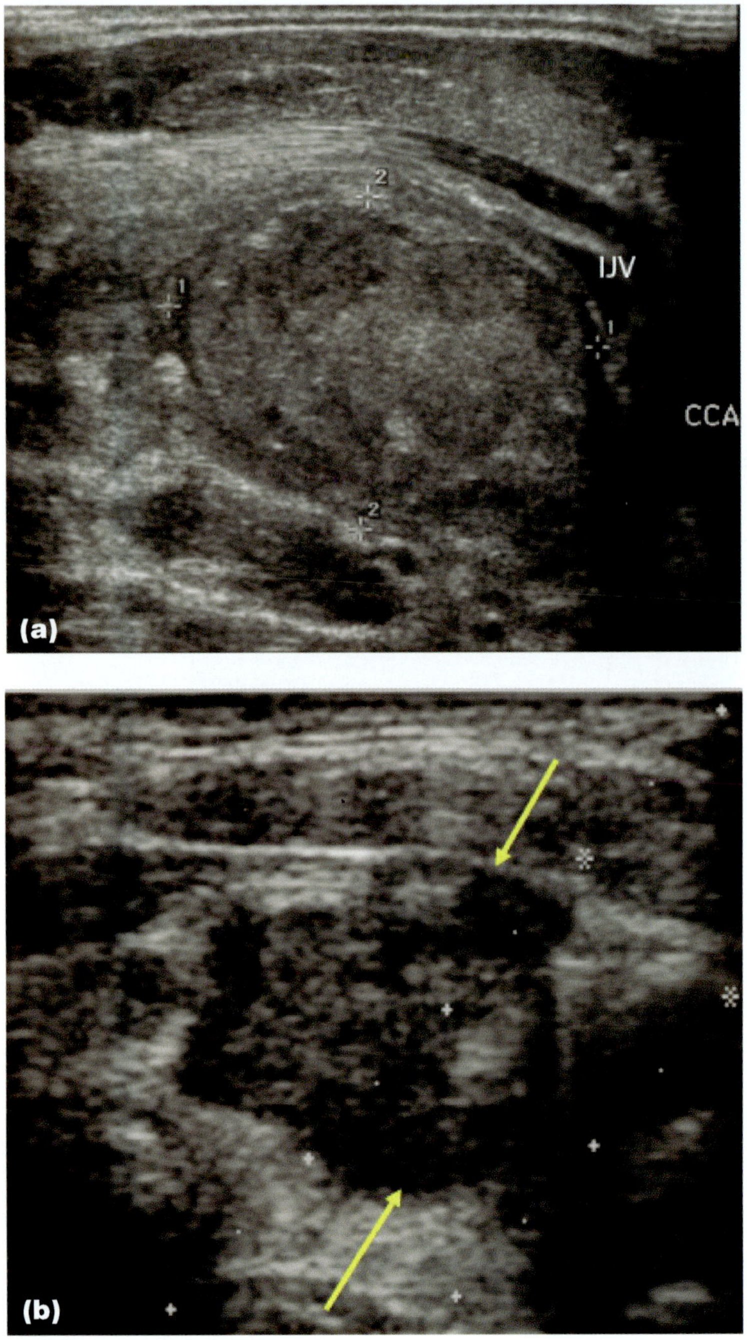

Figure 2.23 — Thyroid Metastases, Spectrum of Sonographic Appearances. (a) Large solid mass in the right thyroid lobe (between calipers) represents a metastasis from esophageal carcinoma on FNAB. IJV = Internal Jugular Vein. CCA = Common Carotid Artery. (b) Large heterogeneous mass in the left thyroid lobe (arrows) represents metastatic melanoma on FNAB.

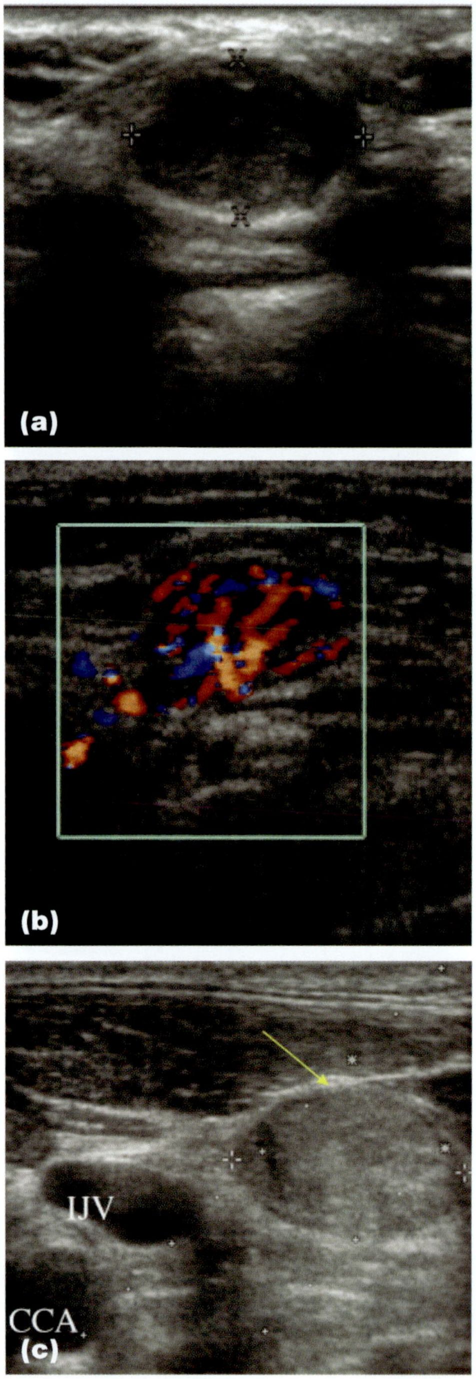

Figure 2.24 — Recurrence of Papillary Thyroid Carcinoma in Neck LNs. (a) Grayscale image of a bulky abnormal LN in the right thyroid bed- level VI (between calipers). (b) CDUS of the LN demonstrates markedly abnormal vascularity. (c) Bulky abnormal LN in left level IV LN (arrow). IJV = Internal Jugular Vein. CCA = Common Carotid Artery.

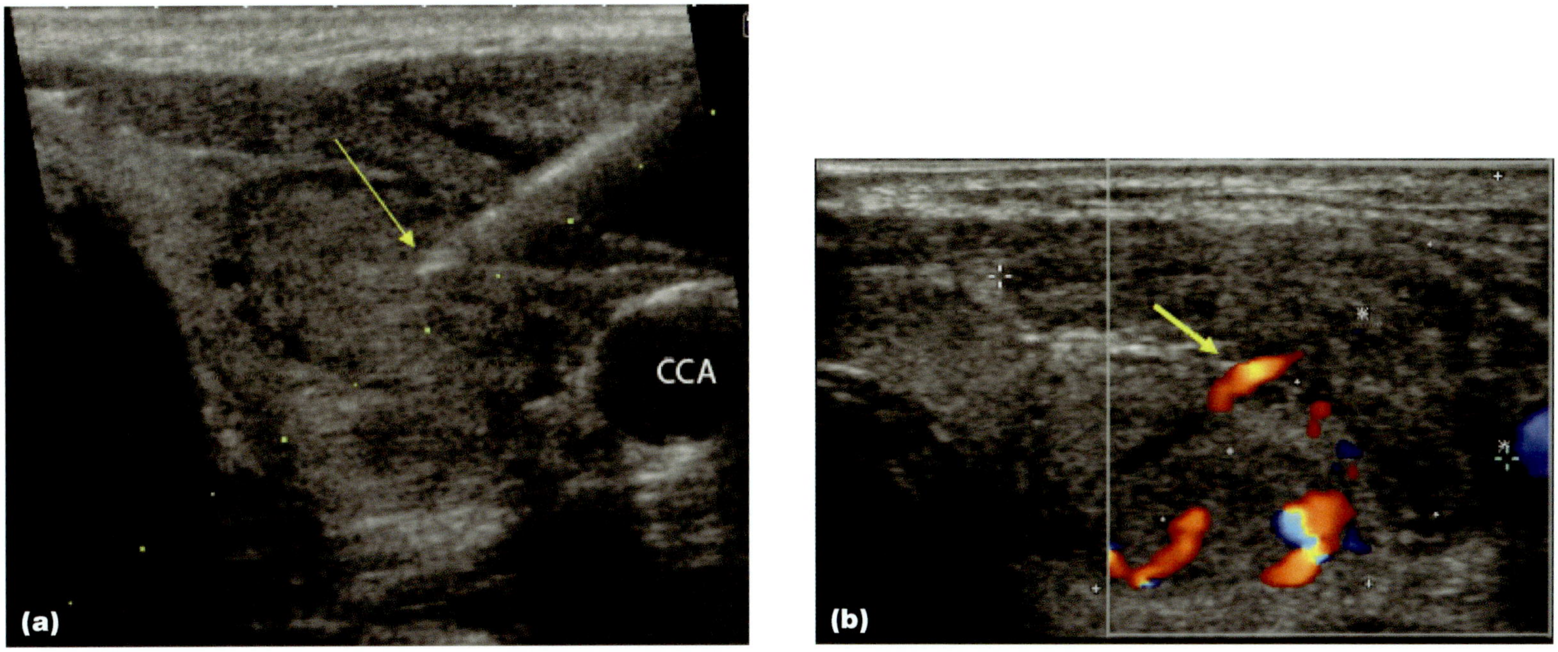

Figure 2.25 — US Guided FNAB. (a) The echogenic tip of the biopsy needle (arrow) is seen in the center of this left thyroid nodule. CCA = Common Carotid Artery. (b) An isoechoic hematoma (between calipers) developed after the biopsy and resolved with conservative therapy. The actively bleeding vessel is seen on CDUS (arrow).

3

Nonneoplastic Nodules and Cysts

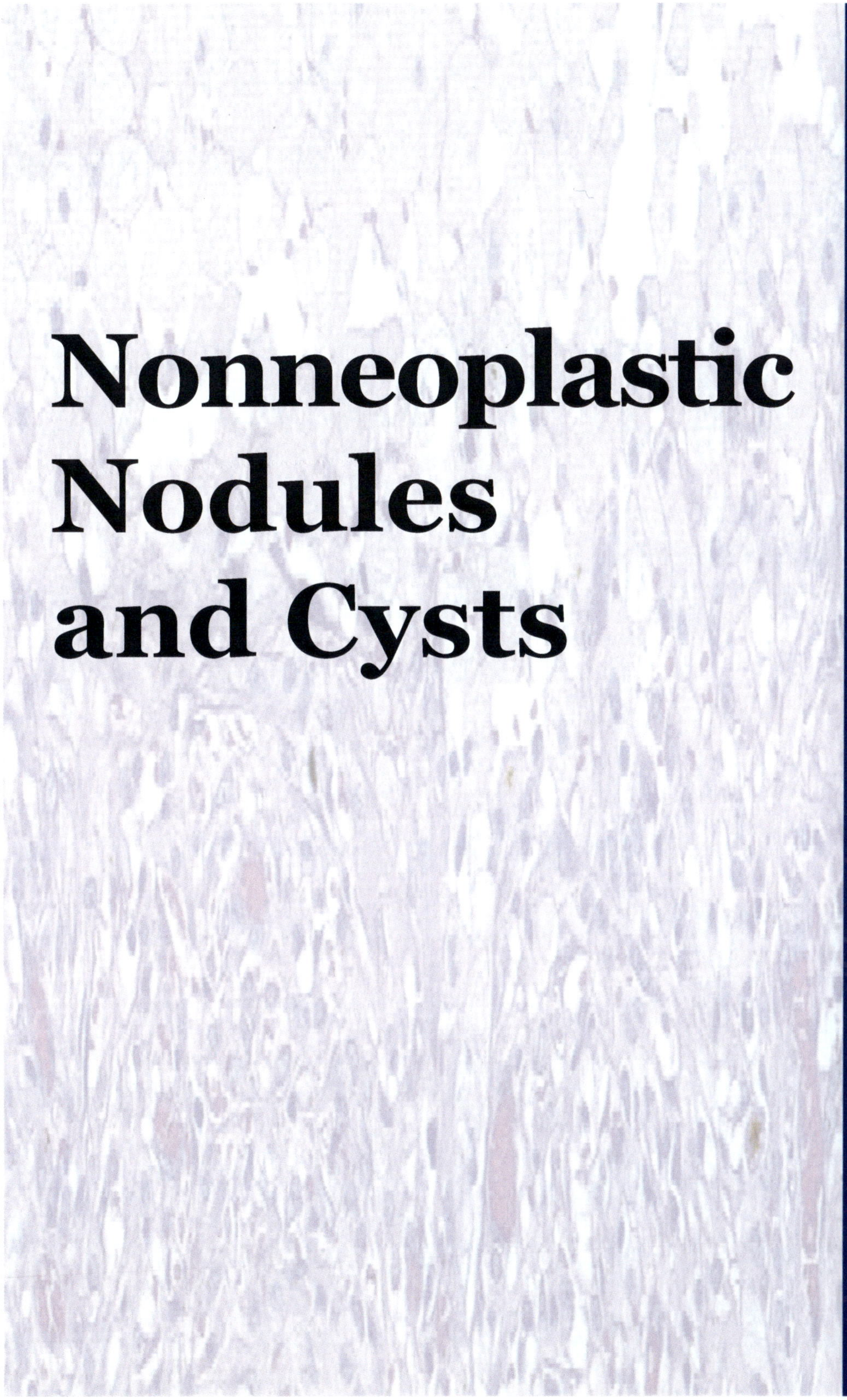

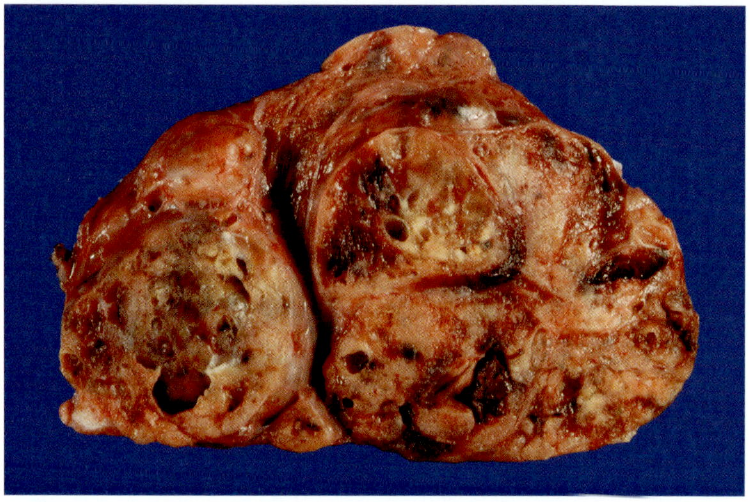

Figure 3.1 — Multinodular Adenomatoid Hyperplasia, Gross Appearance. This misshapen lobe of the thyroid is distorted by the presence of multiple ill-defined nodules. The nodules vary in size and shape replacing most of the normal thyroid parenchyma. Secondary degenerative changes include cyst formation and intranodular hemorrhage. The multiplicity and size of the hyperplastic nodules tends to dominate the gross appearance and may mask the presence of less conspicuous thyroid cancers.

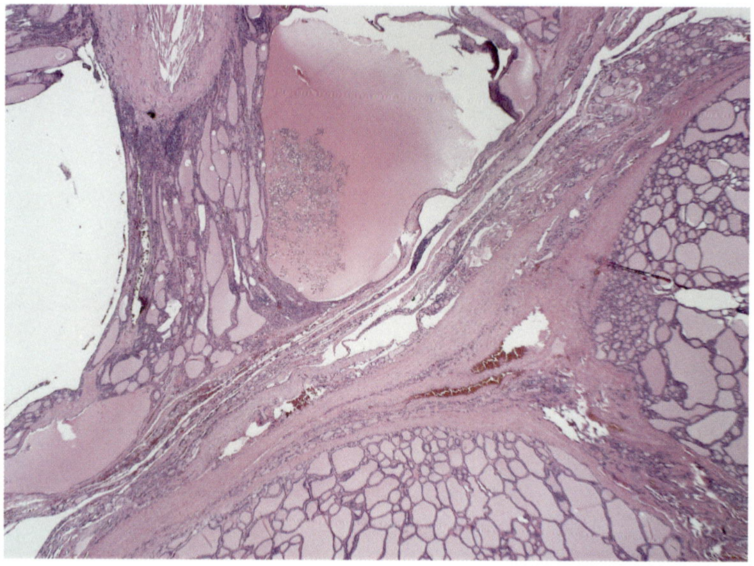

Figure 3.2 — Multinodular Adenomatoid Hyperplasia, Histologic Section. The microscopic appearance of multinodular hyperplasia reflects its gross characteristics. In this low power view, several ill-defined nodules are separated by an irregular zone of fibrosis. Compared to true follicular neoplasms, the follicles exhibit much more variation in size and shape and often become markedly dilated to form colloid-filled cysts. The presence of hemosiderin, scarring, and calcification are commonly encountered degenerative changes. (H&E stain)

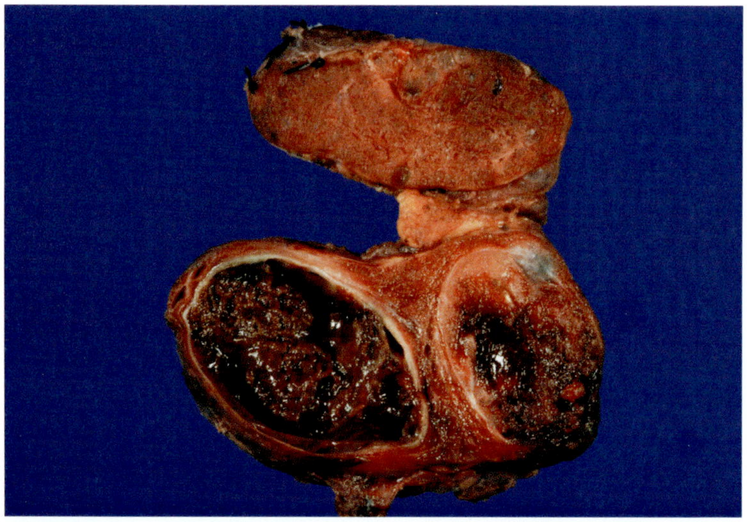

Figure 3.3 — Adenomatoid Nodules With Cystic Degeneration, Gross Appearance. The right lobe of the thyroid harbors two partially encapsulated nodules. The larger nodule shows prominent cystic degeneration. The cyst cavity is lined by clotted blood.

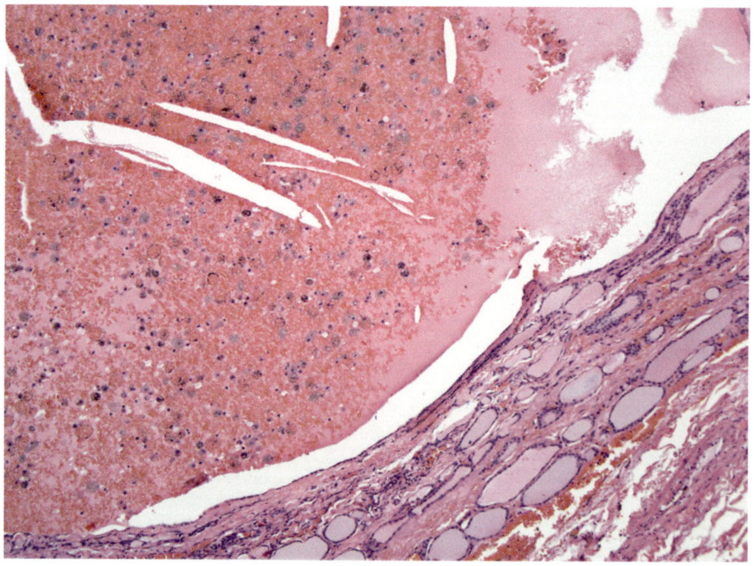

Figure 3.4 — Colloid Cyst, Histologic Section. This cyst essentially represents a markedly distended follicle. It is lined by flattened follicular epithelial cells and filled with colloid, blood, and histiocytes. (H&E stain)

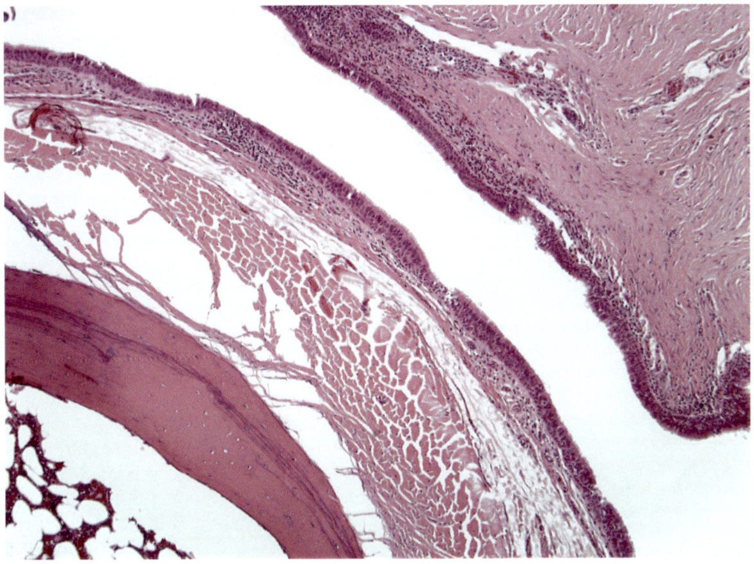

Figure 3.5 — Thyroglossal Duct Cyst, Histologic Section. The thyroglossal duct normally undergoes atrophy during postfetal development. Its abnormal persistence and cystic dilatation results in a thyroglossal duct cyst along the midline of the neck superior to the thyroid isthmus. The cyst is closely associated with the hyoid bone. It is lined by a ciliated columnar epithelium, but this epithelium frequently undergoes squamous metaplasia, particularly in the setting of inflammation. The presence of thyroid follicles is a variable finding and is not required to establish the diagnosis. (H&E stain)

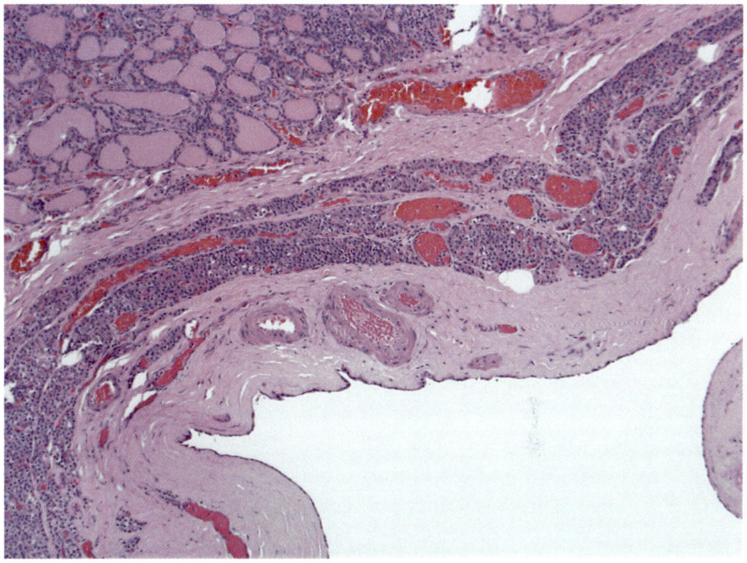

Figure 3.6a — Parathyroid Cyst, Histologic Section. Due to the anatomic proximity of the parathyroid glands, a parathyroid cyst can be clinically mistaken for a cyst of the thyroid. The fluid filling the cyst is usually watery and clear to straw-colored. The cysts do not usually extend into the thyroid parenchyma, but tend to be adhered to the surface of the thyroid and separated by a partitioning zone of fibrosis. The presence of parathyroid tissue within the cyst wall is very helpful in confirming the parathyroid nature of this cyst. (H&E stain)

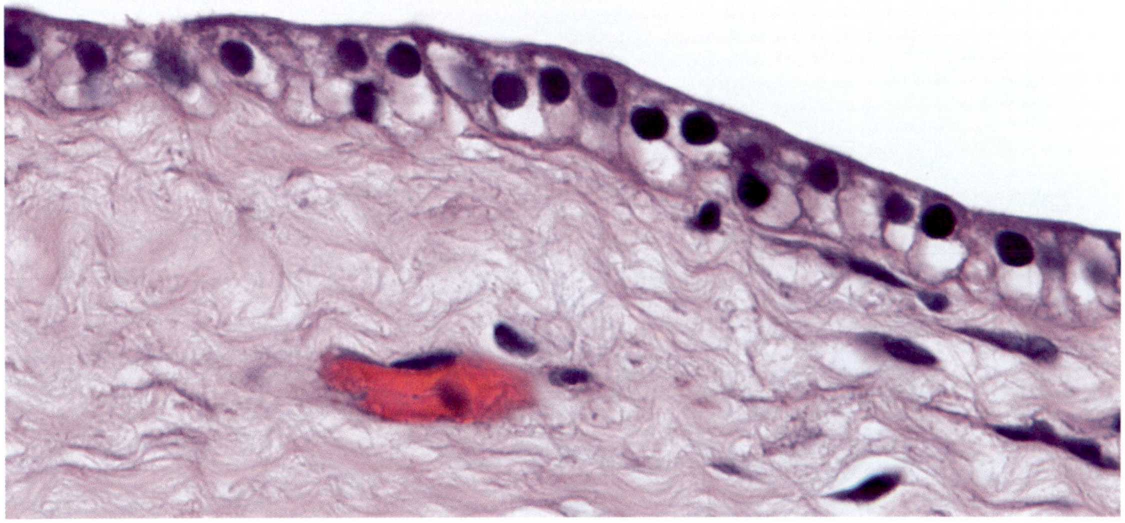

Figure 3.6b — Parathyroid Cyst, Histologic Section. The chief cells lining the cyst tend to be cuboidal with clear cytoplasm. (H&E stain)

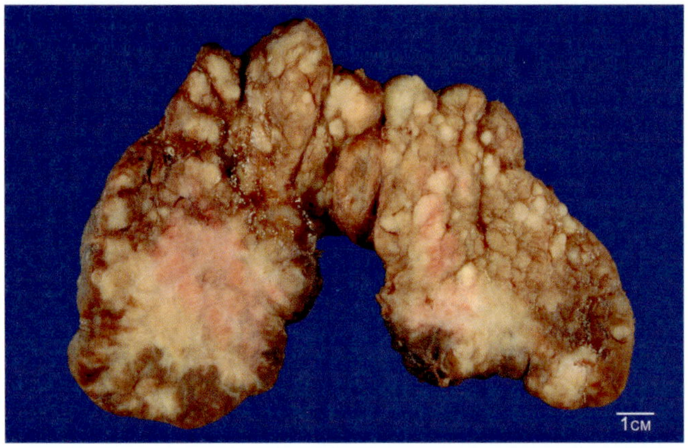

Figure 3.7 — Hashimoto Thyroiditis With Sclerosis, Gross Appearance. The thyroid gland is symmetrically enlarged. Its cut surface is pale and has a distinct cobblestone appearance. The cobblestoning reflects infiltration of chronic inflammatory cells in and around expanded thyroid lobules. Further expansion of one or several of these lobules may give rise to discrete dominant nodules (ie, nodular Hashimoto thyroiditis). The lobules are separated by bands of fibrosis. In areas, the bands become thickened and confluent resulting in broad zones of fibrosis effacing the thyroid architecture. Unlike Riedel disease, the fibrosis is confined by the thyroid capsule and does not extend beyond the thyroid into perithyroidal soft tissues.

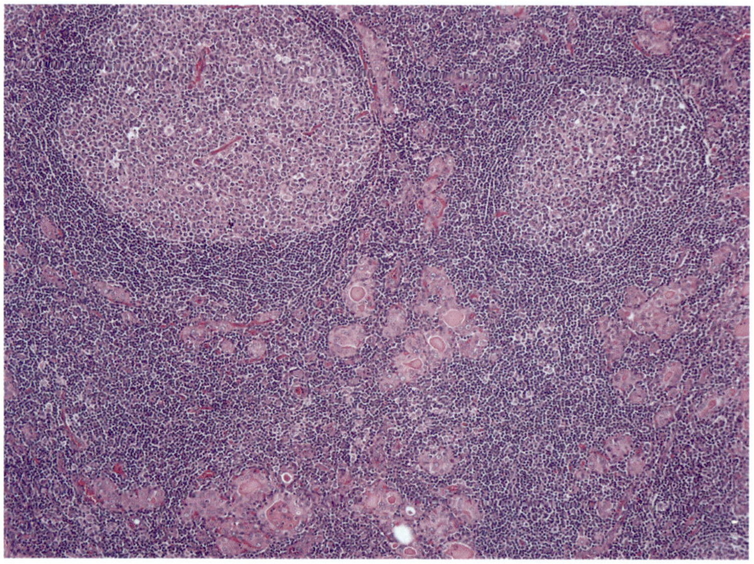

Figure 3.8a — Hashimoto Thyroiditis, Histologic Section. At low power, the thyroid stroma is infiltrated by a dense infiltrate of lymphocytes and plasma cells. Germinal centers are usually present and well developed. On occasion, the lymphoid component is so well developed that it is mistaken as a lymph node harboring metastatic thyroid cancer. The degree of follicular atrophy and replacement fibrosis is highly variable. (H&E stain)

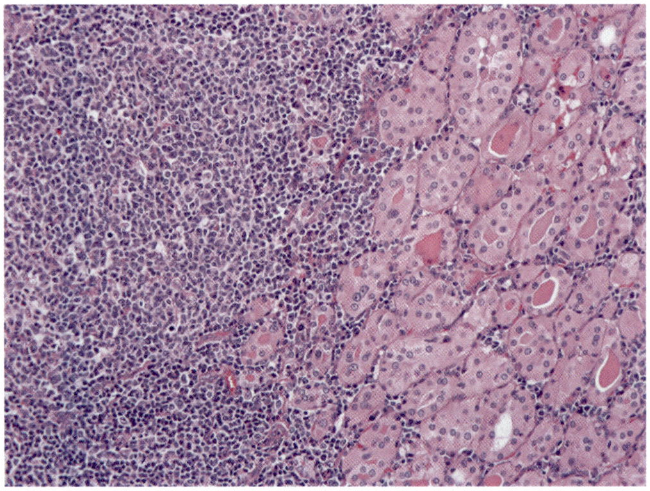

Figure 3.8b — Hashimoto Thyroiditis, Histologic Section. The follicular epithelium in Hashimoto thyroiditis often demonstrates oxyphilic change characterized by a cytoplasm that is abundant, eosinophilic and granular, and nuclei that are enlarged and vesicular with prominent nucleoli. The nuclear changes are most pronounced in those areas heavily enveloped by the lymphoplasmacytic infiltrate. Caution must be used not to mistake these reactive nuclear alterations for the nuclear atypia of papillary carcinoma. (H&E stain)

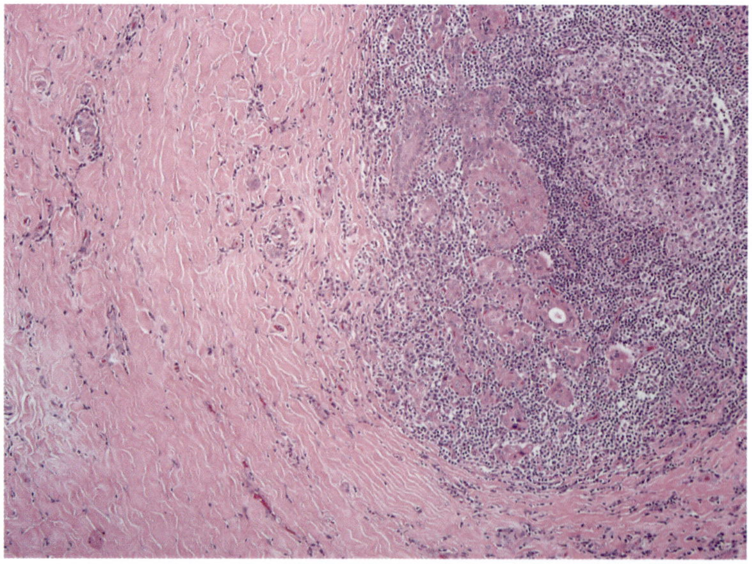

Figure 3.9 — Hashimoto Thyroiditis, Sclerosing Variant, Histologic Section. The sclerosing variant of Hashimoto thyroiditis is characterized by severe follicular atrophy and large zones of replacement fibrosis. (H&E stain)

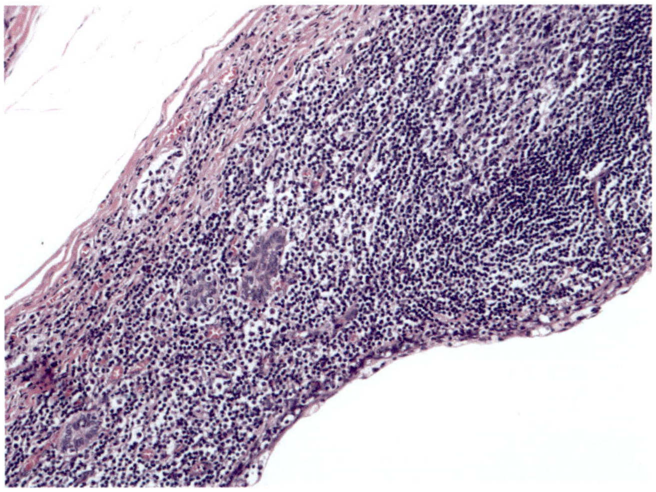

Figure 3.10 — Lymphoepithelial Cyst Arising in Hashimoto Thyroiditis, Histologic Section. Lymphoepithelial cysts of the thyroid are usually encountered in the setting of chronic lymphocytic thyroiditis. They show some resemblance to branchial cleft cysts of the lateral neck. The cyst is lined by a squamous epithelium, and its wall is heavily infiltrated by lymphocytes with scattered germinal centers. In this case, a few entrapped thyroid follicles with early squamous metaplasia are present within the lymphoid infiltrate. (H&E stain)

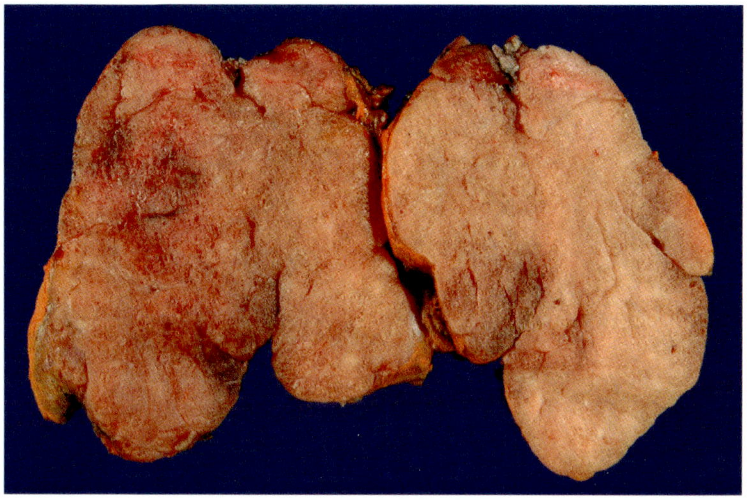

Figure 3.11 — Graves Disease, Gross Appearance. In Graves disease, the thyroid is diffusely and symmetrically enlarged. The presence of macronodularity and fibrosis are not common findings in untreated forms of Graves disease.

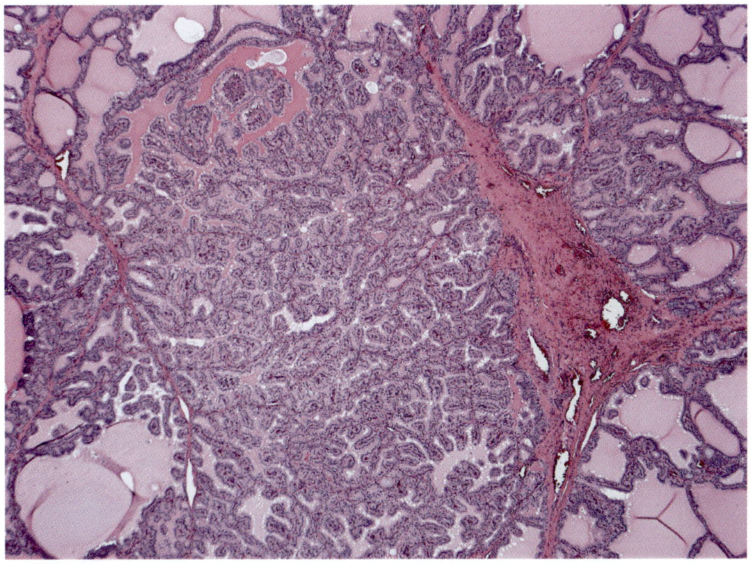

Figure 3.12a — Graves Disease, Histologic Section. Accentuated thyroid lobules are separated by thin fibrous bands. The degree of cellularity and the amount of colloid depends on the state of the disease. In untreated Graves disease, the thyroid parenchyma is highly cellular and much of the colloid is depleted. Papillary infoldings into the follicles by hyperplastic follicular cells is a common finding. (H&E stain)

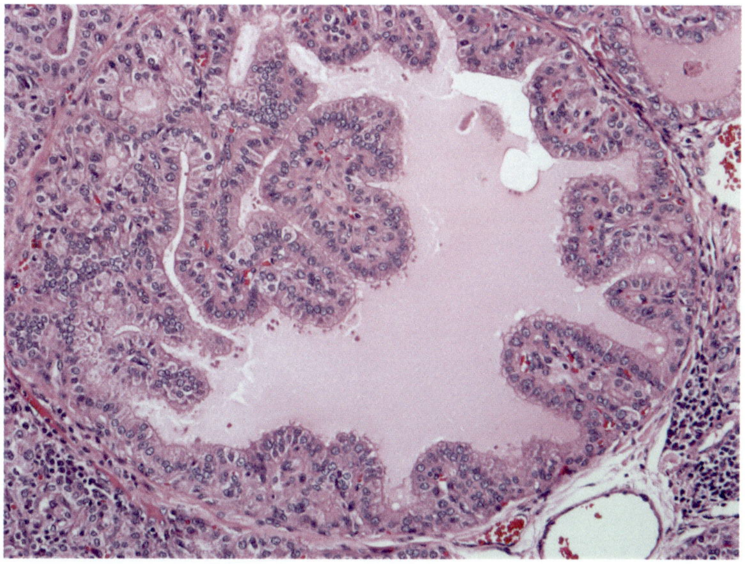

Figure 3.12b — Graves Disease, Histologic Section. Papillary hyperplasia is a common finding in Graves disease, and one that may cause confusion with papillary thyroid carcinoma. The presence of nuclear enlargement with chromatin clearing may further contribute to the confusion. Unlike papillary carcinoma, the benign papillae in Graves disease are consistently broad-based, have short stubby projections that point to the center of the follicles, lack complex branching, and tend to be a diffuse rather than localized finding. (H&E stain)

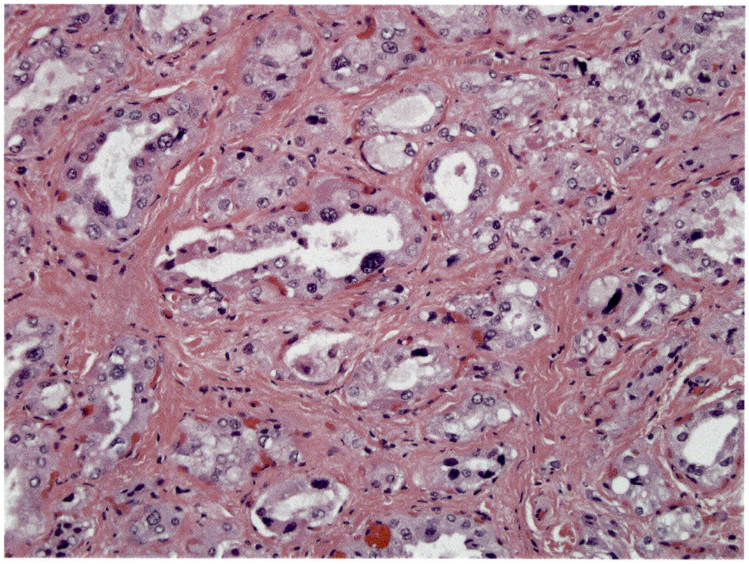

Figure 3.12c — Graves Disease, Histologic Section. The histologic picture of Graves disease may dramatically shift with some forms of treatment. In particular, radioiodine treatment causes involution of the thyroid with progressive follicle atrophy and fibrosis. The cells lining the follicles often show nuclear enlargement with hyperchromasia. This is a degenerative form of atypia related to the radioiodine. (H&E stain)

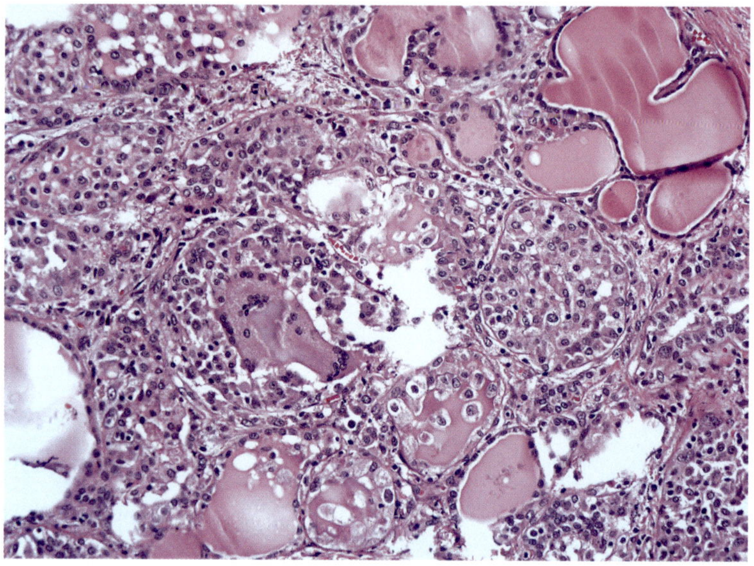

Figure 3.13 — Granulomatous (Subacute) Thyroiditis, Histologic Section. The thyroid is involved by a patchy infiltrate comprised mostly of histiocytes. The histiocytic infiltrate is centered on individual thyroid follicles. Destruction of the follicular epithelium results in a rim of histiocytes and giant cells surrounding residual droplets of colloid. Unlike palpation granulomas, the inflammatory process spills into the surrounding thyroid parenchyma. (H&E stain)

Figure 3.14 — Amyloid Goiter, Histologic Section. Amyloid deposition causing clinical enlargement of the thyroid is known as amyloid goiter. The deposition of pink amyloid material in the interfollicular areas causes atrophy and replacement of the thyroid follicles. As amyloid deposition is a common finding in medullary thyroid carcinoma, the presence of amyloid should prompt a careful microscopic evaluation to rule out the possibility of tumor-associated amyloid deposition. Conversely, zones of dense acellular hyalinization are often present in the center of follicular adenomas and hyperplastic nodules, often in a perivascular distribution. These areas of collagen deposition should not be confused with amyloid. A Congo Red stain for amyloid is helpful in those cases where the distinction is not readily apparent on histologic grounds. (H&E stain)

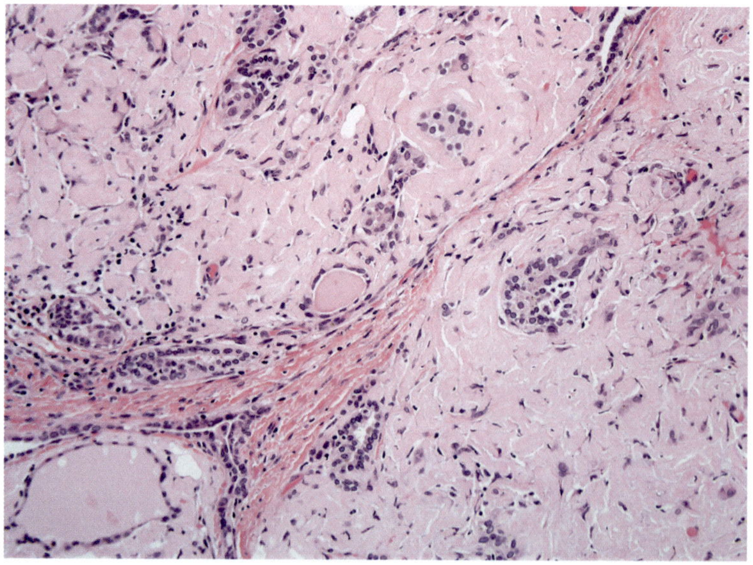

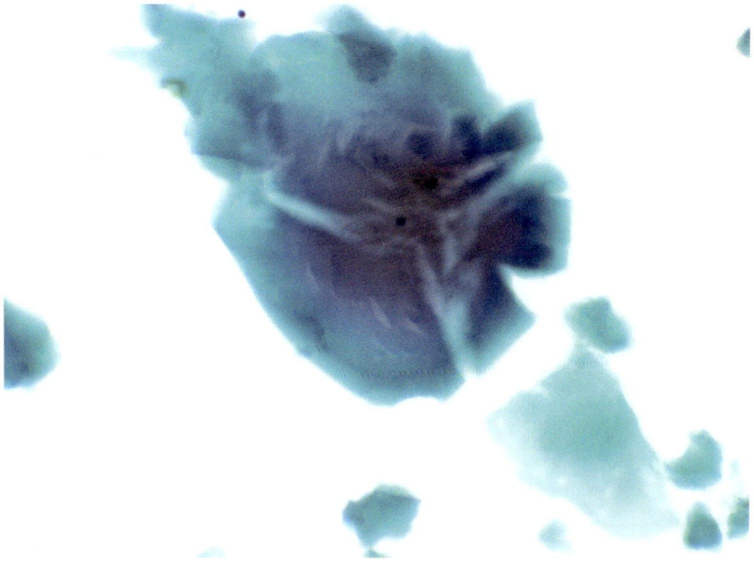

Figure 3.15a — Colloid, Fine Needle Aspiration (FNA). Benign follicular nodules are comprised of varying proportions of follicular epithelium and colloid. Colloid may have a variety of appearances, but most frequently appears as dense green to pink droplets on Papanicolaou stained preparations. These droplets frequently have jagged edges with cracks and bubbles evident within the substance of the colloid. Degenerated or the so-called "watery" colloid can be confused on both Diff Quik and Papanicolaou stains with serum in bloody specimens. Helpful clues are the recognition of cracking and folding in colloid, as well as its tendency to surround follicular cells, whereas serum accumulates at the edges of the slide and around platelets, fibrin, and blood clots. (Papanicolaou stain)

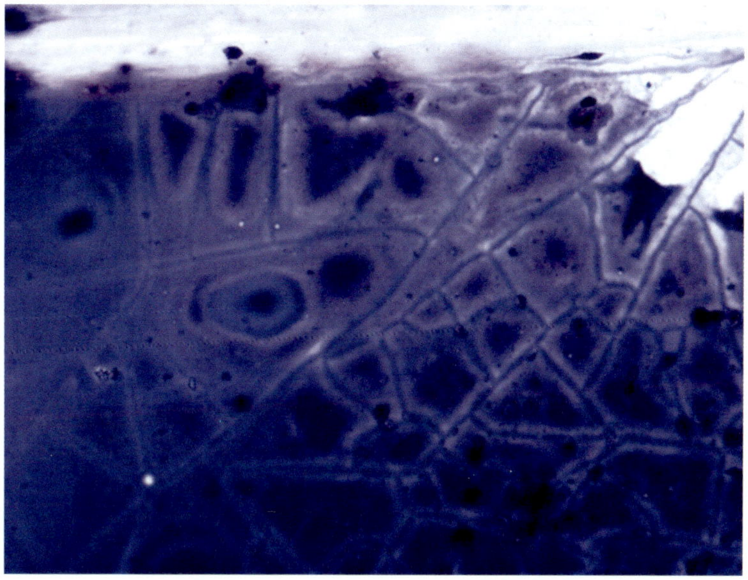

Figure 3.15b — Colloid, FNA. On air dried direct smear preparations, colloid aspirated from benign nodules may show a characteristic artifact with linear or crisscrossing lines frequently referred to as a "broken glass" appearance. This appearance is not specific for colloid and can occasionally be seen with precipitated serum in a bloody aspirate. Colloid appears dark blue or violet or magenta on Diff Quik stain and assumes a green to orange/pink color with the Papanicolaou stain. (Diff Quik stain)

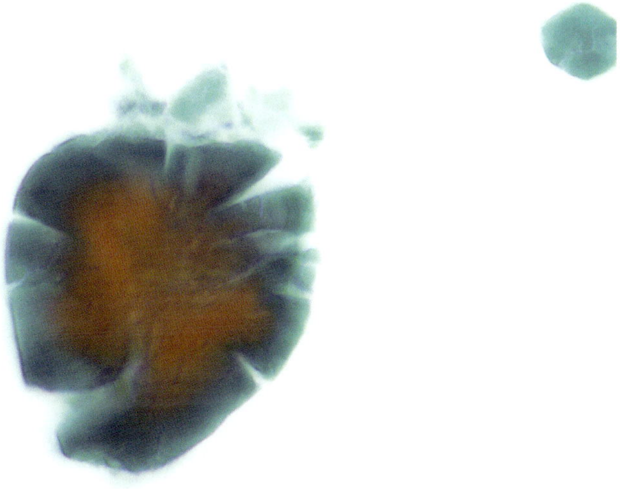

Figure 3.16a — Colloid, FNA. At high power, the cracking artifact characteristic of colloid is easily appreciated. The staining quality of skeletal muscle can closely resemble colloid at low power. At high power, skeletal muscle exhibits striations in contrast to the features seen here. On gross examination, colloid appears as shiny, viscous and light yellow or gold colored substance (resembling honey or varnish) when expelled from the needle onto the glass slide. (Liquid based preparation, Papanicolaou stain)

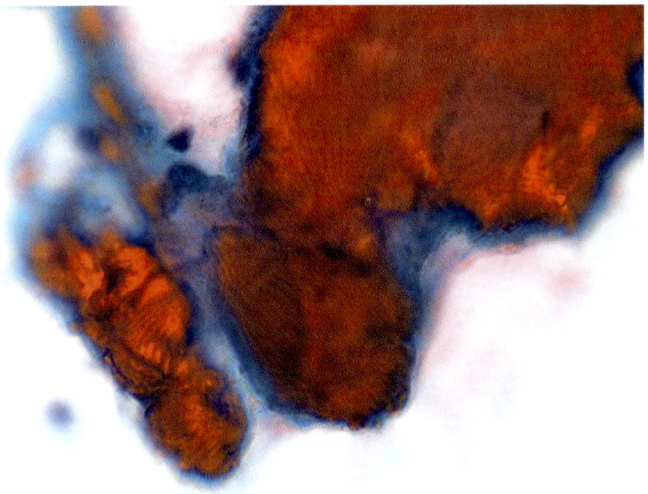

Figure 3.16b — Skeletal Muscle, FNA. Although at low power, these fragments of skeletal muscle can resemble colloid aspirated from a thyroid lesion, higher magnification will almost always display the characteristic cross striations (as seen here). Needle penetration of sternocleidomastoid muscle can occur in small thyroid nodules located laterally in the lobe. The patient may complain of significant pain when the needle traverses a segment of muscle, often occluding the needle's lumen and usually resulting in a nondiagnostic aspirate. (Papanicolaou stain)

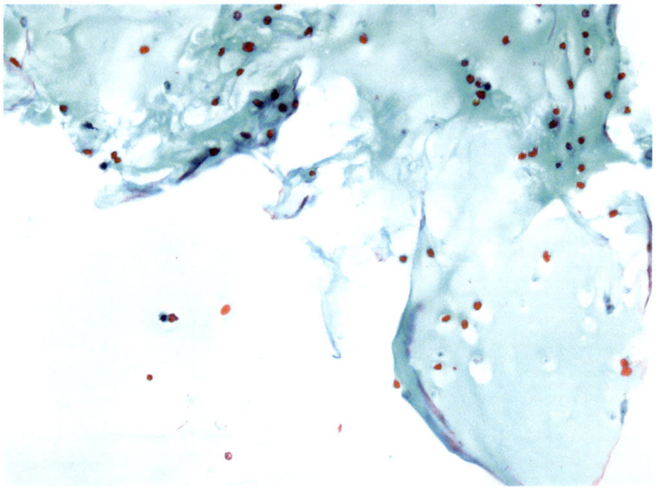

Figure 3.17a — Liquid Colloid, FNA. In smears, colloid may present with a thin, filmy quality. Focal holes or bubbles appear to be embedded within the colloid. The presence of abundant colloid increases the likelihood that the sample represents a benign thyroid nodule. Specimens consisting of abundant colloid only, with very few or no follicular cells, are considered benign and may be reported as being suggestive of or consistent with a colloid nodule. (Papanicolaou stain)

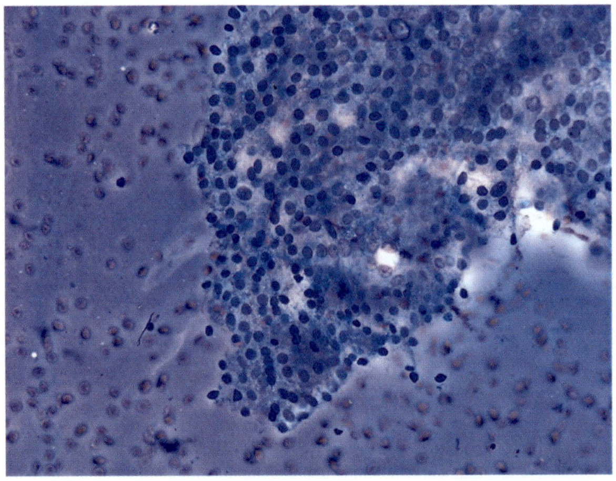

Figure 3.17b — Adenomatoid Nodule, FNA. In this direct smear preparation, abundant colloid and associated follicular epithelium are characteristic findings. Occasionally, it becomes difficult to distinguish colloid from precipitated serum on Wright-Giemsa staining. Because most thyroid nodules are benign, a benign result is the most common FNA interpretation (approximately 65% of all cases). Note the relationship of colloid to follicular epithelium as it surrounds the tissue fragment. (Diff Quik stain)

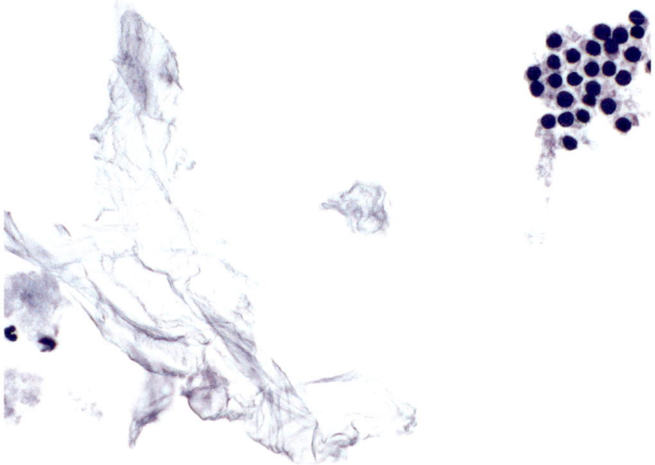

Figure 3.18 — Liquid Colloid, FNA. In liquid based preparations, liquid colloid may also form thin, filmy collections that stain a pale blue to grey color. There are irregular folds within the colloid conferring a tissue paper-like quality to the colloid. Fibrin aggregates may mimic this appearance at low power, but are comprised of thin fibrin strands when examined at higher power. A small sheet of benign follicular cells is present at upper right. (Liquid based preparation, Papanicolaou stain)

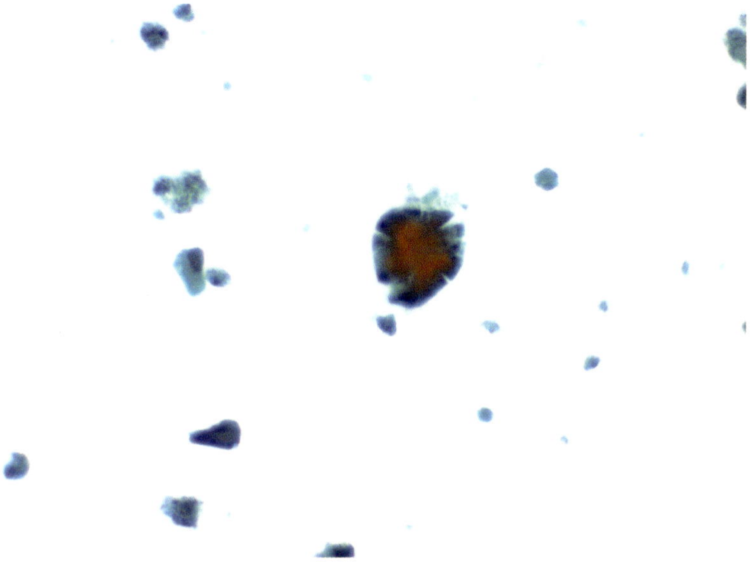

Figure 3.19 — Colloid Nodule, FNA. Even in the absence of follicular cells, the presence of abundant colloid implies sampling of a macrofollicular nodule and should be interpreted as benign rather than nondiagnostic. The adequacy criteria for a benign adenomatoid nodule (6 groups of follicular cells with 10 or more cells per group) does not apply to such cases with an abundance of colloid and these aspirates can be deemed adequate with far few follicular cells. Same case as in Figure 3.16a. (Liquid based preparation, Papanicolaou stain)

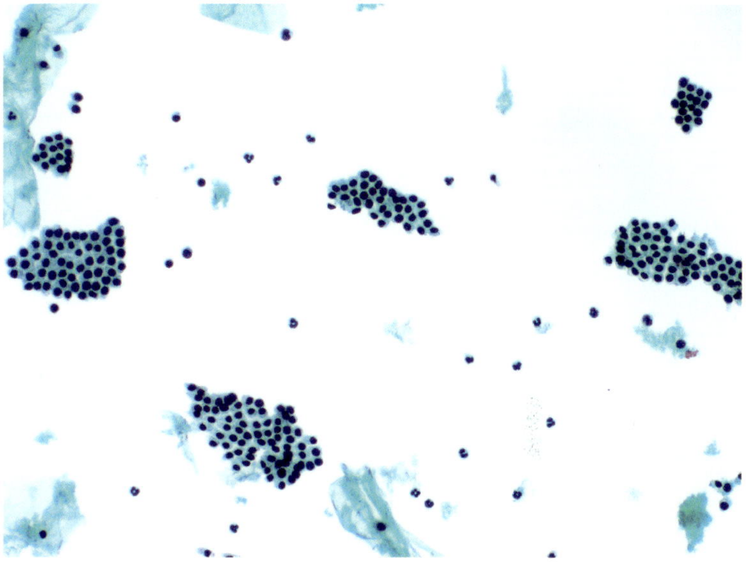

Figure 3.20a — Normal Follicular Epithelium, FNA. Benign thyroid nodules, including hyperplastic nodules and macrofollicular adenomas, are recognizable on FNA by a predominance of macrofollicles. In most instances, macrofollicles are not removed intact. Colloid is released from the ruptured follicle while the macrofollicular epithelium is seen as large flat sheets of cohesive follicular cells. (Liquid based preparation, Papanicolaou stain)

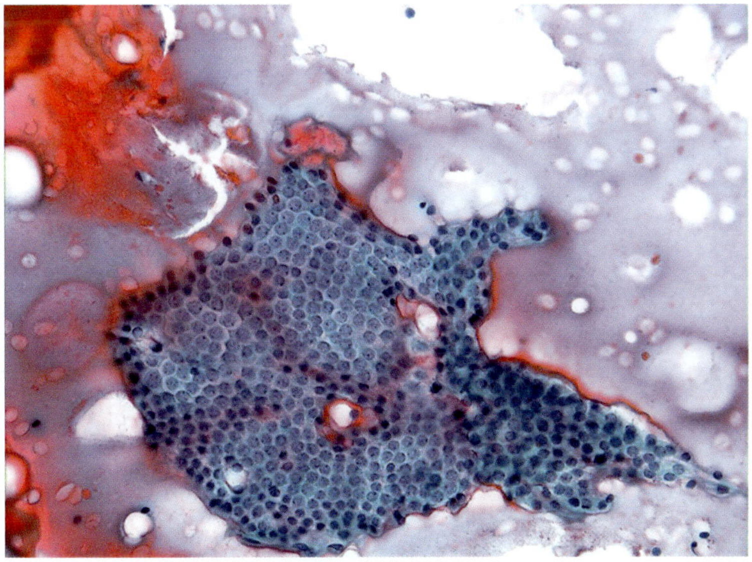

Figure 3.20b — Adenomatoid Nodule, FNA. Flat honey-combed sheets of follicular epithelium represent portions of ruptured macrofollicles. Abundant colloid is usually present in the smear background. Lack of nuclear features (grooves, intranuclear inclusions, oval nuclear shapes) distinguishes these benign fragments from papillary thyroid carcinoma. Adenomatoid nodule or nodular goiter is the most common benign diagnosis in thyroid cytopathology. Benign cytopathology is associated with a very low risk of malignancy and patients are usually followed conservatively with periodic clinical and radiologic examinations. (Papanicolaou stain)

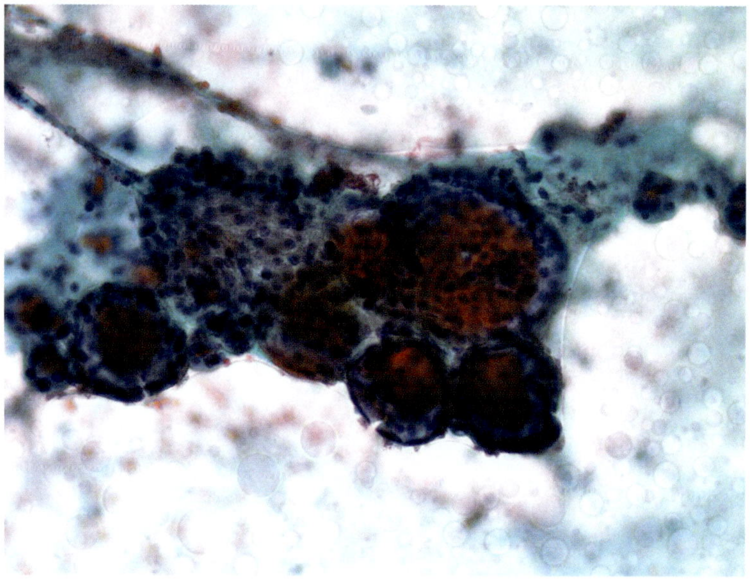

Figure 3.20c — Adenomatoid Nodule, FNA. In adenomatoid nodules, the specimens are sparsely to moderately cellular showing a polymorphous architectural pattern characterized by mostly macrofollicles of varying sizes containing colloid. Free colloid is also present in the smear background. To report benign thyroid FNA results, the term "benign" is preferred over other terms such as "negative for malignancy" and "nonneoplastic." (Papanicolaou stain)

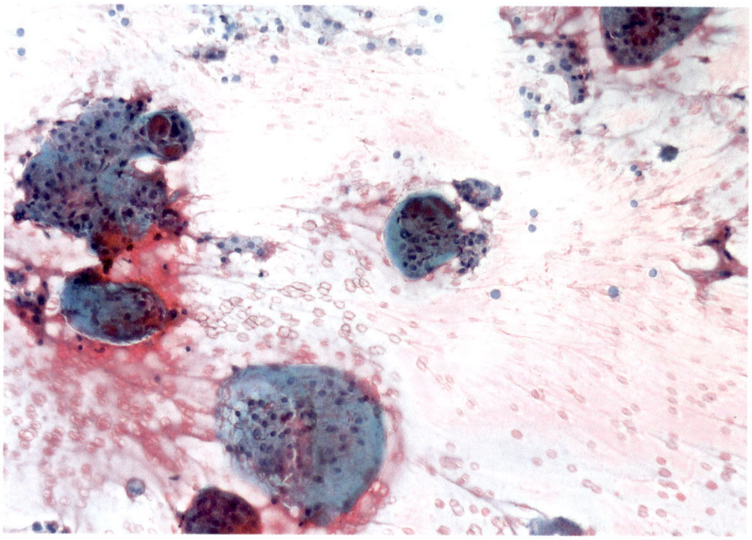

Figure 3.20d — Adenomatoid Nodule, FNA. Multinucleated giant cells are commonly present in benign nodules with cystic changes (as seen in this direct smear preparation). Such cases occasionally raise the possibility of papillary thyroid carcinoma, cystic variant as the latter tumor may contain similar giant cells. Presence of abundant background colloid (as seen here) would be unusual for papillary carcinoma. (Papanicolaou stain)

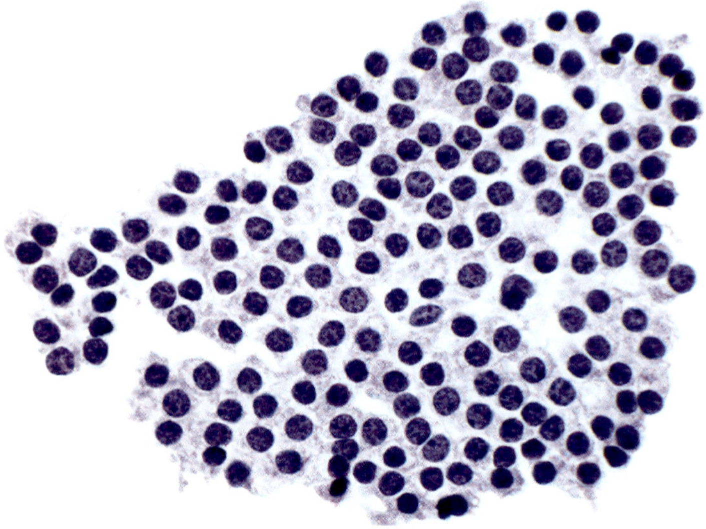

Figure 3.21 — Normal Follicular Epithelium, FNA. Macrofollicular sheets have a honeycombed appearance with regular spacing between cells. The follicular cells have relatively sparse, clear to slightly granular cytoplasm. Nuclei are round, small (about the size of a red blood cell), and uniform in appearance. Scattered microfollicles may be present. (Liquid based preparation, Papanicolaou stain)

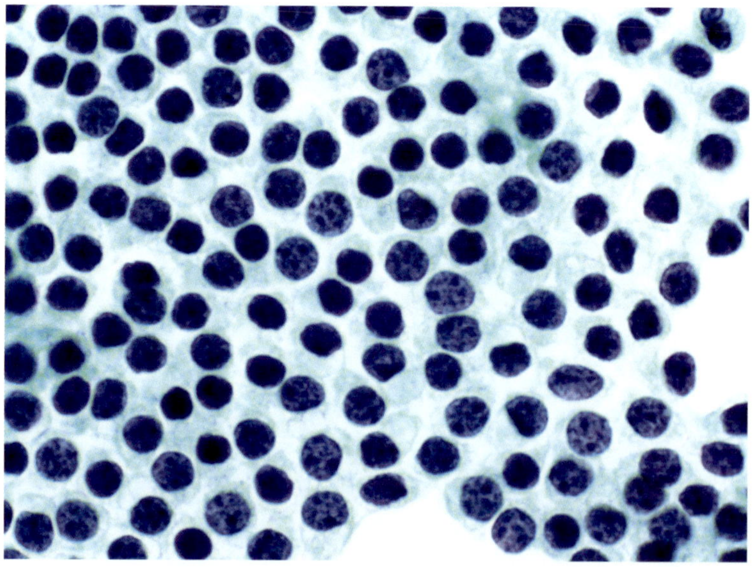

Figure 3.22 — Normal Follicular Epithelium, FNA. At high power, the uniformity of the cellular spacing is evident. Nuclei are round with coarse, granular chromatin. The follicular cells have scant or moderate amounts of delicate cytoplasm. Focal anisonucleosis may be appreciated in some cases, but there is no significant pleomorphism or nuclear atypia. (Liquid based preparation, Papanicolaou stain)

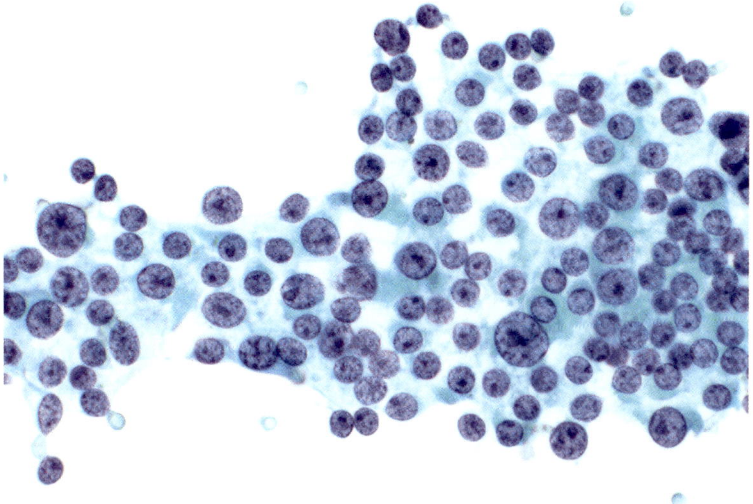

Figure 3.23 — Normal Follicular Epithelium, FNA. Occasionally, benign follicular cells will exhibit more pronounced variation in nuclear size as demonstrated here. Although spacing is somewhat irregular, the nuclei do not crowd and overlap one another as is often seen in papillary carcinoma. Nuclear chromatin is coarse and granular with round nuclear contours. The cytoplasm, although not abundant, has some of the granularity of Hürthle cells, which may account in some part for the nuclear variability. Isolated nuclear size variation in a macrofollicular sheet does not warrant an atypical diagnosis. (Papanicolaou stain)

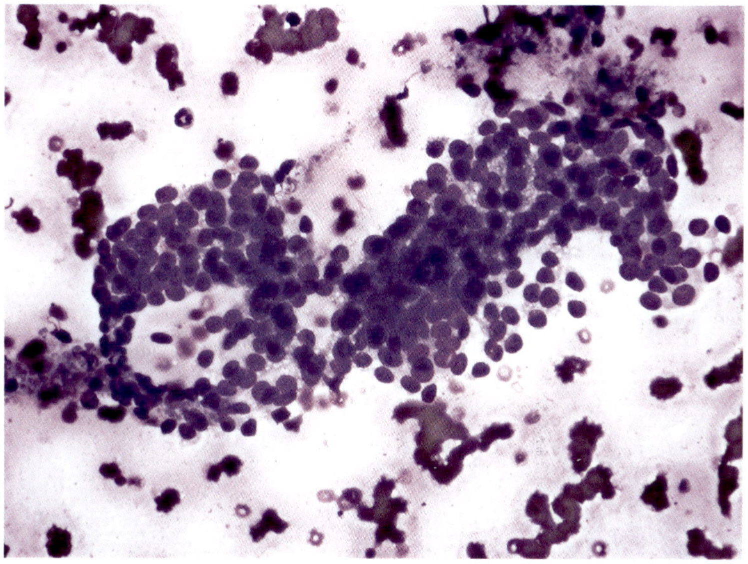

Figure 3.24 — Normal Follicular Epithelium, FNA. Macrofollicular sheets sometimes fold upon themselves which creates the impression of slight cellular crowding. A papillary-like pattern (without fibrovascular cores) is an uncommon architectural variation and reflects papillary hyperplasia in an adenomatoid nodule. (Diff Quik stain)

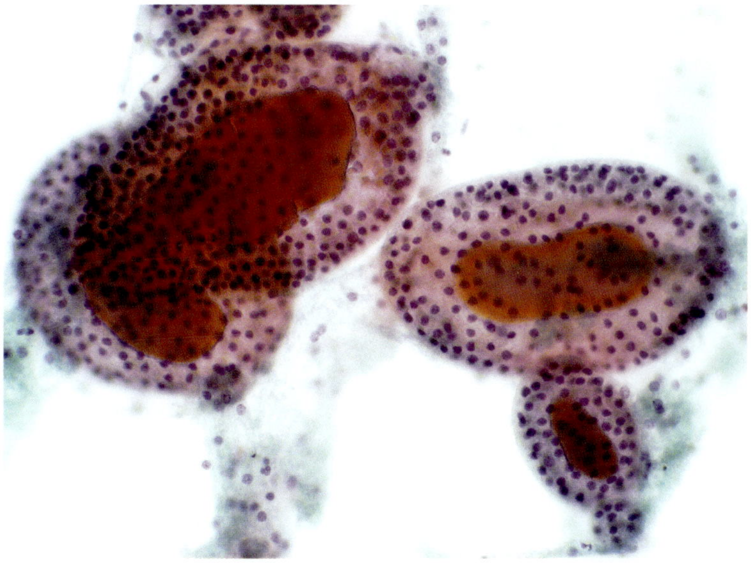

Figure 3.25a — Normal Follicular Epithelium, FNA. Occasionally intact macrofollicles are aspirated in which the spherical quality of the follicles can be appreciated and centrally located colloid with associated cracking artifact is present. Although most of the intact follicles here are variably sized macrofollicles, a microfollicle can be seen at the lower right. A predominance of macrofollicles is indicative of a benign thyroid nodule. (Liquid based preparation, Papanicolaou stain)

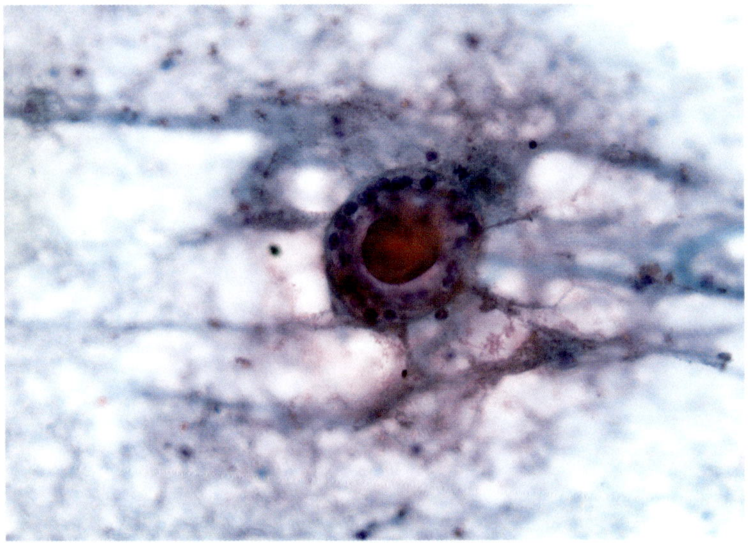

Figure 3.25b — Normal Follicular Epithelium, FNA. An intact macrofollicle is seen in this direct smear preparation comprising of a well-defined ring of follicular epithelium enclosing a globular aggregate of centrally located colloid. (Papanicolaou stain)

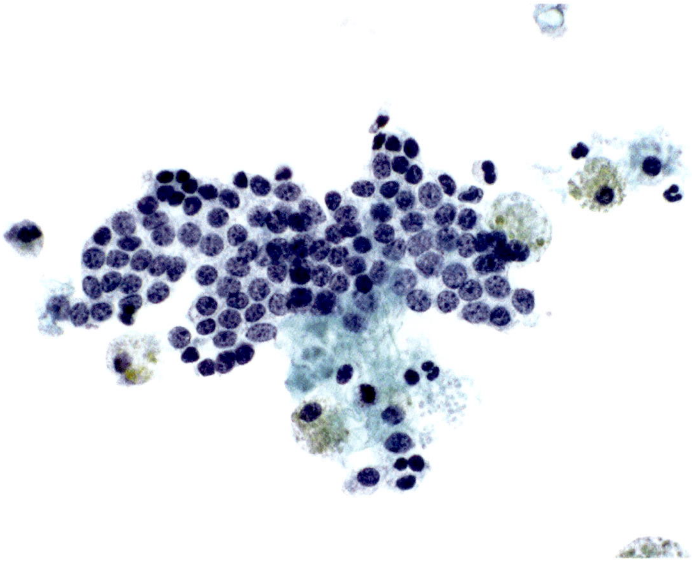

Figure 3.26 — Benign Nodule With Cystic Degeneration, FNA. Some degree of cystic degeneration occurs frequently in benign thyroid nodules. In addition to a macrofollicular sheet of epithelial cells, several hemosiderin-laden macrophages are present indicative of the presence of cystic degeneration. (Liquid based preparation, Papanicolaou stain)

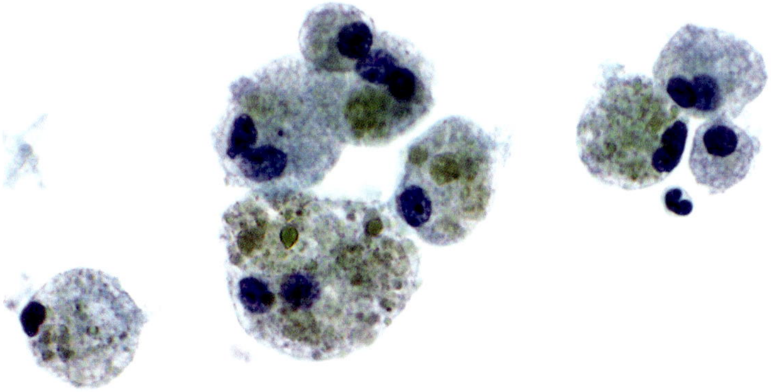

Figure 3.27a — Hemosiderin-Laden Macrophages, FNA. Macrophages are present as individual cells. The cells have abundant granular cytoplasm with refractile greenish-brown hemosiderin pigment. Cystic degeneration can occur with both benign and malignant nodules. When epithelial elements are not adequately represented (less than 6 groups of follicular cells with at least 10 cells per group), the specimen should be reported as nondiagnostic representing cyst contents. (Liquid based preparation, Papanicolaou stain)

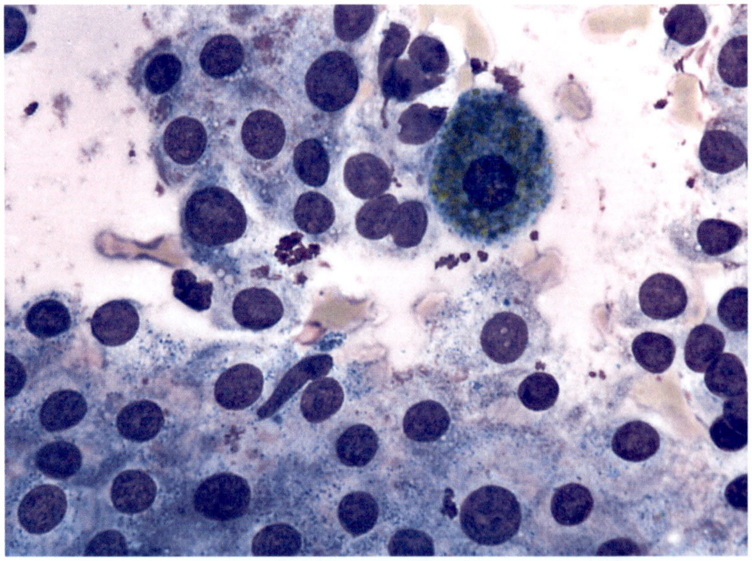

Figure 3.27b — Hemosiderin-Laden Macrophage, FNA. In this direct smear image, a single hemosiderin-laden macrophage is seen alongside abundant Hürthle cells. The thin cystic walls often contain fragile capillary vessels which are prone to bleeding and hence the presence of hemosiderin-laden macrophages signifies hemorrhage into a cystic nodule. (Diff Quik stain)

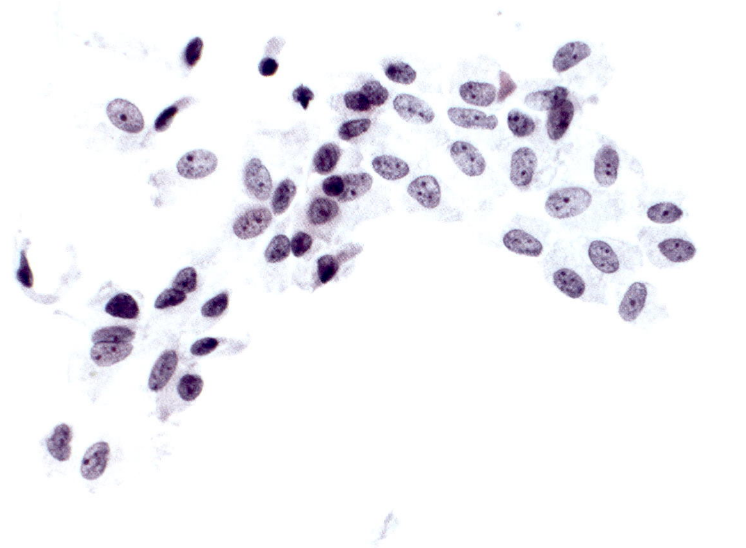

Figure 3.28a — Cyst Lining Cells, FNA. With cystic degeneration, a population of reparative cyst lining cells may be seen. These cells have abundant cytoplasm and may have a rounded or spindled shape. Nuclei are round, oval, or spindled with pale chromatin. Nuclear grooves may be present raising concern for papillary carcinoma when the nuclear changes are pronounced or the cyst lining origin is uncertain. (Liquid based preparation, Papanicolaou stain)

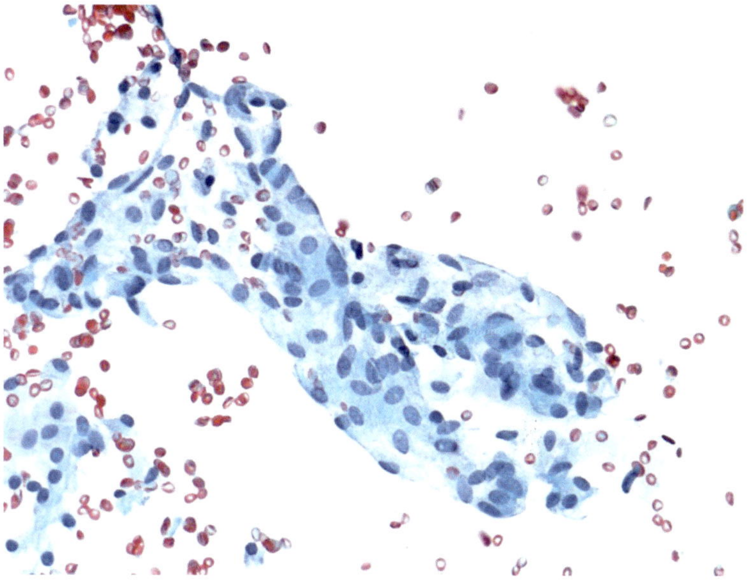

Figure 3.28b — Cyst Lining Cells, FNA. Bland cells with mostly uniform oval-shaped nuclei are seen on a direct smear preparation. Occasionally these cells may display longitudinal nuclear grooves and may be classified as Atypia of Undetermined Significance (AUS) in a limited sample. (Papanicolaou stain)

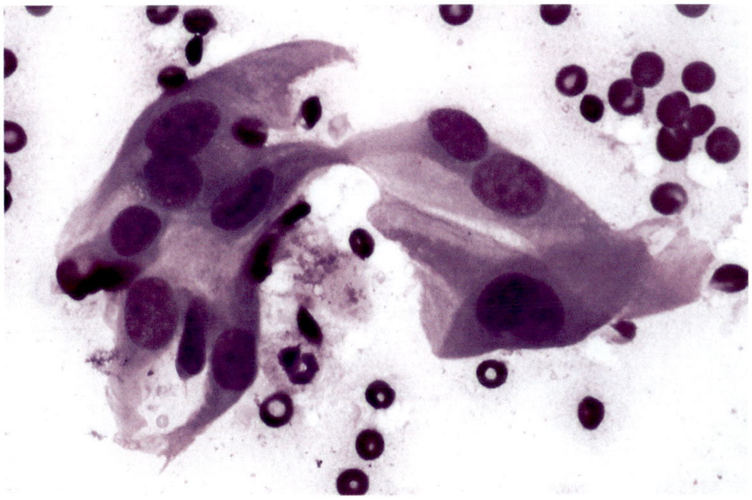

Figure 3.29 — Cyst Lining Cells, FNA. In this example of cyst lining cells, the reparative quality of the cells is more apparent than the prior images. Spindled cells with abundant cytoplasm form a streaming sheet. (Diff Quik stain)

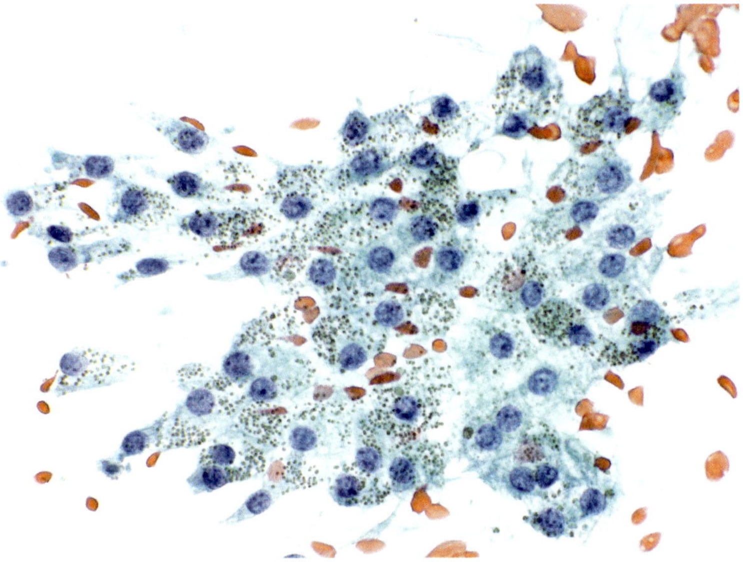

Figure 3.30 — Black Thyroid, FNA. Follicular cells may contain pigment such as hemosiderin in the presence of cystic degeneration. In patients on long-term therapy with antibiotics such as minocycline, pronounced deposition of dark brown pigment can be seen within follicular cells. These deposits can result in the gross appearance of a "black thyroid." Ultrastructural examinations of black thyroid glands display lysosomal accumulations of lipofuscin-like pigment and granular electron-dense material. Hypothyroidism has been reported in severe cases of black thyroid. (Papanicolaou stain)

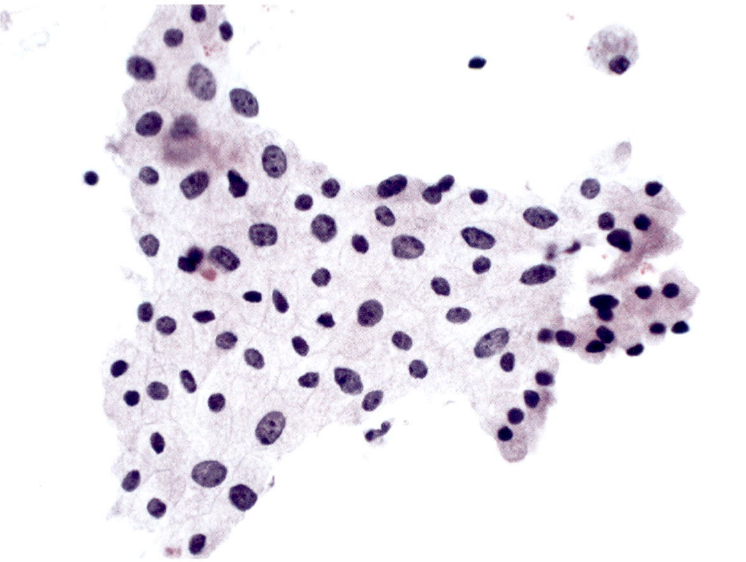

Figure 3.31a — Hürthle Cells, FNA. Hürthle cells are present as a component of many benign nodules. The cells are large, polygonal, and have abundant granular cytoplasm. In benign nodules, the presence of Hürthle cell change is typically a focal finding. The Hürthle cells usually occur in cohesive clusters as seen in this example. (Liquid based preparation, Papanicolaou stain)

Figure 3.31b — Adenomatoid Nodule With Hürthle Cell Change, FNA. The anisonucleosis seen in this direct smear preparation is an expected finding. Hürthle cells are large, polygonal cells with abundant granular cytoplasm, a large nucleus, and often prominent nucleolus. Hürthle cells can be seen as cohesive sheets or as single dissociated cells. (Diff Quik stain)

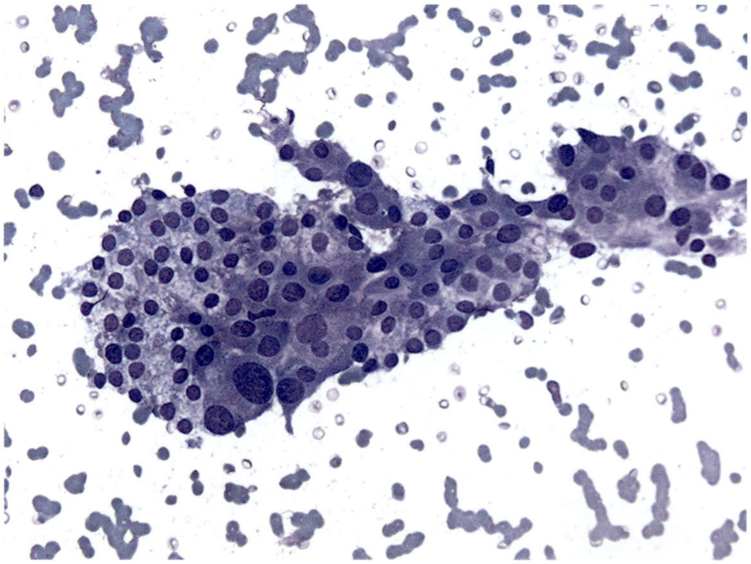

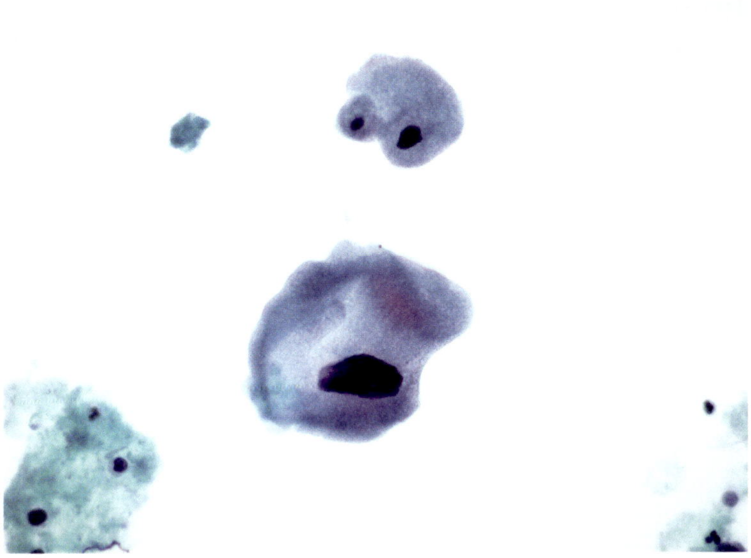

Figure 3.32 — Hürthle Cells, FNA. Hürthle cells with abundant granular cytoplasm may also occur as single cells. Marked nuclear size variation, as seen here, is a common finding in nonneoplastic Hürthle cells. Morphometric studies measuring cell size, nuclear size, and nucleolar prominence have failed to identify a single feature that can reliably distinguish a metaplastic from a neoplastic Hürthle cell. (Liquid based preparation, Papanicolaou stain)

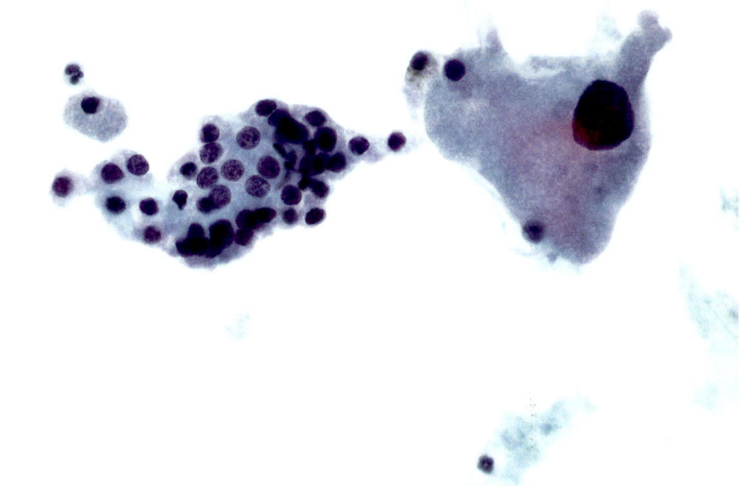

Figure 3.33a — Hürthle Cells, FNA. Hürthle cells in benign aspirates occur in a mixed background with benign appearing follicular cells as seen here. Often there are cells exhibiting a spectrum of changes with some cells lacking any Hürthle cell features, others having modestly increased amounts of oncocytic cytoplasm and still others with abundant granular cytoplasm. (Liquid based preparation, Papanicolaou stain)

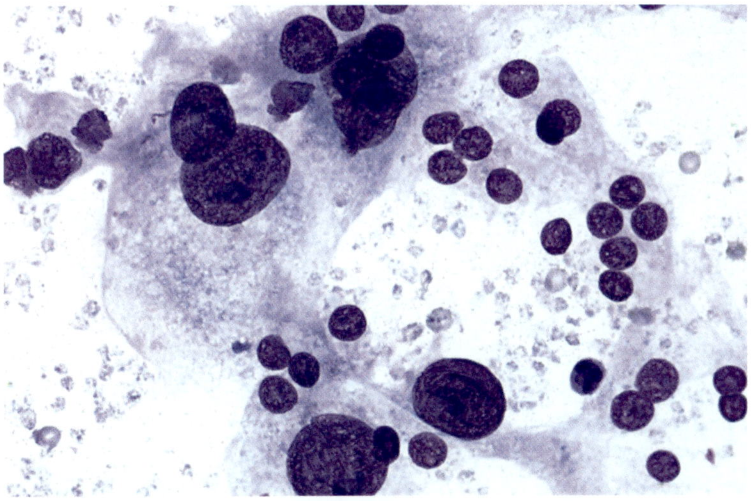

Figure 3.33b — Hürthle Cells, FNA. A similar appearance as in the previous image is seen on this direct smear preparation of an adenomatoid nodule. Note the presence of significant anisonucleosis, macronucleoli, and naked nuclei. Such anisonucleosis is fairly common in adenomatoid nodules with Hürthle cell metaplasia and is a common source of an overcall of these cases as AUS. (Diff Quik stain)

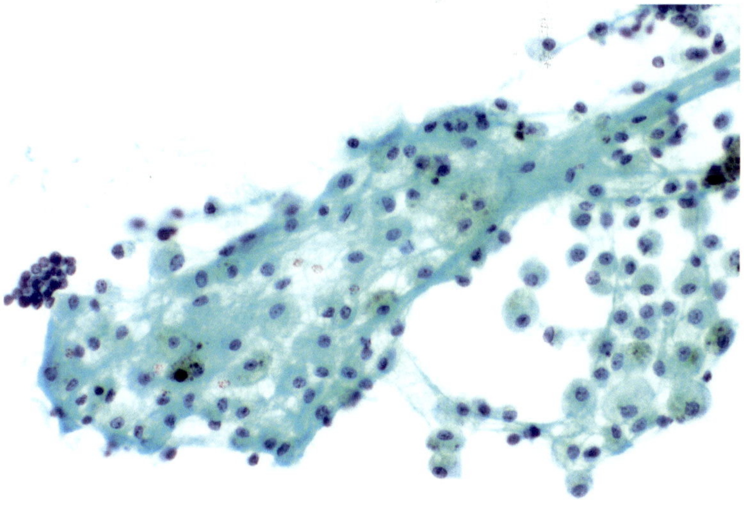

Figure 3.34 — Macrophages Mimicking Hürthle Cells, FNA. Hürthle cells may be difficult to distinguish from macrophages, especially when the Hürthle cells are present in isolation or the macrophages are clustered. In this case, macrophages entrapped in fibrin are artificially clustering. At low power, the cells have abundant slightly granular cytoplasm that could be mistaken for Hürthle cells. (Papanicolaou stain)

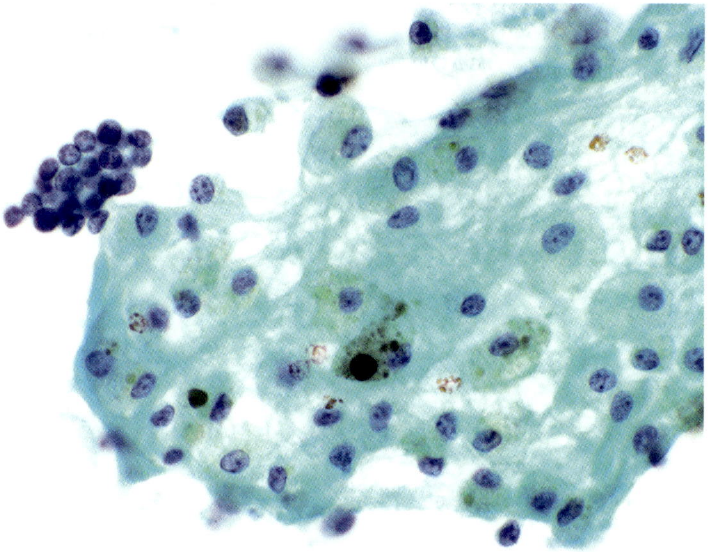

Figure 3.35 — Macrophages Mimicking Hürthle Cells, FNA. At higher power, the cells from the previous image are more easily appreciated as being macrophages. The macrophages have somewhat vacuolated cytoplasm in contrast to the uniform, dense, granular cytoplasm of Hürthle cells. Several of the macrophages also contain hemosiderin. The oval, occasionally slightly folded, contour of the macrophage nucleus is also a helpful distinguishing feature. (Papanicolaou stain)

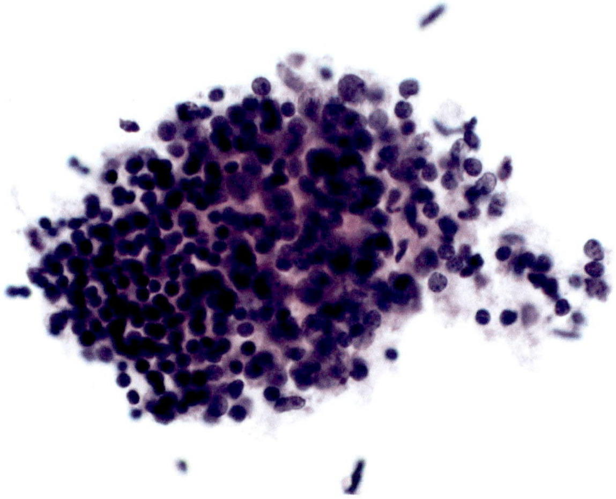

Figure 3.36a — Lymphocytes in Hashimoto (Lymphocytic) Thyroiditis, FNA. Hashimoto thyroiditis is characterized by the presence of benign appearing follicular cells, Hürthle cells, and lymphocytes. Lymphoid cells may be present singly in the background, as single cells percolating through epithelial cell groups, or as isolated lymphohistiocytic aggregates as shown in this image. A polymorphous aggregate of lymphoid cells is present with admixed histiocytes. Anisonucleosis of Hürthle cells may be prominent in some cases of Hashimoto thyroiditis. Occasionally, mild nuclear atypia is encountered, including scattered nuclear clearing and grooves, and rare intranuclear inclusions. A diagnosis of "Atypia of Undetermined Significance" is not unusual in cases of Hashimoto thyroiditis. (Liquid based preparation, Papanicolaou stain)

Figure 3.36b — Lymphocytes and Hürthle Cells in Hashimoto (Lymphocytic) Thyroiditis, FNA. Lymphocytic thyroiditis most commonly affects middle-aged women but is also frequent in adolescents. In this air dried direct smear preparation, a more characteristic biphasic (or bimodal) appearance is evident with an intimate admixture of polymorphous lymphocytes and Hürthle cells. In Hashimoto thyroiditis the smears are usually hypercellular, but advanced cases with fibrosis may decrease the apparent cellularity. It is important to remember that an interpretation of lymphocytic thyroiditis does not require a minimum number of follicular/Hürthle cells for specimen adequacy. (Diff Quik stain)

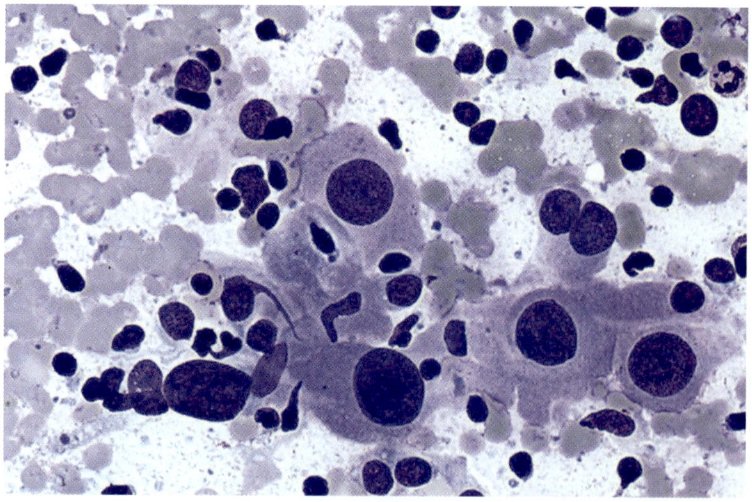

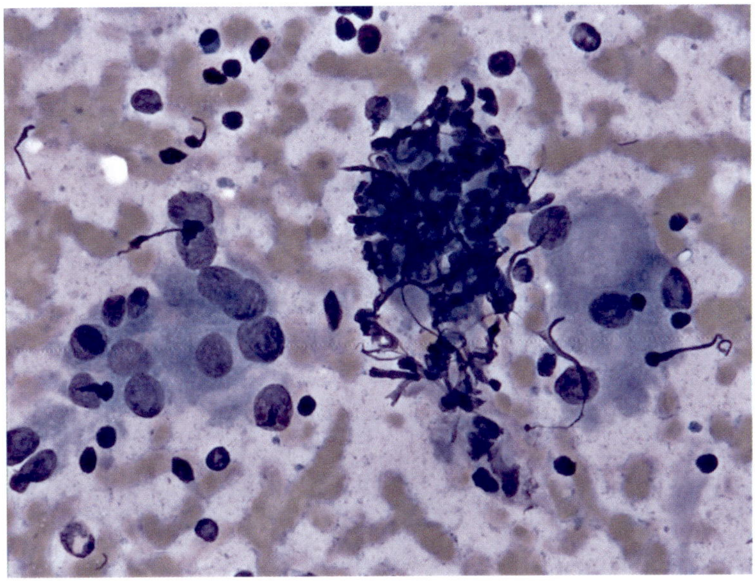

Figure 3.36c — Hashimoto (Lymphocytic) Thyroiditis, FNA. Crushed lymphoid tangles are extremely helpful in the diagnosis of chronic lymphocytic thyroiditis. In this case abundant metaplastic Hürthle cells were also observed. Hashimoto thyroiditis patients often develop diffuse thyroid enlargement, but are referred for FNA only when they develop nodularity or an increasing thyroid volume to exclude the possibility of carcinoma (most often a papillary thyroid carcinoma). (Diff Quik stain)

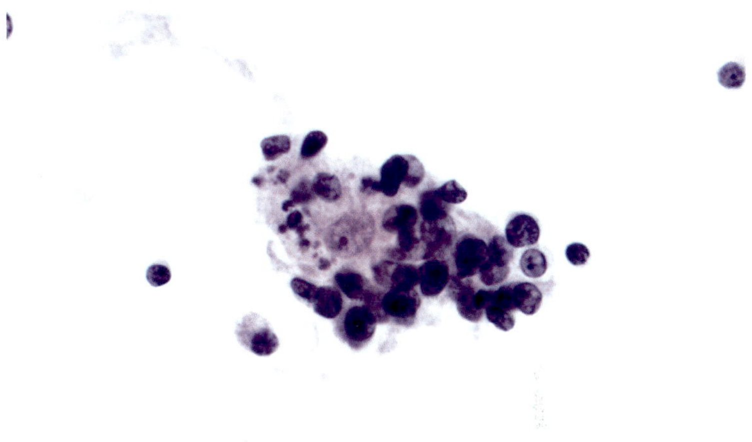

Figure 3.37a — Lymphocytes in Hashimoto (Lymphocytic) Thyroiditis, FNA. In this image from a case of Hashimoto thyroiditis, an aggregate of polymorphous lymphoid cells is seen in association with a tingible body macrophage containing apoptotic cellular fragments from a germinal center. Hashimoto thyroiditis is most often associated with circulating antibodies to thyroglobulin, thyroperoxidase (microsomal antigen), colloid antigen, and thyroid hormones. (Liquid based preparation, Papanicolaou stain)

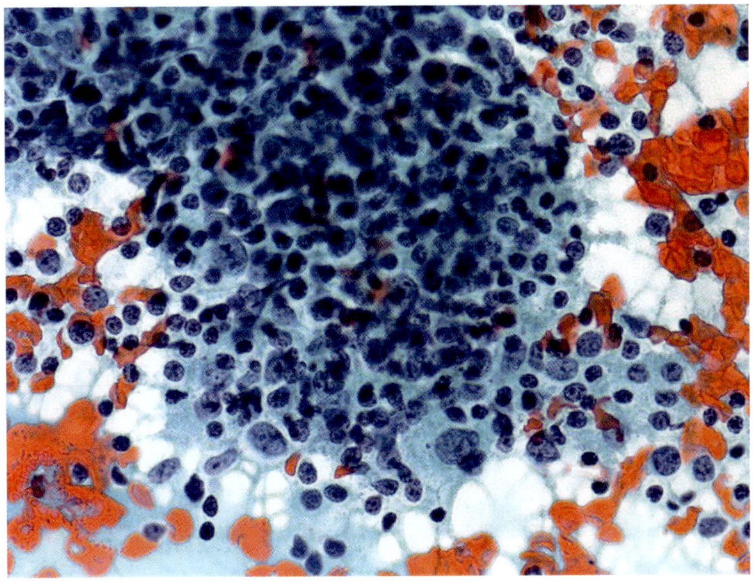

Figure 3.37b — Lymphocytes in Hashimoto (Lymphocytic) Thyroiditis, FNA. Occasionally, the diagnosis of Hashimoto thyroiditis is made with only polymorphous lymphocytes and few or no follicular cells, as long as the patient has clinical or serologic evidence of the disease. A large aggregate of lymphoid cells is seen here with few embedded tingible body macrophages on this direct smear preparation. (Papanicolaou stain)

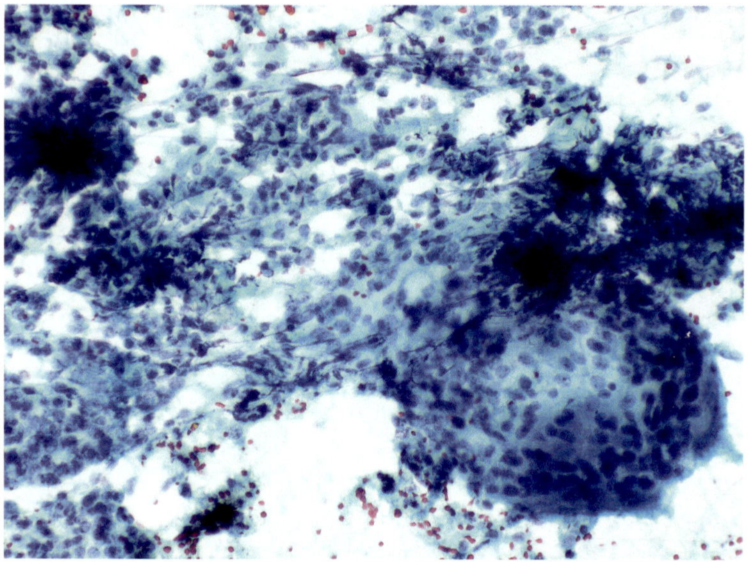

Figure 3.38a — Granulomatous (Subacute, De Quervain) Thyroiditis, FNA. This cellular aspirate had numerous granulomas comprised of aggregates of epithelioid histiocytes as well as frequent multinucleated giant cells. Depending on the stage of this self-limited inflammatory disease, the findings may more closely resemble acute thyroiditis with prominent neutrophils and/or eosinophils or be hypocellular in later stages. (Papanicolaou stain)

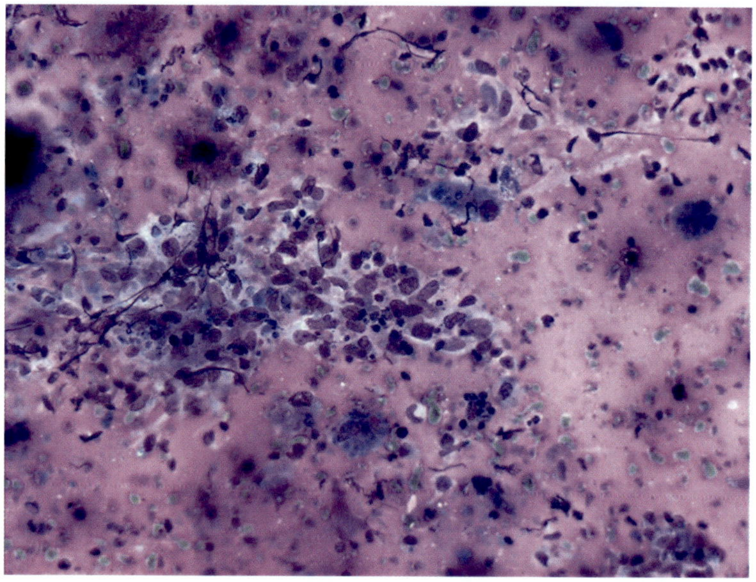

Figure 3.38b — Granulomatous (Subacute, De Quervain) Thyroiditis, FNA. The cellularity is variable and depends on the stage of disease. The FNA procedure may be quite painful for the patient, preventing adequate sampling of the thyroid nodule. A loose aggregate of epithelioid histiocytes is observed here consistent with granuloma formation. In the absence of granulomas, the cytologic findings are nonspecific in this condition. Background shows cystic changes and scattered inflammatory cells. Granulomatous thyroiditis is a self-limited inflammatory disease of the thyroid that is usually diagnosed clinically. (Diff Quik stain)

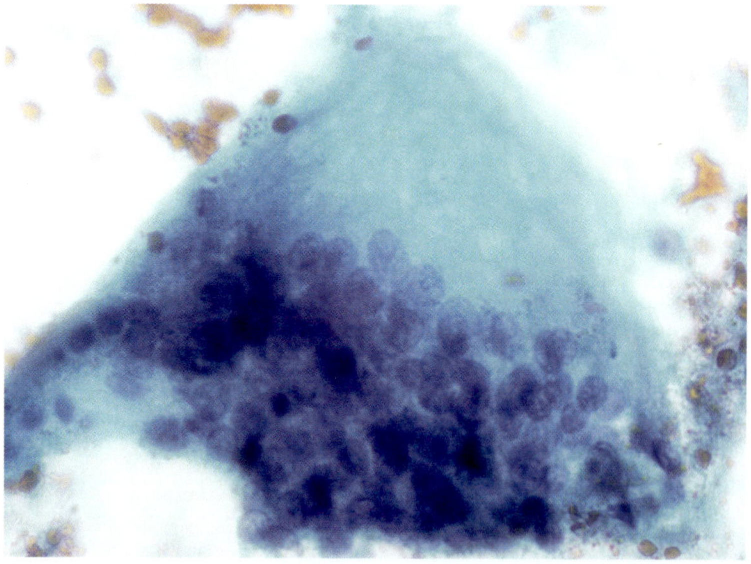

Figure 3.39 — Granulomatous (Subacute, De Quervain) Thyroiditis, FNA. Multinucleated giant cells, frequently with unusual shapes and numerous nuclei, are a characteristic feature of granulomatous thyroiditis. True granulomas are often more difficult to identify than these large giant cells. In later stages of the disease, the smears are hypocellular and the diagnosis is more challenging. FNA is generally performed in this condition only if there is a distinct nodularity that raises the possibility of a coexisting malignancy. (Papanicolaou stain)

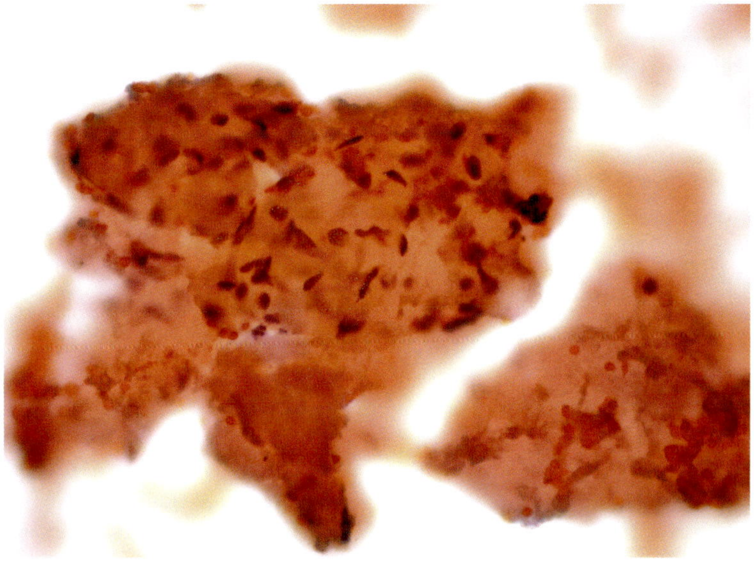

Figure 3.40 — Amyloid Goiter, FNA. Amyloid goiter is characterized by extensive amyloid deposits within the thyroid, typically in patients with a predisposition to systemic amyloidosis. The amyloid has a dense, waxy quality that is extremely difficult to distinguish from colloid. The cells often associated with the amyloid are inconspicuous spindled fibroblasts as seen in this image that are present within the fibrous connective tissue of the gland. In spite of the extensive infiltration of the gland by amyloid, thyroid function usually remains euthyroid. (Papanicolaou stain)

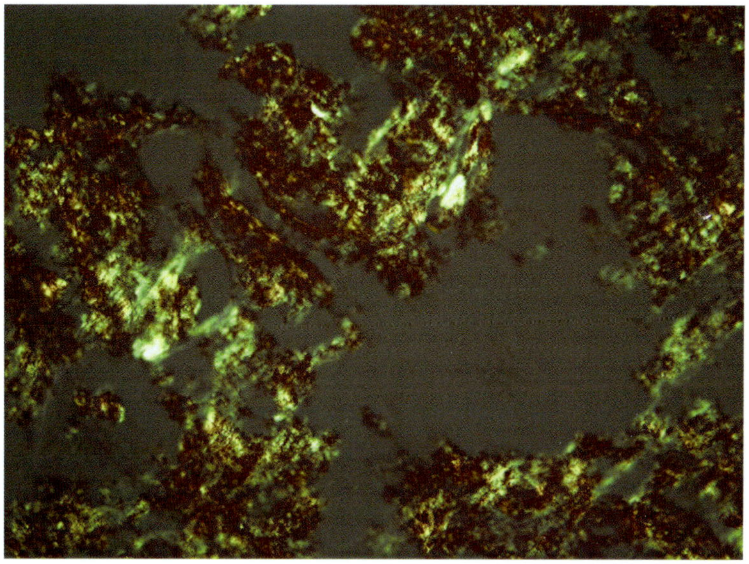

Figure 3.41 — Amyloid Goiter, FNA. The characteristic apple green birefringence is readily appreciated when viewed with polarized light. The preoperative diagnosis of amyloid goiter should be clinically suspected in patients with longstanding predisposing diseases who present with a rapidly growing diffuse thyroid nodule and are functionally euthyroid. Amyloid goiter usually occurs as one of the unusual manifestations of systemic amyloidosis. Special stains for amyloid are needed to distinguish the extensive amyloid deposits from colloid. (Congo Red stain)

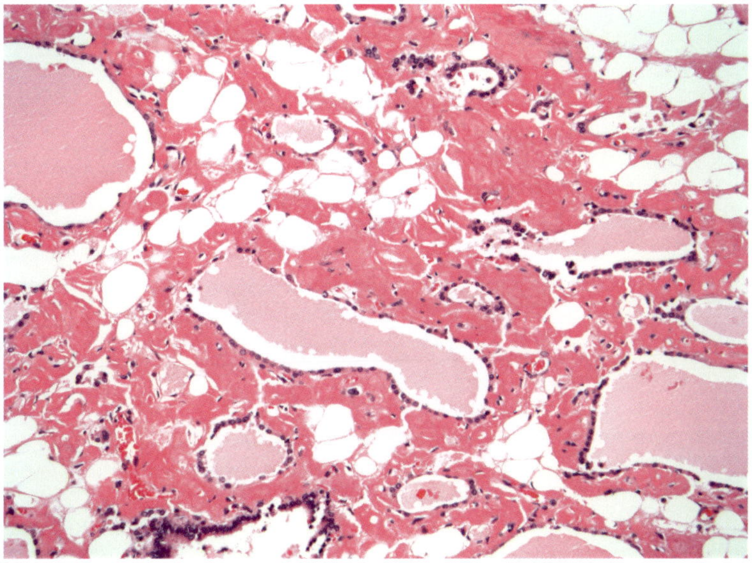

Figure 3.42 — Amyloid Goiter, Histologic Section. Amyloid goiter is extremely rare and presents more frequently as an incidental autopsy finding than in surgically resected material. On histology, abundant amorphous eosinophilic amyloid deposits are seen distributed in the interstitial fibroconnective tissue between sparse atrophic thyroid follicles. Occasionally in amyloid goiter, the rapid growth associated with local pressure symptoms (such as dyspnea, dysphagia, and/or hoarseness) suggests malignancy, prompting the FNA procedure. Amyloid deposition in thyroid can also be seen in medullary carcinoma and other conditions such as multiple myeloma or solitary plasmacytoma, Familial Mediterranean fever (FMF), certain infections, and rheumatoid arthritis. (H&E stain)

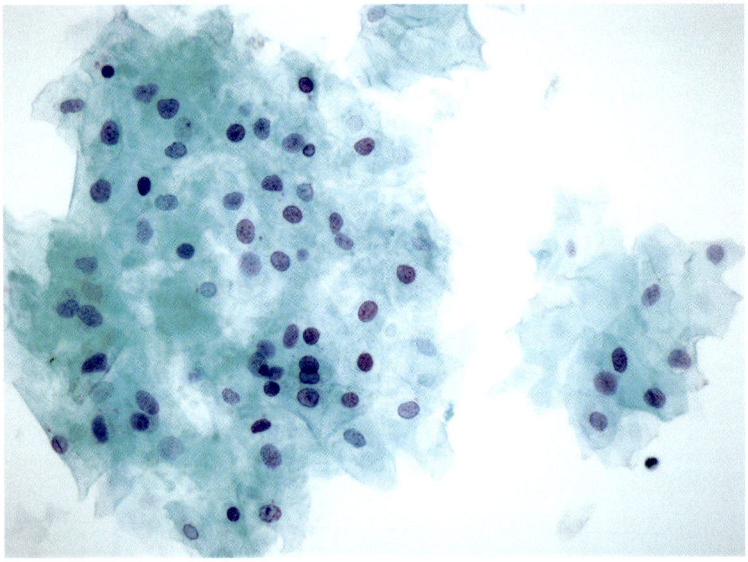

Figure 3.43a — Thyroglossal Duct Cyst (TDC), FNA. Thyroglossal duct cyst may present in any part of the thyroglossal tract commonly beneath the hyoid, in the region of the thyroid cartilage and above the hyoid bone. The cysts are usually painless neck swellings in the midline which characteristically move upward on protrusion of the tongue as well as on swallowing (due to the attachment of the tract to the foramen caecum). This aspirate from a cystic isthmus lesion revealed numerous benign appearing squamous cells as well as anucleate squames. The findings, although nonspecific, suggest the presence of a thyroglossal duct cyst. Differential diagnosis involves branchial cleft cyst, lymphoepithelial cyst, thyroid gland lesions, and lymphadenopathy (of various etiologies). (Liquid based preparation, Papanicolaou stain)

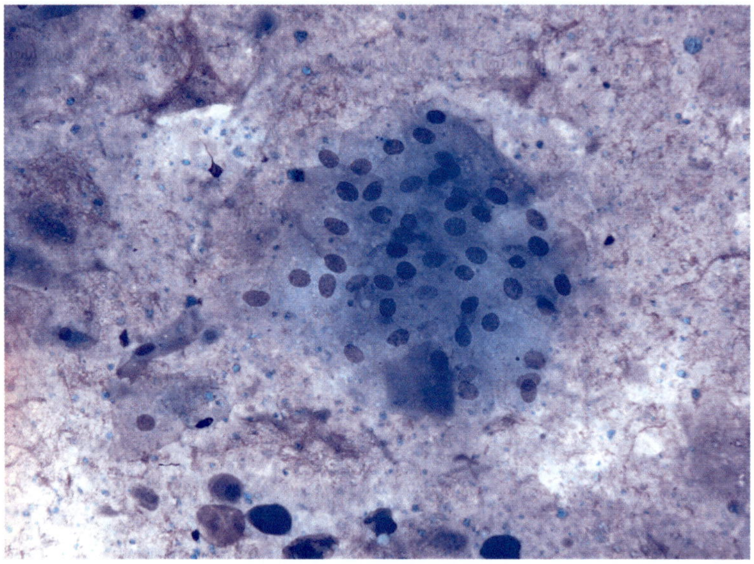

Figure 3.43b — Thyroglossal Duct Cyst, FNA. Similar features, as in the previous case, are seen on a direct smear preparation. Additionally, this case displays abundant degenerated background colloid. Thyroglossal duct cysts occur with equal frequency in males and females and are the most common mass found in the midline of the neck in children. Thyroglossal duct cyst results from the failure of obliteration of the thyroglossal duct which forms a bridge between the base of the tongue and the thyroid gland. (Diff Quik stain)

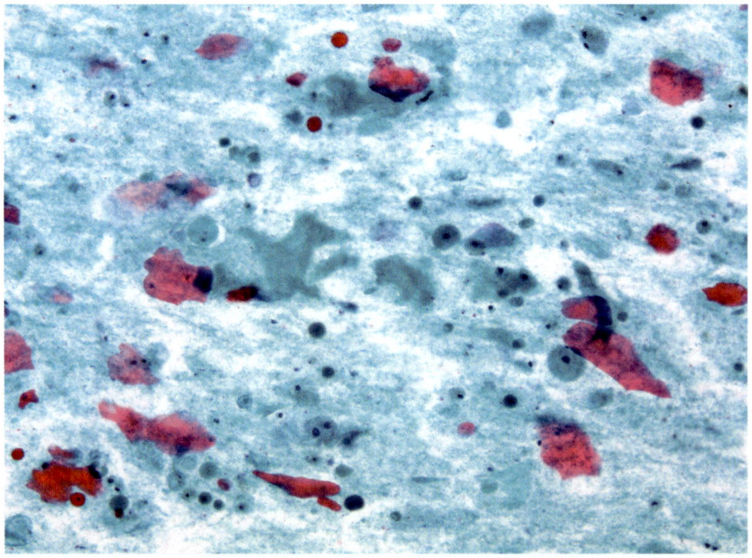

Figure 3.43c — Thyroglossal Duct Cyst, FNA. This direct smear preparation displays abundant cystic debris, colloid, and metaplastic/keratinized squamous cells. No follicular epithelium was noticed in this case. Thyroglossal duct cyst is a common congenital anomaly. TDC may cause a midline neck mass, which occasionally may become infected, and rarely gives rise to carcinoma. Abundant colloid, most often with ciliated columnar epithelium, is the predominant cytopathologic finding. Thyroid epithelium is rarely identified. The coexistence of carcinomas in thyroglossal duct cysts is extremely rare, with most being papillary carcinomas. The diagnosis of a thyroglossal duct cyst carcinoma can be missed due to its rarity. (Papanicolaou stain)

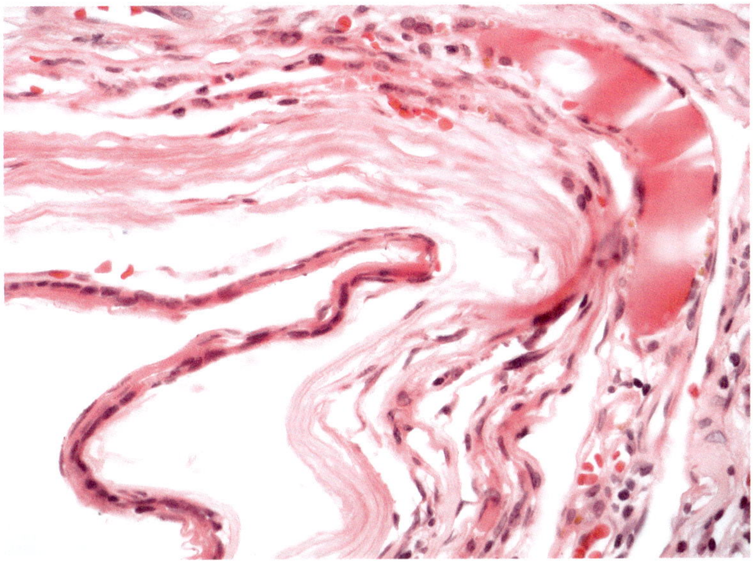

Figure 3.44 — Thyroglossal Duct Cyst, Histologic Section. The histologic correlate to the aspirate shown in the prior figure confirms the diagnosis of a thyroglossal duct cyst. An attenuated cyst lining comprised of benign squamous epithelium is present in the lower left-hand portion of the image. A benign thyroid follicle can be seen in the adjacent tissue at right. Sistrunk's procedure is often considered the surgical treatment of choice for thyroglossal duct cysts as it significantly reduces the risk of recurrence. This procedure involves an excision of the thyroglossal duct tract and the middle third of the hyoid bone. (H&E stain)

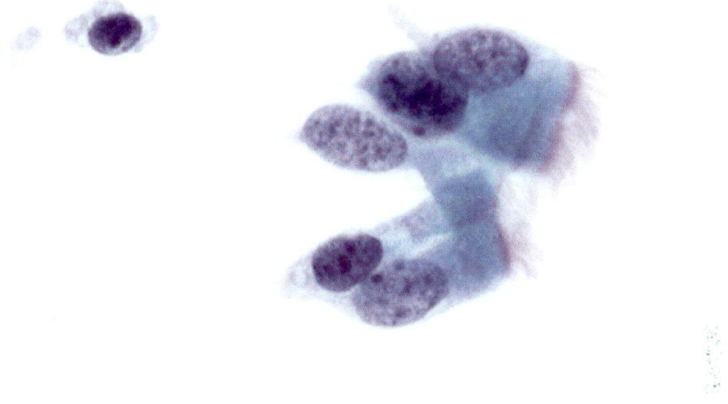

Figure 3.45 — Normal Tracheal Epithelium, FNA. These ciliated cells from the respiratory tract are indistinguishable from the ciliated columnar cells that might be obtained from a thyroglossal duct cyst. Lack of other cellular elements (ie, metaplastic squamous cells, anucleate squames, macrophages, and inflammatory cells) is not usually seen in cases of inadvertent sampling of airway. When the aspiration needle transgresses the airway, the patient will cough reflexively. However, this incidental finding poses no clinical risk. (Papanicolaou stain)

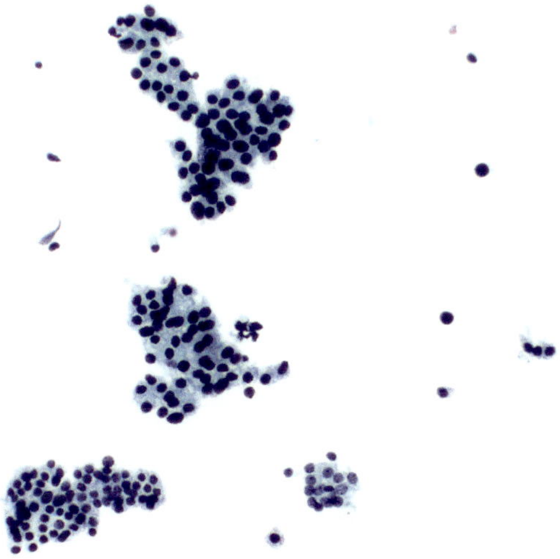

Figure 3.46a — Parathyroid, FNA. Parathyroid can be cytologically indistinguishable from thyroid follicular cells. This low power image provides subtle clues to the distinction. Cells are in tightly arranged, somewhat trabecular, groups. Colloid is completely absent. When the possibility of parathyroid sampling is a consideration, clinical correlation is essential. Serum parathyroid hormone levels can help confirm the presence of a parathyroid adenoma. (Liquid based preparation, Papanicolaou stain)

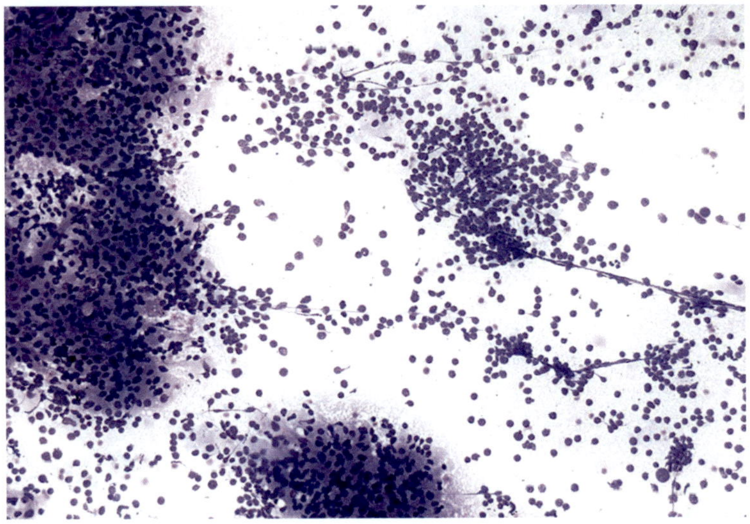

Figure 3.46b — Parathyroid, FNA. This direct smear preparation depicts a cellular smear with an extremely monotonous population of small-sized cells forming partially intact fragments. Abundant naked nuclei and a granular smear background are characteristic of parathyroid tissue. Unsuspected sampling of parathyroid tissue or parathyroid lesions in fine needle aspirations directed at "thyroid" or "neck" lesions can result in diagnostically challenging specimens. (Diff Quik stain)

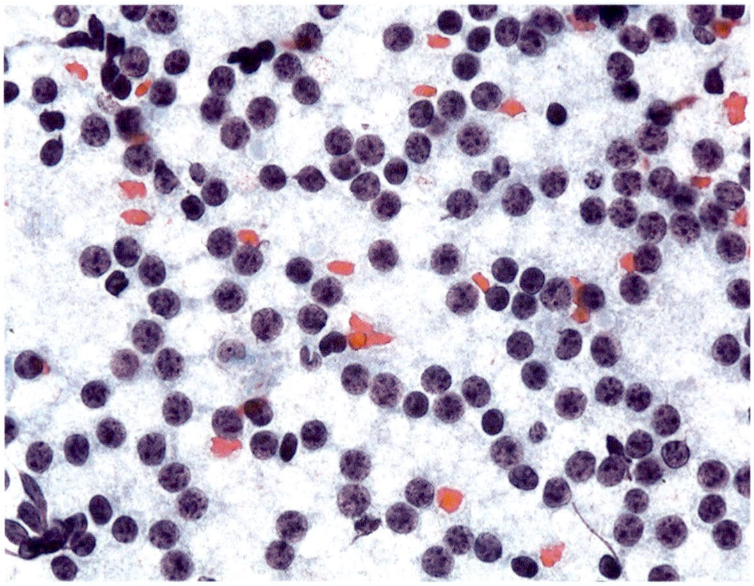

Figure 3.46c — Parathyroid, FNA. A uniform population of small "lymphocyte-like" cells is seen in a distinctly granular background. Cellular specimens with features not typical for thyroid lesions should be triaged for parathyroid hormone level in the needle rinse fluid. Routine use of the latter technique results in appropriate triage of patients to less aggressive excisional biopsies rather than unnecessary thyroidectomy. Aspirates of parathyroid lesions are often cellular and have considerable morphologic overlap with virtually every common primary thyroid tumor. (Papanicolaou stain)

Figure 3.46d — Parathyroid, FNA. Mostly naked nuclei with small nucleoli are observed in this case, which also displays a characteristic "foamy" slide background. Cytomorphologic features of parathyroid tissue include cohesive cellular sheets, cords, and occasional microfollicles. Often, the predominant pattern is a single cell (or naked nuclear) population, as seen in this case. The cells are distinctly smaller, monotonous, and generally show neuroendocrine-type features (uniformly round nuclei, granular chromatin, occasional cytoplasmic granules). (Diff Quik stain)

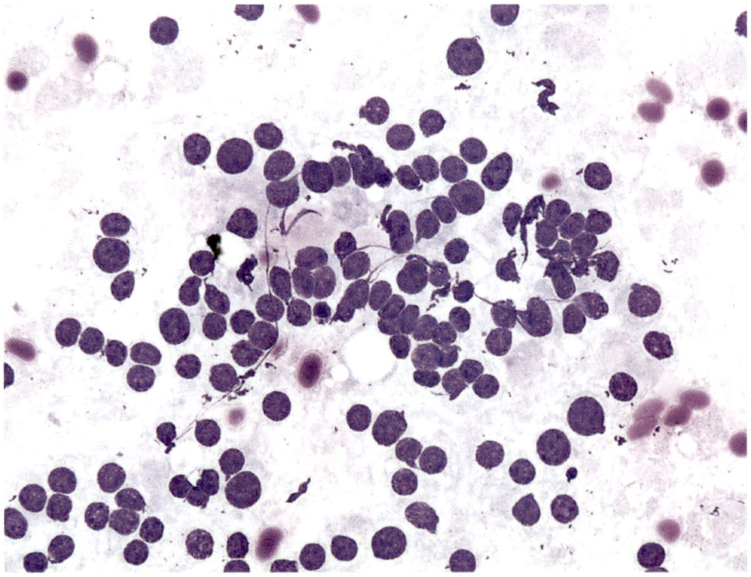

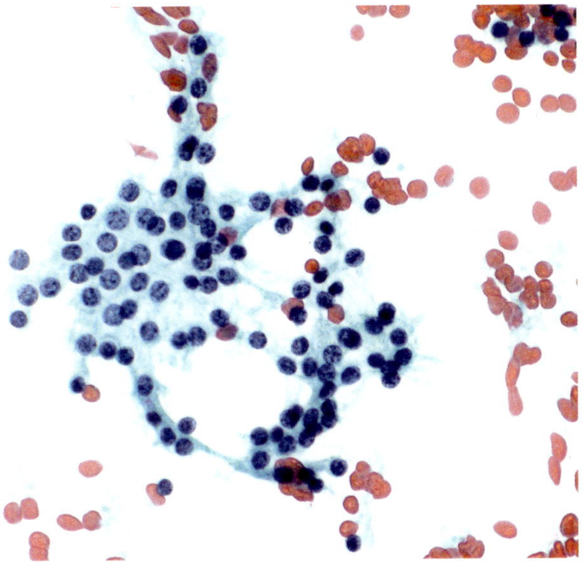

Figure 3.47 — Parathyroid, FNA. This lesion was subsequently shown to be a parathyroid adenoma, but the cytologic appearance is indistinguishable from a benign macrofollicular sheet of follicular cells. (Papanicolaou stain)

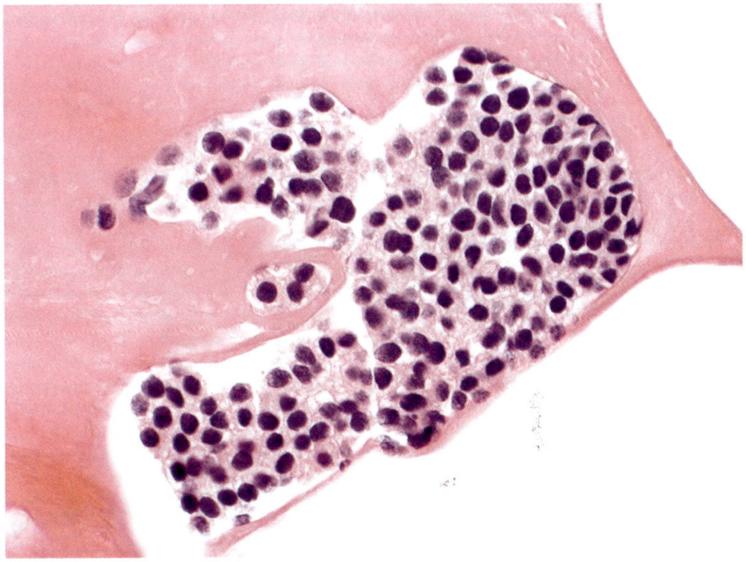

Figure 3.48 — Parathyroid, FNA. If the aspirator suspects a parathyroid adenoma, fluid from the needle rinse can be sent for parathyroid hormone testing. If the cytopathologist has concern for the diagnosis, immunocytochemistry can resolve the issue. A cell block preparation was prepared from residual material in the ThinPrep® vial in this aspirate. (Cell block, H&E stain)

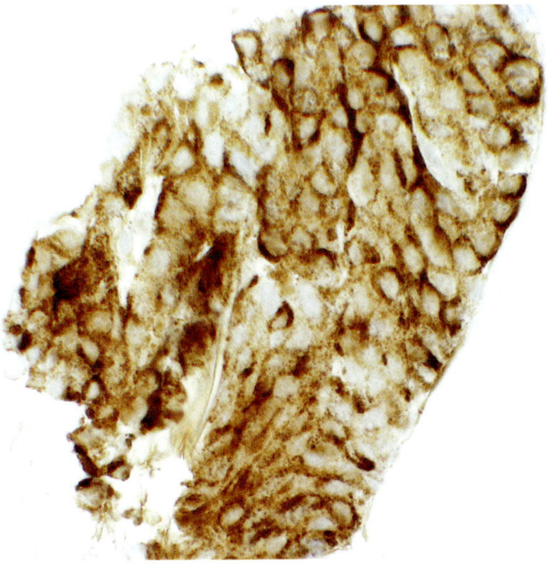

Figure 3.49 — Parathyroid, FNA. Immunocytochemistry for parathyroid hormone was strongly positive supporting the diagnosis of a parathyroid adenoma. Stains for TTF-1 and thyroglobulin were negative. (Parathyroid hormone immunostain)

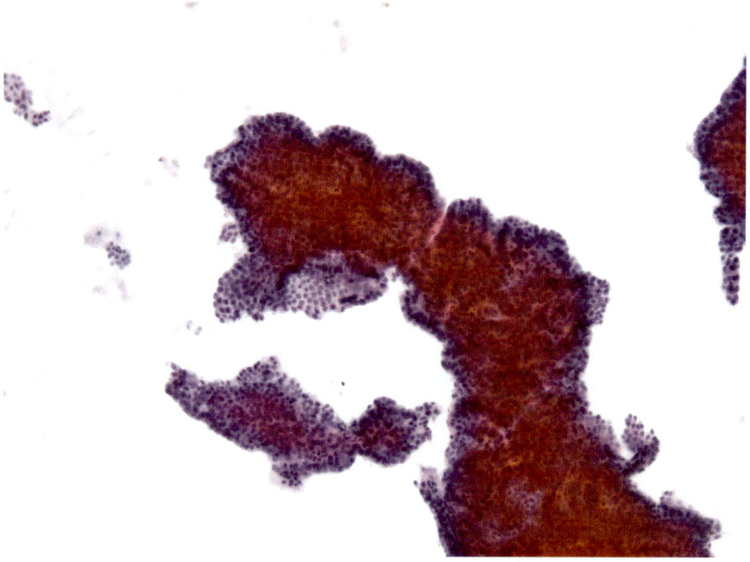

Figure 3.50a — Benign Papillary Hyperplasia, FNA. This liquid-based smear displays a large fragment of benign follicular epithelium with a papillary-like architecture. Note the absence of fibrovascular cores and lack of nuclear features of papillary carcinoma. When cellular, these cases can often be over-called as "suspicious for papillary carcinoma." (Papanicolaou stain)

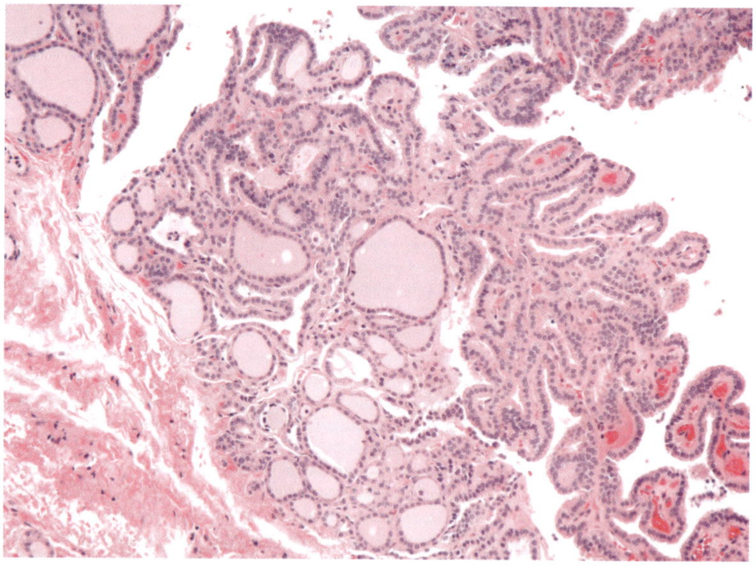

Figure 3.50b — Benign Papillary Hyperplasia, FNA. The papillary hyperplasia is nicely depicted in this section and shows beautiful correlation with the corresponding cytology in the previous image. Papillary hyperplasia is simply a phenotypic architectural variation in an adenomatoid nodule. Distinction from papillary carcinoma is essential and is dependent on the absence of the characteristic nuclear features of papillary carcinoma. (H&E stain)

4

Atypia of Undetermined Significance (AUS)/Follicular Lesion of Undetermined Significance (FLUS)

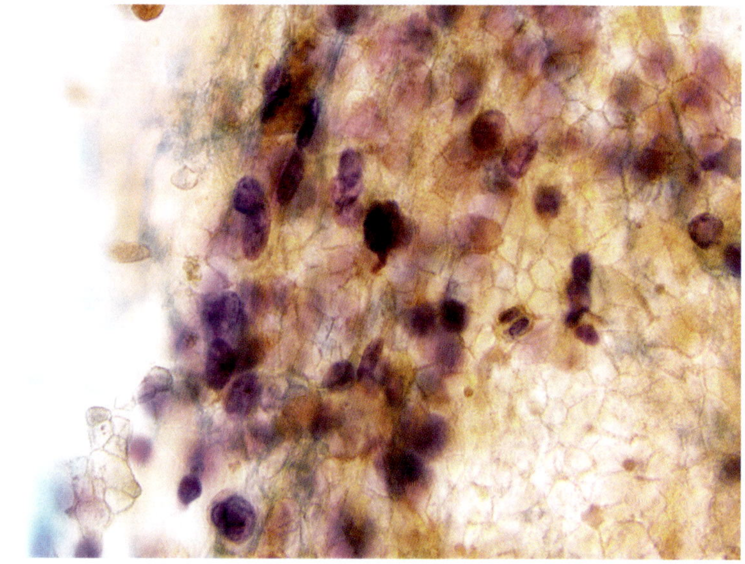

Figure 4.1 — Atypia of Undetermined Significance (AUS)/ Follicular Lesion of Undetermined Significance (FLUS), Fine Needle Aspiration (FNA). AUS with obscuring blood. The Bethesda System category of Atypia of Undetermined Significance (AUS)/Follicular Lesion of Undetermined Significance (FLUS) is reserved for aspirates containing cells with atypia exceeding that of clearly benign aspirates but insufficient to warrant a suspicious or malignant diagnosis. Inevitably, this is a heterogeneous category. Many AUS aspirates are compromised in some fashion as in this case with extensively obscuring blood. The follicular cells have slightly enlarged nuclei with pale chromatin, but are not well visualized within the clotted blood. Clotting also creates artificial crowding of follicular cells. Excessive blood and clotting may distort and obscure the follicular cells to an extent that warrants a nondiagnostic designation. (Papanicolaou stain)

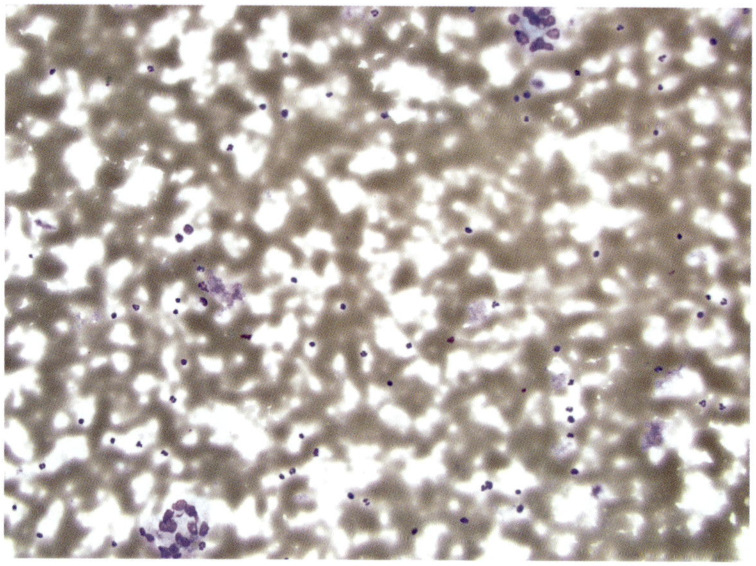

Figure 4.2 — Atypia of Undetermined Significance (AUS)/ Follicular Lesion of Undetermined Significance (FLUS), FNA. The classification of "indeterminate" lesions (those not clearly benign or malignant) in thyroid cytopathology has long been a significant source of confusion and frustration for both pathologists and clinicians. This case illustrates an AUS with rare microfollicles. A rare atypical finding in a sparsely cellular specimen may prompt an AUS diagnosis. In this instance, rare microfollicles are visible in the upper and lower portions of the image. The findings raise the possibility of a follicular neoplasm, but the sparse cellularity is insufficient to justify the Follicular Neoplasm/Suspicious for a Follicular Neoplasm diagnosis. A single AUS stratifies to a low risk of malignancy estimated to be in the 5% to 15% range. A repeat aspirate is appropriate follow-up for most patients after an initial AUS. Most cases resolve to a more definitive diagnostic category on repeat FNA. Repeat AUS will usually prompt surgical excision. (Papanicolaou stain)

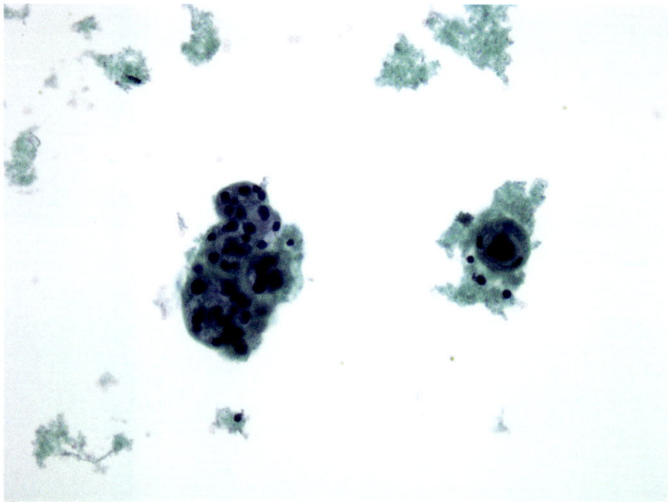

Figure 4.3 — Atypia of Undetermined Significance (AUS)/Follicular Lesion of Undetermined Significance (FLUS), FNA. The Bethesda system defines Atypia of Undetermined Significance (AUS) as FNA specimens that contain cells (follicular, lymphoid, or other) with nuclear and/or architectural atypia that is not sufficient to be classified as suspicious for a follicular neoplasm, suspicious for a Hürthle cell neoplasm, suspicious for malignancy, or malignant. This example depicts an AUS with rare microfollicles. As in the previous image, the specimen is sparsely cellular but exclusively comprised of follicular cells arranged in microfollicles and trabeculae. The excised nodule was diagnosed as a follicular adenoma. (Liquid based preparation, Papanicolaou stain)

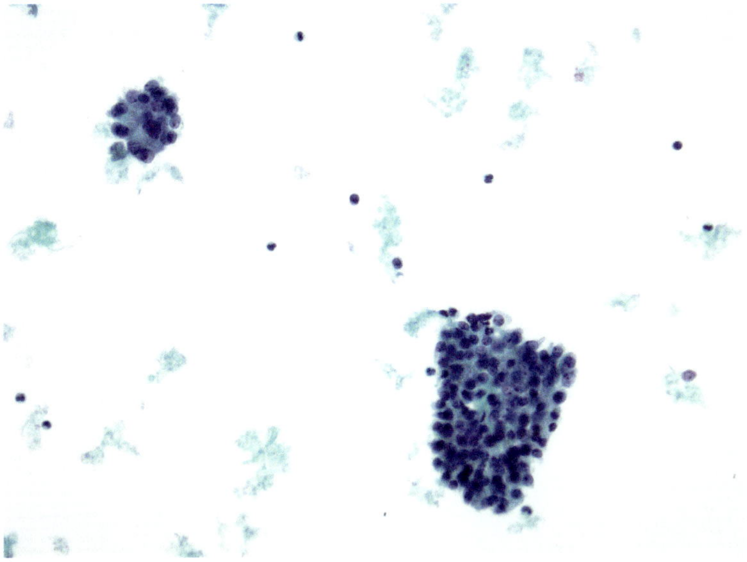

Figure 4.4 — Atypia of Undetermined Significance (AUS)/ Follicular Lesion of Undetermined Significance (FLUS), FNA. This example shows AUS with mild architectural atypia. The architectural alterations in these slightly crowded and three-dimensional groups of follicular cells raise some concern for a follicular neoplasm, but these subtle findings are best classified as AUS. The diagnosis was follicular adenoma on surgical excision. AUS preferably should be considered a category of last resort and should not be used indiscriminately. (Liquid based preparation, Papanicolaou stain)

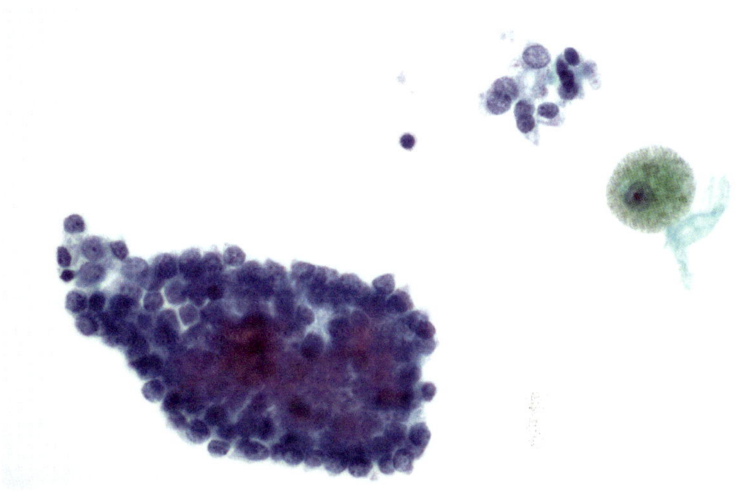

Figure 4.5 — Atypia of Undetermined Significance (AUS)/ Follicular Lesion of Undetermined Significance (FLUS), FNA. AUS with architectural and cytologic atypia. In this case, cellular crowding is more pronounced than in the prior image. Additionally, nuclei at the periphery of the crowded group and in the smaller cluster at upper right appear enlarged with powdery chromatin. These findings were focally present in a background of benign appearing follicular cells. On resection, a follicular variant of papillary carcinoma was identified. (Liquid based preparation, Papanicolaou stain)

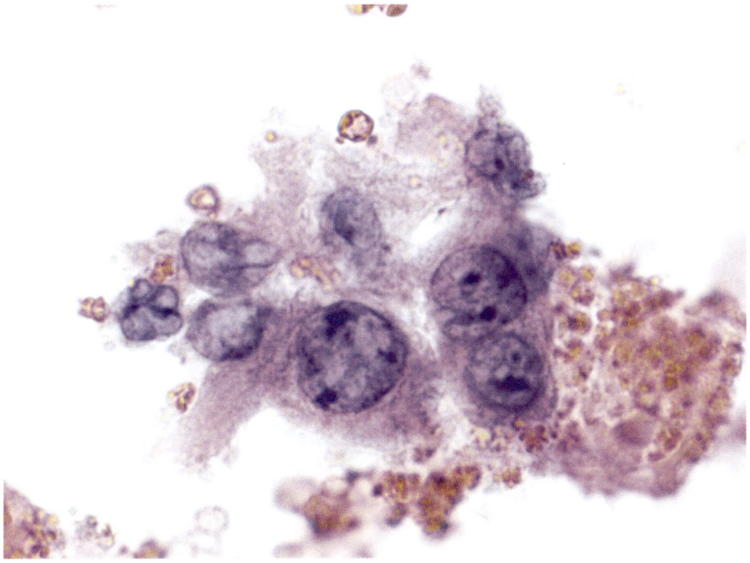

Figure 4.6 — Atypia of Undetermined Significance (AUS)/Follicular Lesion of Undetermined Significance (FLUS), FNA. Focal findings suggestive of papillary carcinoma. This otherwise benign appearing aspirate has a single small group of cells with nuclear features suggestive of papillary carcinoma. Nuclei are enlarged with pale chromatin and nuclear grooves. Aspirates with focal findings worrisome for papillary carcinoma may carry higher risk of papillary carcinoma than other AUS diagnoses. Such cases are more appropriately classified as suspicious for papillary carcinoma unless the findings are limited to rare cells as in this case. (Liquid based preparation, Papanicolaou stain)

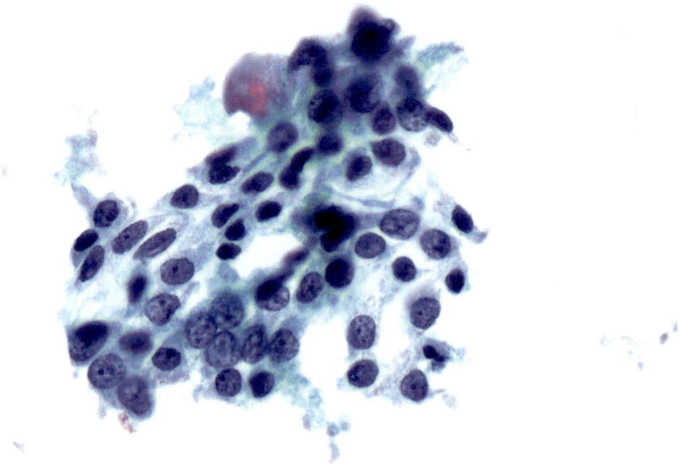

Figure 4.7 — Atypia of Undetermined Significance (AUS)/ Follicular Lesion of Undetermined Significance (FLUS), FNA. Focal mild cytologic atypia. Some cells in this group (particularly those on the left) have slightly enlarged nuclei with pale chromatin, slight nuclear contour irregularity, a small distinct nucleolus, and nuclear grooves. The findings are not sufficiently prominent to warrant a diagnosis of suspicious for papillary carcinoma. Instead, the diagnosis was AUS. (Liquid based preparation, Papanicolaou stain)

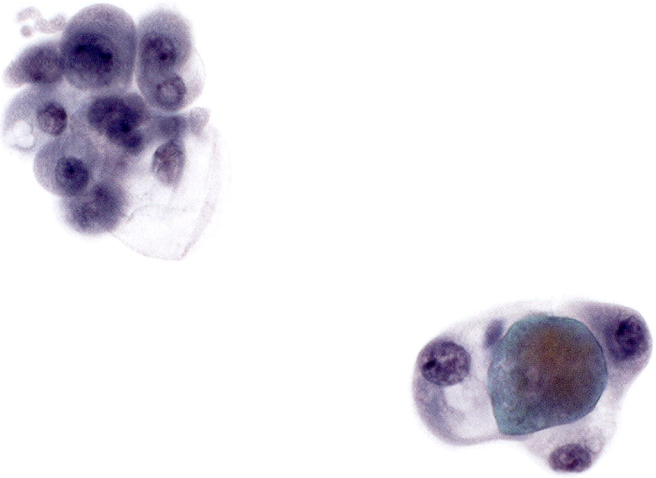

Figure 4.8 — Atypia of Undetermined Significance (AUS)/ Follicular Lesion of Undetermined Significance (FLUS), FNA. Histiocytoid cells. In rare cases of papillary carcinoma, cells such as those illustrated here may be the only abnormal finding. Although these cells are of follicular origin, they superficially resemble histiocytes with their abundant vacuolated cytoplasm. Nuclei are enlarged, but do not have classic cytologic features of papillary carcinoma. Chromatin is coarse with occasional prominent nucleoli. Nuclear grooves are absent. There may be a suggestion of intranuclear cytoplasmic pseudoinclusions as can be seen here. While these cells have been reported to be specific for papillary carcinoma, they may be difficult to distinguish from histiocytes or cyst lining cells. This case was diagnosed as AUS and proved to be papillary carcinoma at surgery. (Liquid based preparation, Papanicolaou stain)

Figure 4.9 — Atypia of Undetermined Significance (AUS)/ Follicular Lesion of Undetermined Significance (FLUS), FNA. Atypical cyst lining cells. These cells have enlarged oval nuclei with chromatin appearing coarse in some cells, but pale in others. Nuclear grooves are evident. Evaluation is hindered by the presence of air drying artifact in some of the cells. The reparative configuration of the cells suggests that these are cyst lining cells, but an AUS diagnosis is appropriate because of some concern for a papillary carcinoma. (Papanicolaou stain)

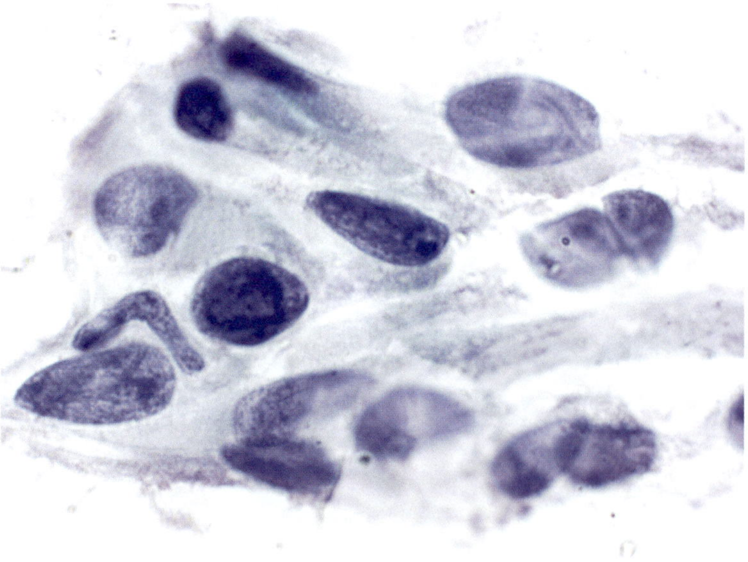

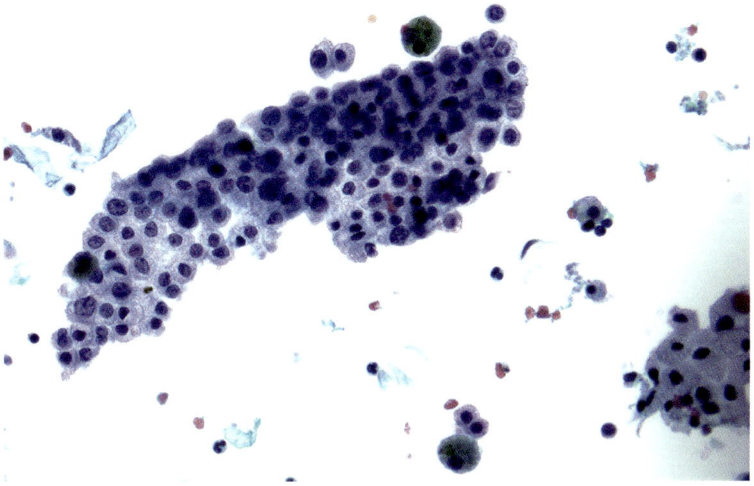

Figure 4.10 — Atypia of Undetermined Significance (AUS)/ Follicular Lesion of Undetermined Significance (FLUS), FNA. Hürthle cells in multinodular goiter. This aspirate is comprised of numerous Hürthle cells. While these findings in a solitary nodule indicate the presence of a Hürthle cell neoplasm, in some clinical situations a hyperplastic Hürthle cell nodule may be more probable. These would include patients with clinically known Hashimoto thyroiditis or a multinodular thyroid. In such cases, AUS is an appropriate diagnosis. Since repeat FNA is likely to yield similar findings, clinical correlation is most appropriate for deciding on appropriate treatment. The AUS diagnosis in such cases provides greater clinical flexibility to avoid lobectomy than would the alternative diagnosis of (suspicious for a) follicular neoplasm, Hürthle cell type. (Liquid based preparation, Papanicolaou stain)

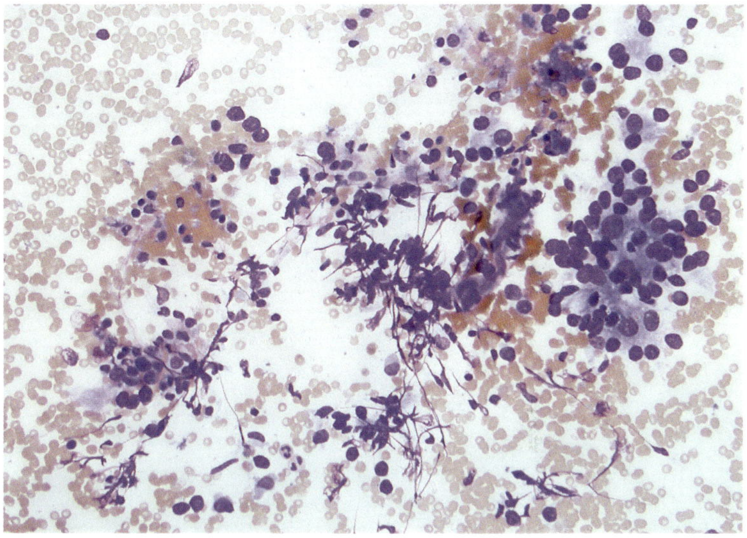

Figure 4.11 — Atypia of Undetermined Significance (AUS)/ Follicular Lesion of Undetermined Significance (FLUS), FNA. Hürthle cells in Hashimoto thyroiditis. Hashimoto thyroiditis can present a variety of vexing findings on FNA that suggest the presence of a coexisting neoplasm. This aspirate shows only a Hürthle cell epithelial component (at right) with few admixed lymphoid cells. When lymphocytes are more prominent than Hürthle cells, the findings are reassuring for Hashimoto thyroiditis. On occasion, a pure population of Hürthle cells is sampled with little or no lymphocytes or follicular cells present. A solitary hyperplastic Hürthle cell nodule in a patient with Hashimoto thyroiditis is most likely, but a Hürthle cell neoplasm cannot be excluded. In the proper clinical context, an AUS diagnosis allows for conservative management as an alternative to surgical excision. (Diff Quik stain)

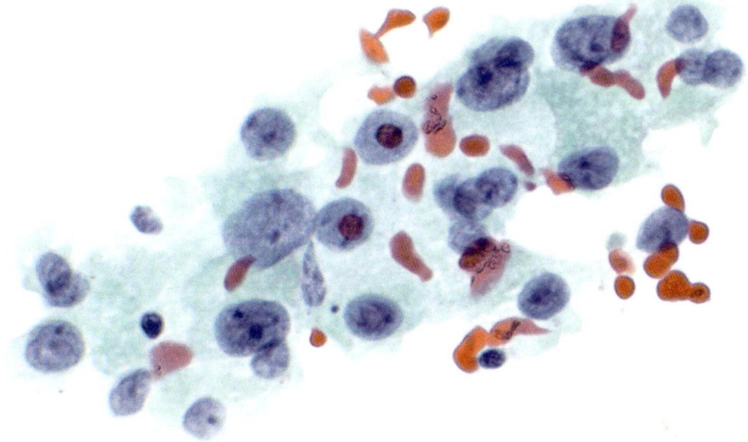

Figure 4.12 — Atypia of Undetermined Significance (AUS)/Follicular Lesion of Undetermined Significance (FLUS), FNA. Hürthle cell atypia in Hashimoto thyroiditis. Hürthle cells often have reactive atypia that may include marked nuclear size variation. Such changes are usually appreciable as being benign. In this case from a patient with Hashimoto thyroiditis, chromatin is also pale with small nucleoli present. These minimal changes raise the possibility of an oncocytic variant of papillary carcinoma, but this concern is mitigated by the presence of Hashimoto thyroiditis. (Papanicolaou stain)

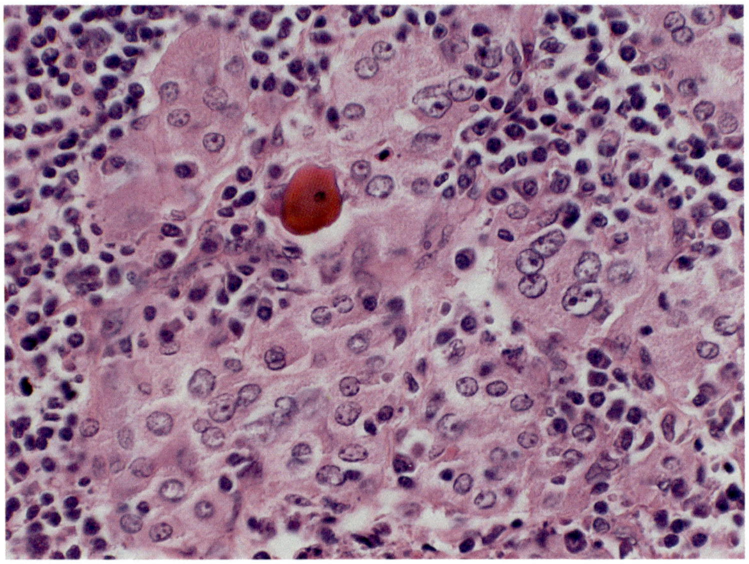

Figure 4.13 — Hashimoto Thyroiditis, Histologic Section. Hürthle cell atypia in Hashimoto thyroiditis. The surgical resection specimen from the case shown in the prior figure demonstrates Hürthle cells in intimate association with a dense lymphoplasmacytic infiltrate. The same nuclear changes noted on FNA can be appreciated, but in context are appreciated as reactive changes. (H&E stain)

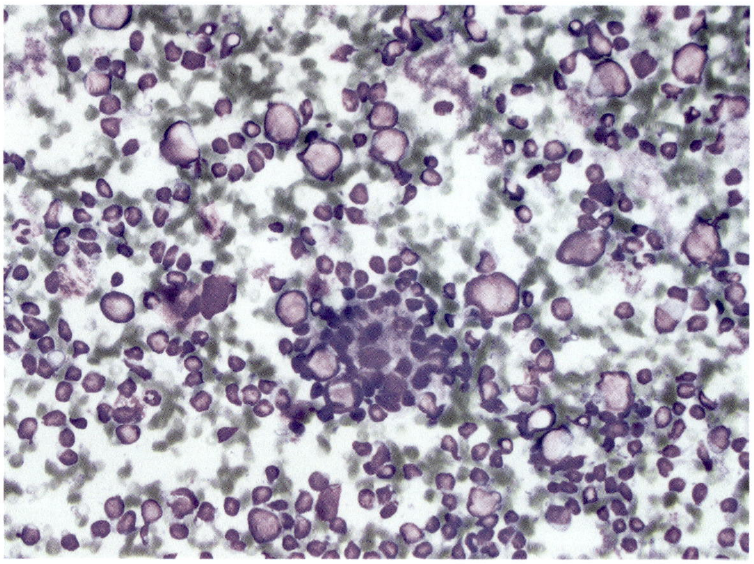

Figure 4.14 — Atypia of Undetermined Significance (AUS), FNA. Lymphoid cells in Hashimoto thyroiditis. Some aspirates from Hashimoto thyroiditis are dominated by the inflammatory component of the process. Such a marked predominance of lymphoid cells raises concern for a lymphoproliferative disorder. The polymorphous nature of this aspirate is reassuring, but may also be seen in MALT lymphoma. In Hashimoto thyroiditis, clonal B cell proliferations may be detected by flow cytometry and can be clinically misleading. Therefore, an AUS diagnosis with immunophenotyping should be reserved for cases where there is clinical suspicion (such as a large or rapidly enlarging mass). If there were a monotonous or markedly atypical lymphoid population evident cytomorphologically, a suspicious diagnosis would be appropriate. (Diff Quik stain)

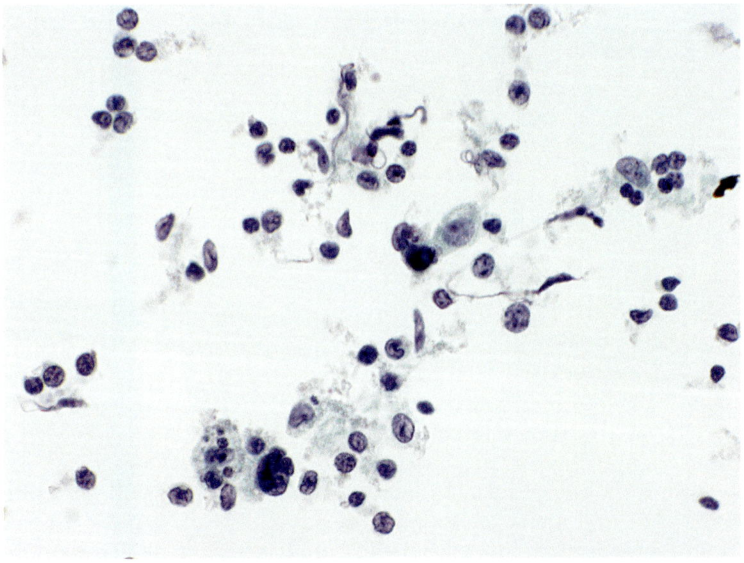

Figure 4.15 — Atypia of Undetermined Significance (AUS), FNA. Atypical lymphoid infiltrate. This patient clinically had a multinodular goiter with multiple nodules that were increasing in size. Aspirates from two nodules both showed similar findings with increased numbers of a polymorphous lymphoid infiltrate including scattered tingible body macrophages (lower left) and small lymphoid cells with irregular nuclei. An atypical diagnosis because of the worrisome clinical scenario resulted in a surgical biopsy that demonstrated a MALT lymphoma (see Figure 4.16). (Liquid based preparation, Papanicolaou stain)

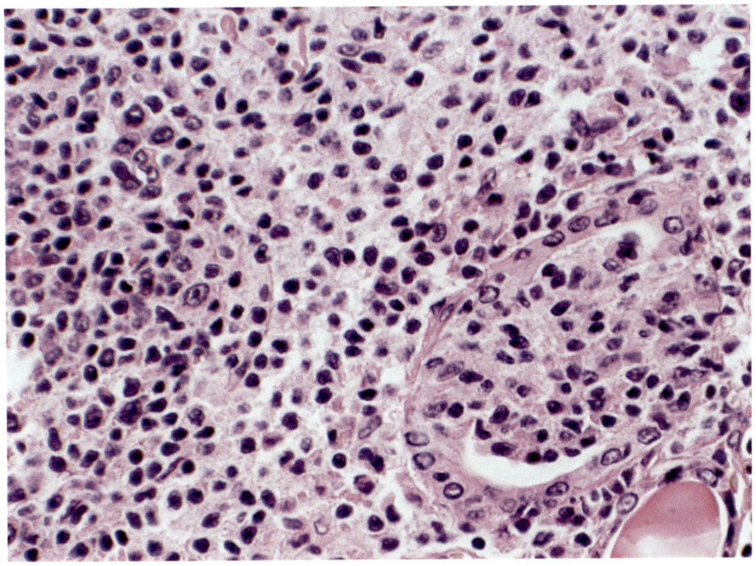

Figure 4.16 — Extranodal Marginal Zone Lymphoma (MALT), Histologic Section. The surgical resection from the aspirate in Figure 4.15 demonstrates a polymorphous lymphoid infiltrate, but with a marked predominance of monocytoid lymphocytes with abundant cytoplasm. At right, a lymphoepithelial lesion is evident in which there is infiltration of a follicle by the lymphoid cells. Immunophenotypically, the neoplastic B cells were negative for CD5, CD10, and CD23. (H&E stain)

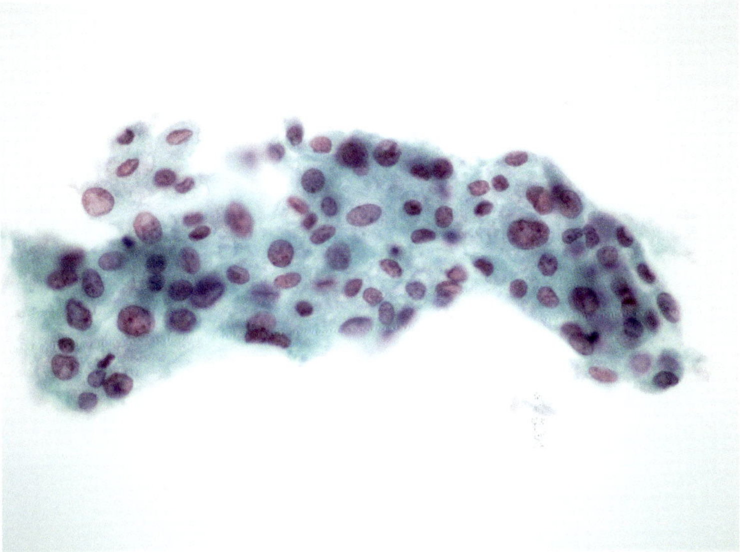

Figure 4.17 — Atypia of Undetermined Significance (AUS)/ Follicular Lesion of Undetermined Significance (FLUS), FNA. Atypia with treated Graves disease. This patient was treated with methimazole (Tapazole®) for Graves disease. Thyroid suppressive pharmaceutical agents as well as radioiodine therapy can produce pronounced nuclear changes, especially nuclear size variation. Anisonucleosis by itself is not indicative of neoplasia in thyroid aspirates. However, the changes shown here also include pale chromatin and rare nuclear grooves that raise the specter of papillary carcinoma. (Liquid based preparation, Papanicolaou stain)

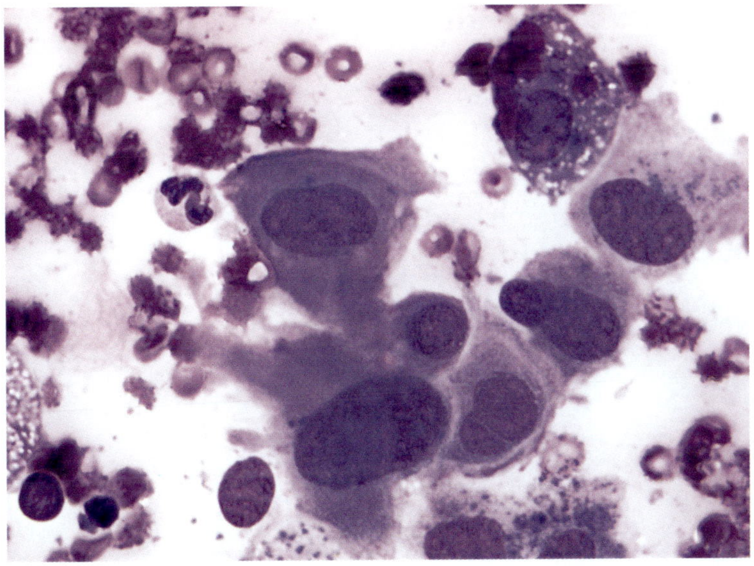

Figure 4.18 — Atypia of Undetermined Significance (AUS)/Follicular Lesion of Undetermined Significance (FLUS), FNA. Radiation atypia. When nuclear size variation is as pronounced as is seen here concern for malignancy, such as metastatic disease, may arise. Knowledge of the patient's history of ionizing radiation to the neck provides reassurance. (Diff Quik stain)

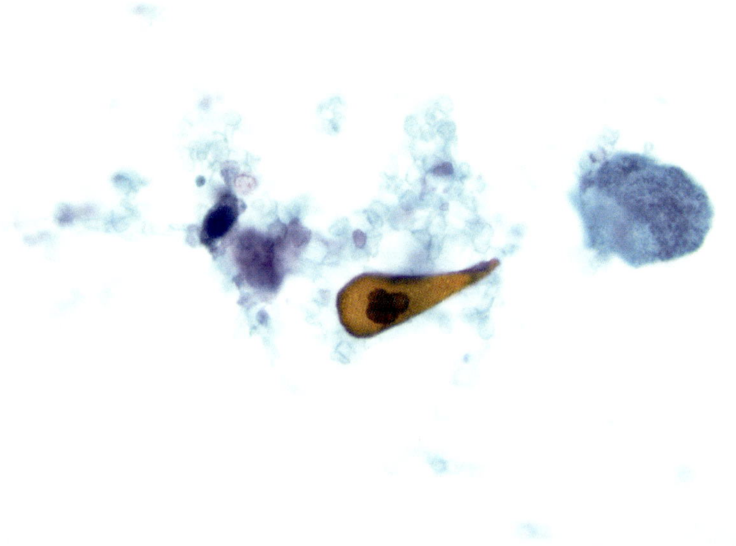

Figure 4.19 — Atypia of Undetermined Significance (AUS)/ Follicular Lesion of Undetermined Significance (FLUS), FNA. Atypical squamous cells. In this extremely sparsely cellular aspirate, an enlarged, but markedly degenerated cell is present at right with smudgy nuclear chromatin. In the center, an atypical squamous cell is present. These findings could arouse suspicion for a metastatic squamous cell carcinoma or an undifferentiated (anaplastic) carcinoma of the thyroid. Conversely, the rarity of the findings and the dubious significance with the poor cell preservation is most suited to the AUS category. (Papanicolaou stain)

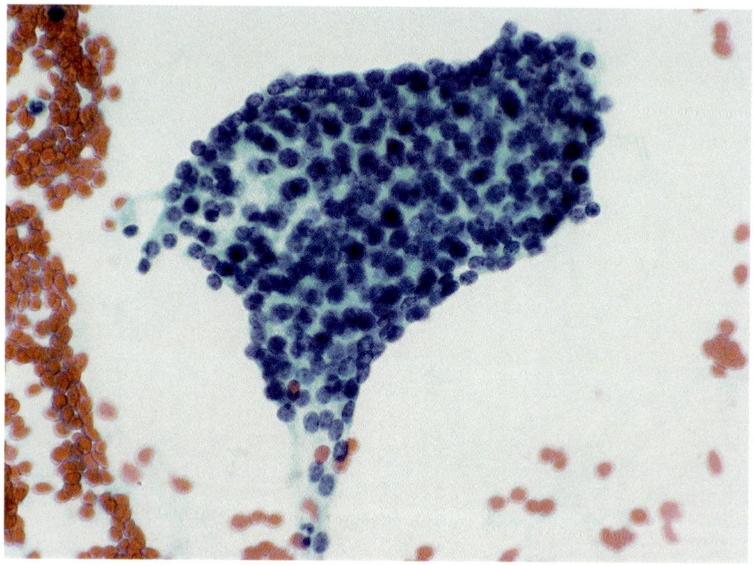

Figure 4.20 — Atypia of Undetermined Significance (AUS)/ Follicular Lesion of Undetermined Significance (FLUS), FNA. Parathyroid adenoma. The image shows a crowded, three-dimensional group of epithelial cells. Cells are uniform in appearance with small round nuclei having coarse chromatin. Colloid is absent. The rest of the aspirate was hypercellular with numerous, identical appearing groups. In the absence of a clinical suspicion, this lesion is likely to be called a follicular neoplasm rather than a parathyroid neoplasm. If there is uncertainty about the origin of the cells, but confirmatory immunocytochemistry or fluid parathyroid hormone levels are not available then a diagnosis of AUS is appropriate. (Papanicolaou stain)

Figure 4.21 — Atypia of Undetermined Significance (AUS)/ Follicular Lesion of Undetermined Significance (FLUS), FNA. Parathyroid adenoma. This thyroid nodule which appeared hypocellular on smears with predominantly blood and rare microfollicles was diagnosed as AUS. No colloid or Hürthle cells were present. Follow-up resection showed an intrathyroidal parathyroid adenoma. In cases with total lack of colloid or other evidence of thyroid tissue, a dedicated needle rinse in 1 mL of Hanks' Balanced Salt Solution (HBSS) should be sent to chemistry for parathyroid hormone analysis to rule out parathyroid sampling. (Diff Quik stain)

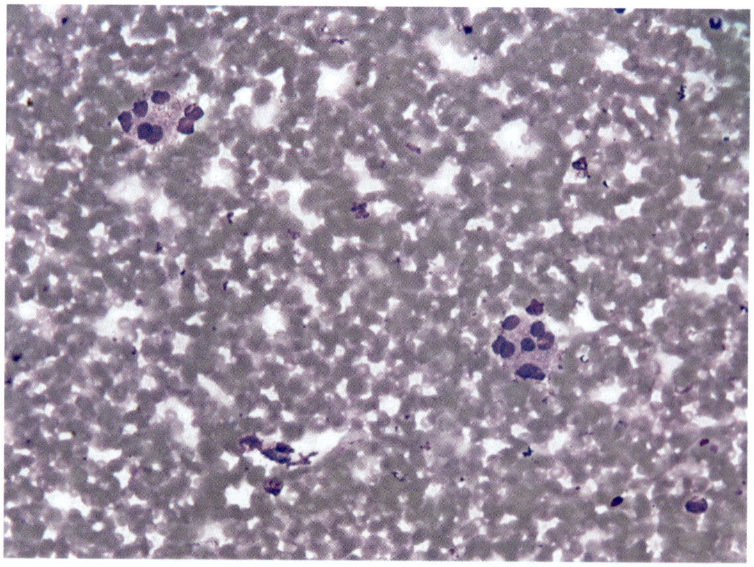

Figure 4.22 — Atypia of Undetermined Significance (AUS)/ Follicular Lesion of Undetermined Significance (FLUS), FNA. Scant with predominantly microfollicles. This was the only smear in the entire case that contained scant follicular cells and the case was flagged with an AUS diagnosis. Most cells displayed microfollicular architecture. No colloid or Hürthle cells were seen. Follow-up revealed a follicular adenoma. (Papanicolaou stain)

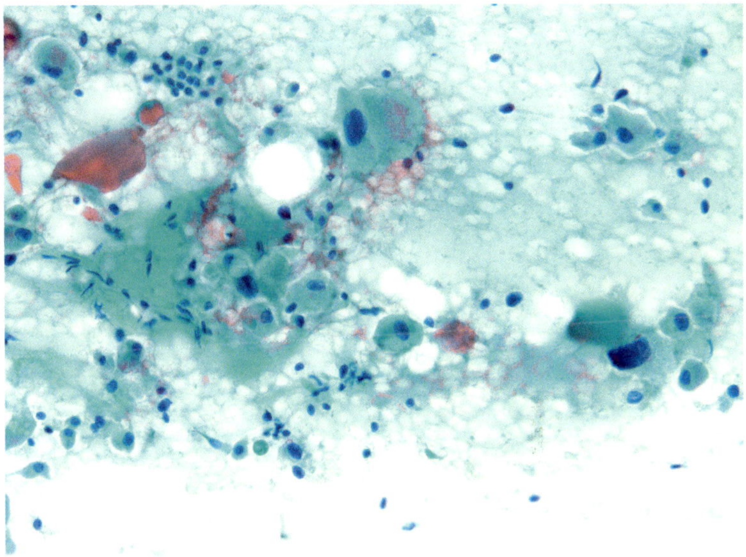

Figure 4.23 — Atypia of Undetermined Significance (AUS)/ Follicular Lesion of Undetermined Significance (FLUS), FNA. Focal nuclear atypia. One of the most common reasons for an AUS diagnosis (often an overcall) is illustrated here, that is, focal anisonucleosis in an adenomatoid nodule with Hürthle cell metaplasia. Notice the abundant colloid in the background and benign-appearing follicle cells. Focal anisonucleosis is an expected finding when Hürthle cell changes are present in a hyperplastic process and should not be diagnosed as "atypical" unless they display other nuclear features (such as grooves, inclusions, or stratification). (Papanicolaou stain)

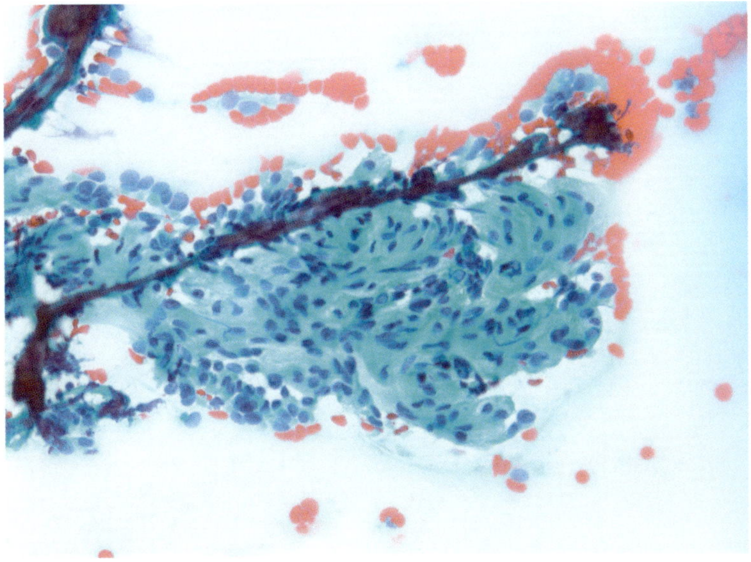

Figure 4.24 — Atypia of Undetermined Significance (AUS)/ Follicular Lesion of Undetermined Significance (FLUS), FNA. Focal nuclear atypia. Cyst lining cells and fibroblasts are admixed with follicular epithelium displaying oval nuclei, pale chromatin, and vague intranuclear inclusions. There is focal air-drying artifact (more noticeable on the left), possibly creating nuclear molding. Follow-up resection showed papillary carcinoma. (Papanicolaou stain)

5

Follicular Neoplasm/ Suspicious for a Follicular Neoplasm

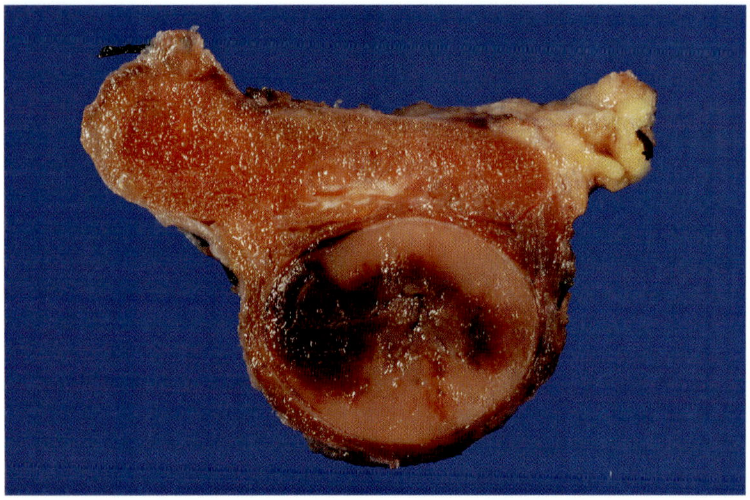

Figure 5.1 — Follicular Adenoma, Gross Appearance. Follicular adenomas are round to oval nodules. They are sharply demarcated from the surrounding thyroid parenchyma by a complete fibrous capsule, but the capsule is usually thin and not easily recognized macroscopically. Follicular adenomas are almost always encountered as grossly visible nodules rather than incidental microscopic findings, but the sizes of these gross nodules vary considerably. The cut surface tends to be solid. Secondary degenerative changes such as cyst formation, calcification, and scarring may occur but not with the high frequency with which they are encountered in adenomatoid nodules. In this case, the presence of a linear tract of hemorrhage likely reflects trauma related to a prior fine needle aspiration. Follicular adenomas tend to have thinner capsules than their malignant counterpart (ie, follicular carcinoma), but the distinction between benign and malignant requires thorough histologic evaluation of the tumor capsule for the presence of invasive tumor growth.

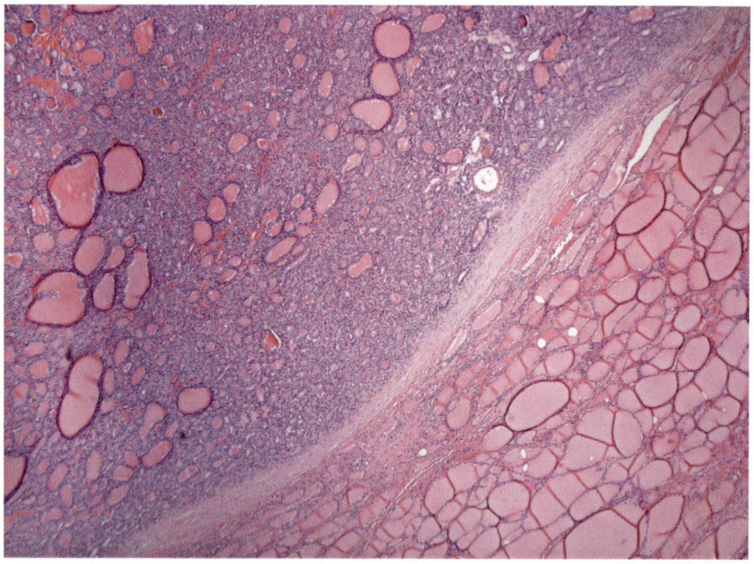

Figure 5.2a — Follicular Adenoma, Histologic Section. Follicular adenomas characteristically exhibit uniformly sized follicles, a surrounding fibrous capsule, and compression (flattening) of adjacent thyroid follicles. This adenoma exhibits a proliferation of microfollicles, but the pattern can vary from macrofollicular to trabecular to even solid growth. The integrity of the tumor capsule is of particular importance in determining malignant potential. In the follicular adenoma, the capsule is usually thin, uniform and completely intact. Penetration of the tumor capsule by neoplastic cells raises the concern of a malignant process (eg, follicular carcinoma). (H&E stain)

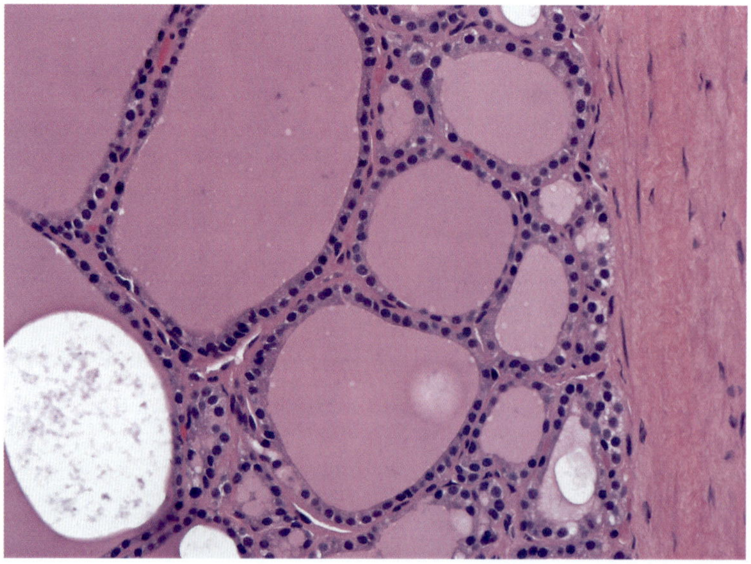

Figure 5.2b — Follicular Adenoma, Histologic Section. The cells lining the follicles have uniformly round to oval nuclei, inconspicuous nucleoli, and they are evenly spaced around the follicles. (H&E stain)

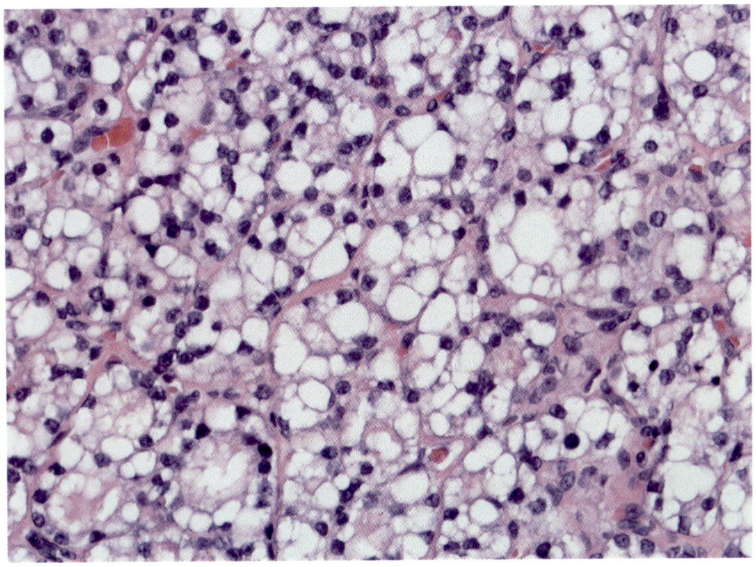

Figure 5.3 — Signet-Ring Follicular Adenoma, Histologic Section. Follicular adenomas sometimes exhibit cytoplasmic clearing. When large clear vacuoles fill the cytoplasm and compress the nucleus, the follicular epithelial cells take on a signet-ring appearance. This change is believed to be due to the cytoplasmic accumulation of thyroglobulin. (H&E stain)

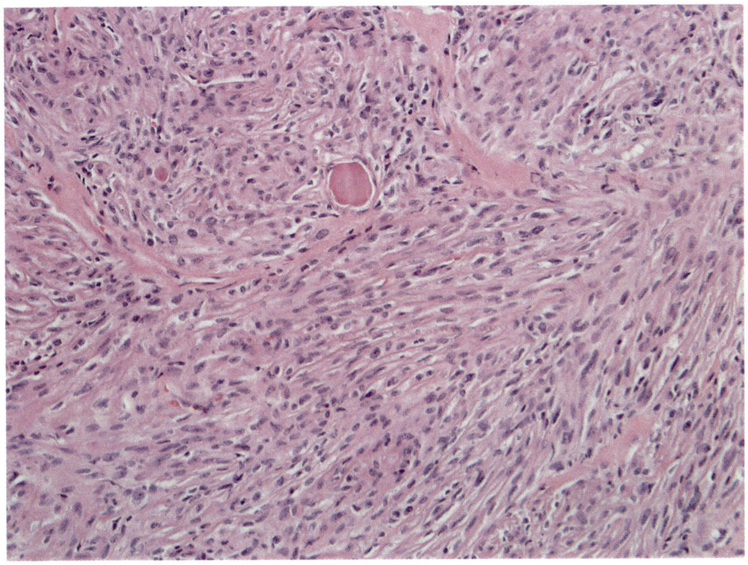

Figure 5.4 — Spindle Cell Follicular Adenoma, Histologic Section. At times the follicular epithelium of follicular adenomas may spindle. The solid proliferation of spindled cells with near total loss of follicle formations may cause confusion with the spindle cell variant of anaplastic carcinoma and various mesenchymal neoplasms. In contrast to anaplastic carcinomas, the cells of these spindled adenomas lack malignant cytologic features. Despite their mesenchymal appearance, these bland follicular epithelial cells retain immunolabeling for cytokeratin and TTF-1. (H&E stain)

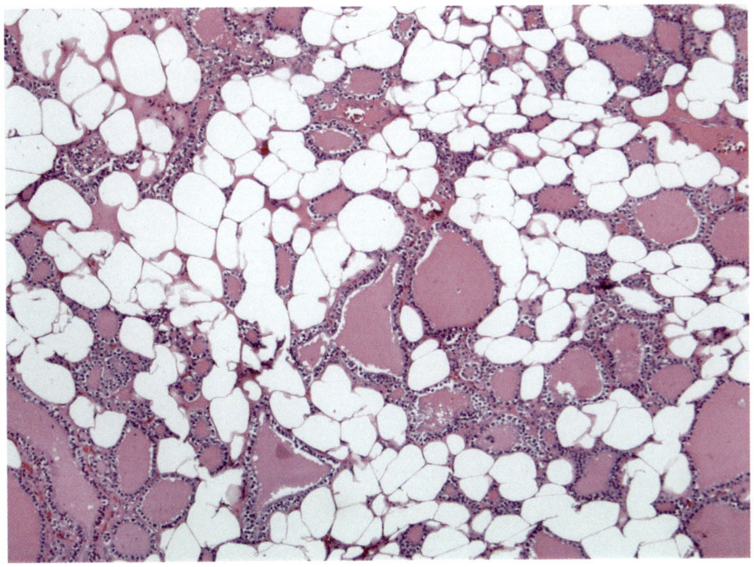

Figure 5.5 — Adenolipoma, Histologic Section. The thyroid stroma can sometimes undergo fatty metaplasia. When the change is prominent, thyroid follicles are widely separated by zones of mature adipose tissue. When this change occurs within a follicular adenoma, the neoplasm is designated as an adenolipoma. (H&E stain)

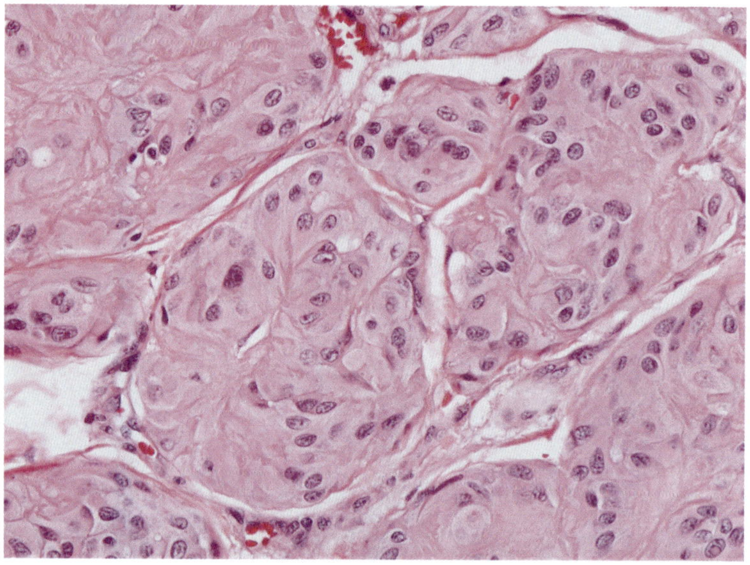

Figure 5.6a — Hyalinizing Trabecular Adenoma, Histologic Section. The hallmark histopathologic features of the hyalinizing trabecular neoplasm are its trabecular pattern of growth and the presence of eosinophilic hyaline material. The hyaline material is deposited within the cytoplasm of the cells and in the extracellular stroma. As the hyaline material accumulates in the center of the trabeculae, it entombs and then displaces the nuclei. The stromal hyaline can undergo calcification. (H&E stain)

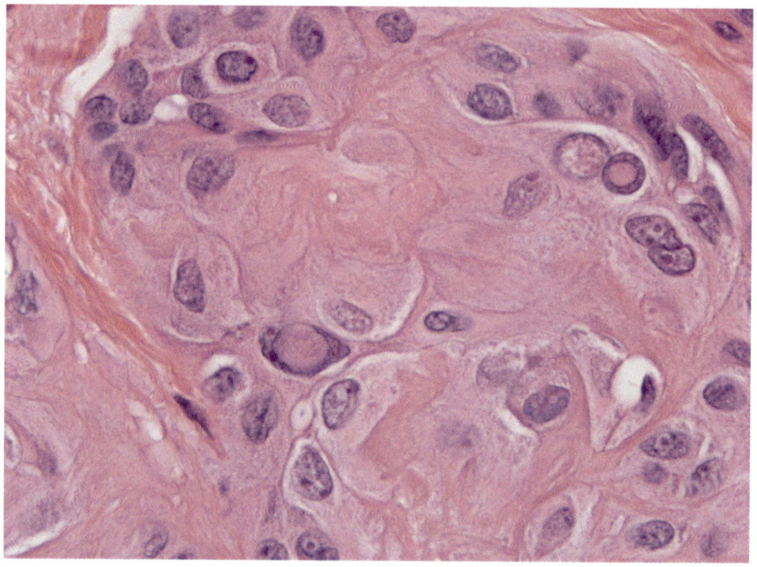

Figure 5.6b — Hyalinizing Trabecular Adenoma, Histologic Section. Hyalinizing trabecular adenoma shows considerable overlap with papillary carcinoma at the cellular level. The nuclei are often enlarged and elongated. Moreover, the nuclei frequently harbor longitudinal grooves and, as is demonstrated in this example, intranuclear pseudoinclusions. The hyalinizing trabecular adenoma often is encountered in the setting of multifocal papillary carcinoma. Reflecting a concern that some hyalinizing trabecular adenomas may in fact represent low grade papillary carcinomas, some pathologists prefer the term hyalinizing trabecular "neoplasm" over "adenoma." (H&E stain)

Figure 5.7 — Follicular Carcinoma, Minimally Invasive, Gross Appearance. Like their benign counterpart the follicular adenoma, the minimally invasive follicular carcinoma presents as a round to oval encapsulated nodule. The presence of invasion of the tumor capsule is usually a microscopic finding that requires thorough histologic evaluation of the tumor capsule. In this case, close inspection of the capsule reveals an area (6 to 7 o'clock position of tumor capsule) where the integrity of the capsule appears compromised. At the microscopic level, this focus corresponded to an area of invasive tumor growth through the tumor capsule.

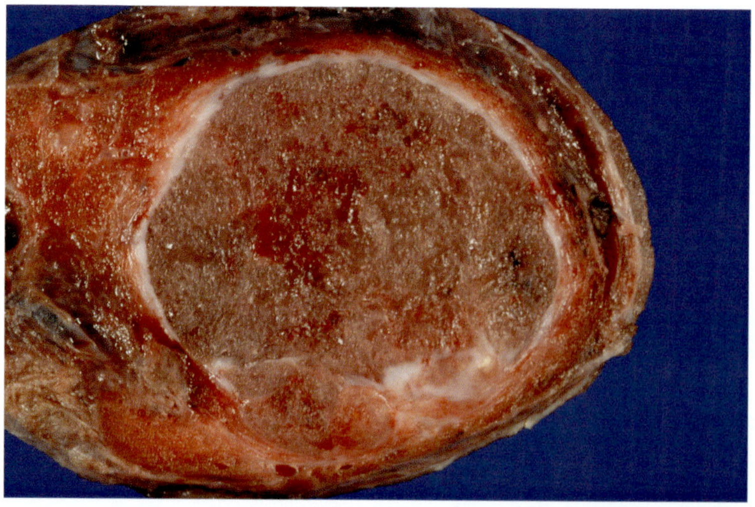

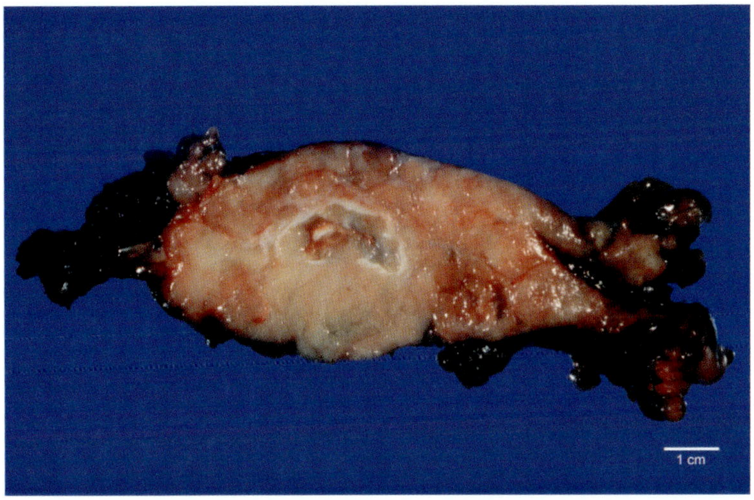

Figure 5.8 — Follicular Carcinoma, Widely Invasive, Gross Appearance. Widely invasive follicular carcinomas are defined by the presence of widespread invasion and destruction of the tumor capsule. In this follicular carcinoma, the skeleton of a tumor capsule is still visible, but the carcinoma extends beyond the tumor capsule to extensively infiltrate the thyroid parenchyma as a firm solid mass.

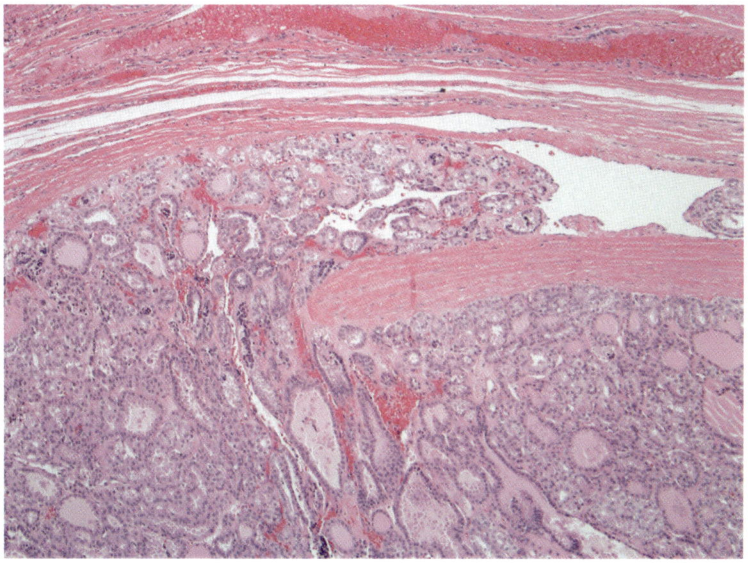

Figure 5.9a — Follicular Carcinoma, Microinvasive, Histologic Section. Most follicular carcinomas are highly cellular neoplasms that exhibit some combination of microfollicular, trabecular and solid growth patterns. The surrounding capsule tends be thicker and more irregular than is usually encountered in follicular adenomas. The diagnosis of malignancy rests on the presence of invasive tumor growth into the tumor capsule and into intracapsular blood vessels. As the carcinoma invades its surrounding tumor capsule, it gains access to the intracapsular blood vessels and extends laterally within the lumen of these intracapsular blood vessels. (H&E stain)

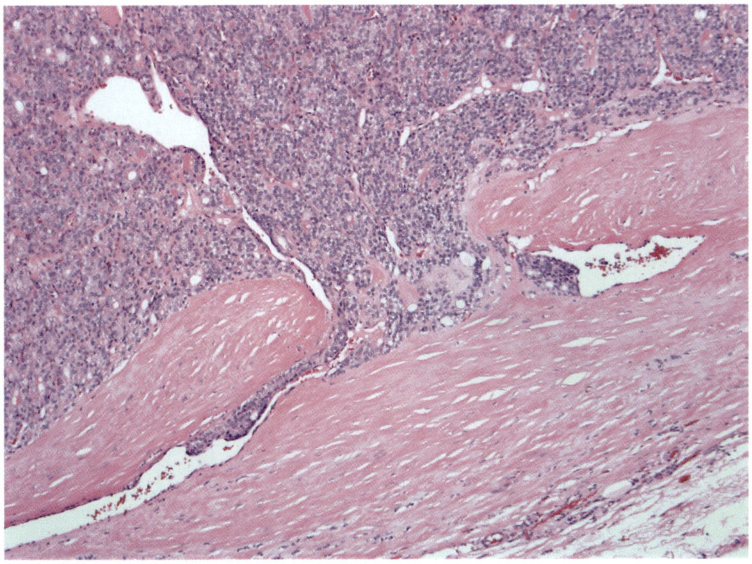

Figure 5.9b — Follicular Carcinoma, Microinvasive, Histologic Section. This linear penetration into the tumor capsule with subsequent lateral extension within intracapsular blood vessels gives rise to a characteristic "mushrooming" or "fish hooking" appearance of the invasive tumor front. (H&E stain)

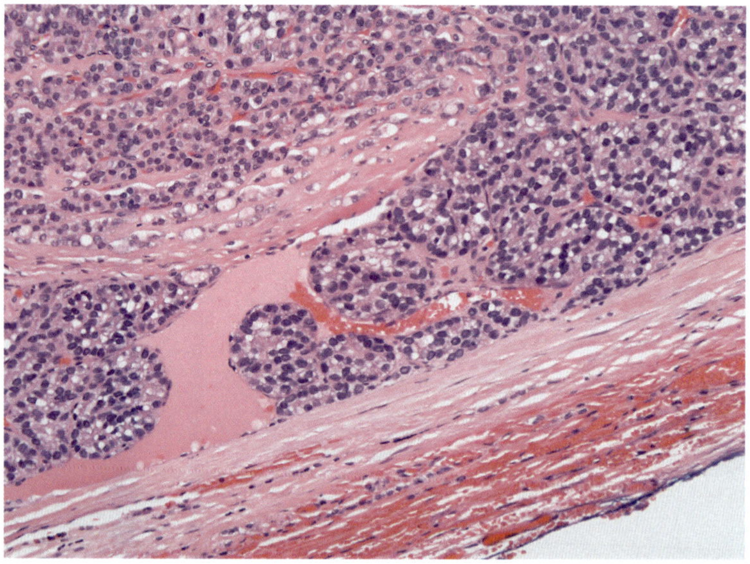

Figure 5.9c — Follicular Carcinoma, Microinvasive, Histologic Section. Vascular invasion is a critical finding in the diagnosis of follicular carcinoma. It is recognized as tumor follicles propagating within the lumen of an intracapsular blood vessel. The tumor must show adhesion to the wall of the blood vessel. The intravascular tumor plugs are often invested by a layer of endothelial cells. When dealing with follicular neoplasms of the thyroid, the finding of "free floating" tumor plugs (ie, tumor follicles that are within vascular spaces but do not show adhesion to the vessel wall) is not to be taken as evidence of true vascular invasion. (H&E stain)

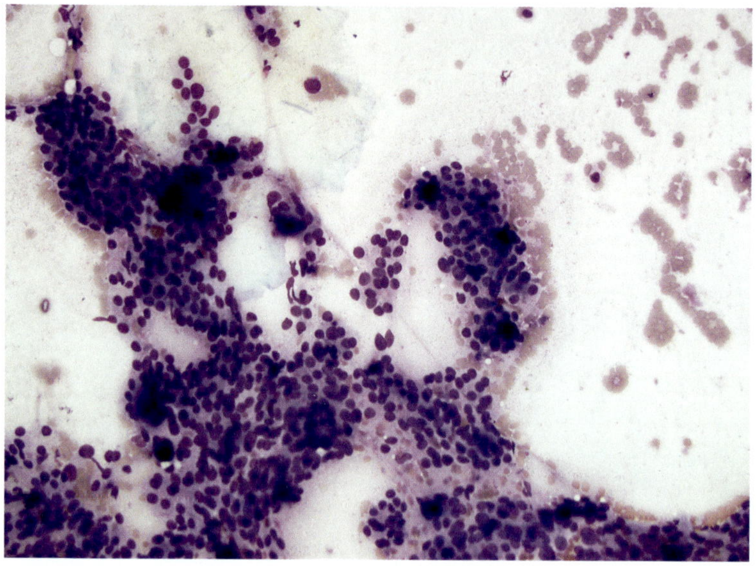

Figure 5.10a — Follicular Neoplasm, FNA. The Bethesda System for Reporting Thyroid Cytopathology (TBSRTC) defines the general diagnostic category of "suspicious for a follicular neoplasm" or "follicular neoplasm" as a cellular aspirate comprised of follicular cells, most of which are arranged in an altered architectural pattern characterized by significant cell crowding and/or microfollicle formation. Cases that demonstrate the nuclear features of papillary carcinoma are excluded from this category. Follicular neoplasms frequently have high cellularity with a predominant microfollicular pattern. Colloid is scant and often inspissated in the center of the microfollicles. (Diff Quik stain)

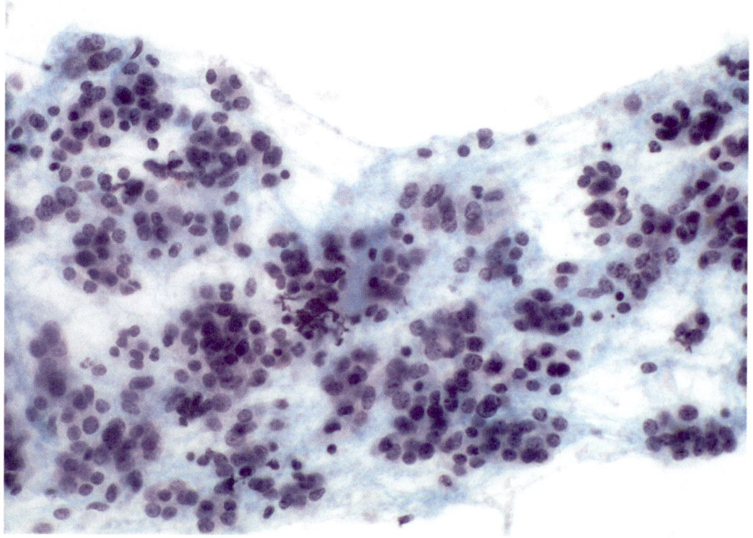

Figure 5.10b — Follicular Neoplasm, Fine Needle Aspiration (FNA). Similar to conventional (direct) smears, liquid-based preparations most often display high cellularity with a predominant population of microfollicles and/or trabeculae. The recommended clinical management of a patient with a diagnosis of follicular neoplasm is surgical excision of the lesion, most often a hemithyroidectomy or lobectomy. Results of the histological examination determine if the patient would need a complete thyroidectomy in cases of follicular carcinoma or follicular variant of papillary carcinoma. (Papanicolaou stain)

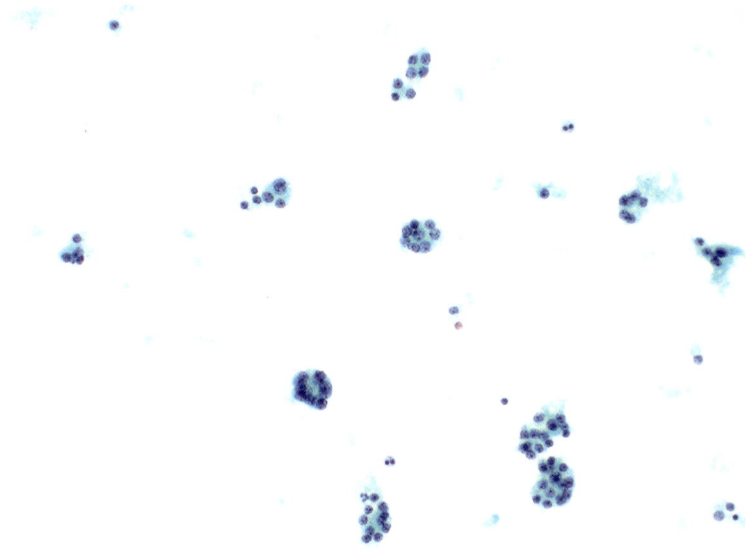

Figure 5.10c — Follicular Neoplasm, FNA. Another appearance of a follicular neoplasm on liquid-based preparation depicting isolated microfollicles having a uniform "equisize" morphology. The goal of the diagnostic category of "suspicious for a follicular neoplasm" or "follicular neoplasm" is to identify all potential follicular carcinomas and refer them for a diagnostic hemithyroidectomy. (Papanicolaou stain)

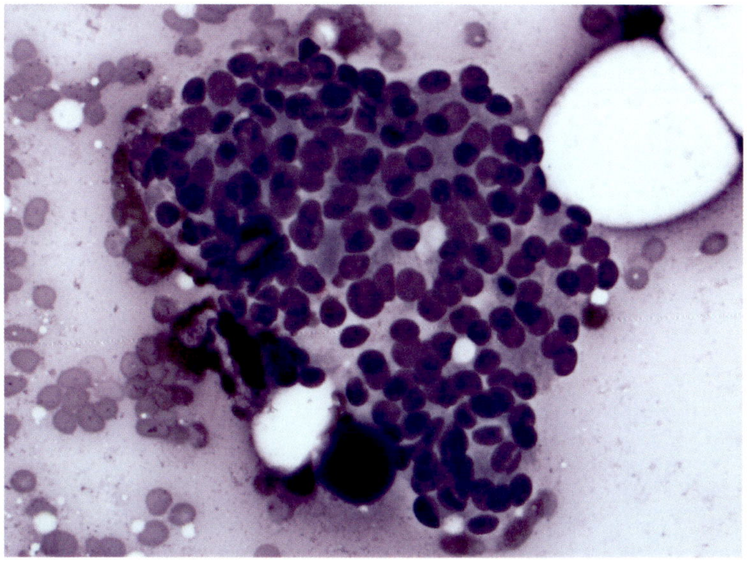

Figure 5.11 — Follicular Neoplasm, FNA. Follicular neoplasm showing round nuclei with nuclear crowding and overlap. Microfollicles can be appreciated. Based on a study by the College of American Pathologists (CAP) Cytopathology Resource Committee, a specific arrangement of cells seems to be consistently classified as a microfollicle. This is a group composed of fewer than 15 cells arranged in a flat circle with a lumen that is at least two-thirds complete. In contrast, small groups of cells arranged either in a row or in flat sheets are more consistently classified as macrofollicular, even when as few as eight cells are present. In between lies a group of cases that are not consistently classified. (Diff Quik stain)

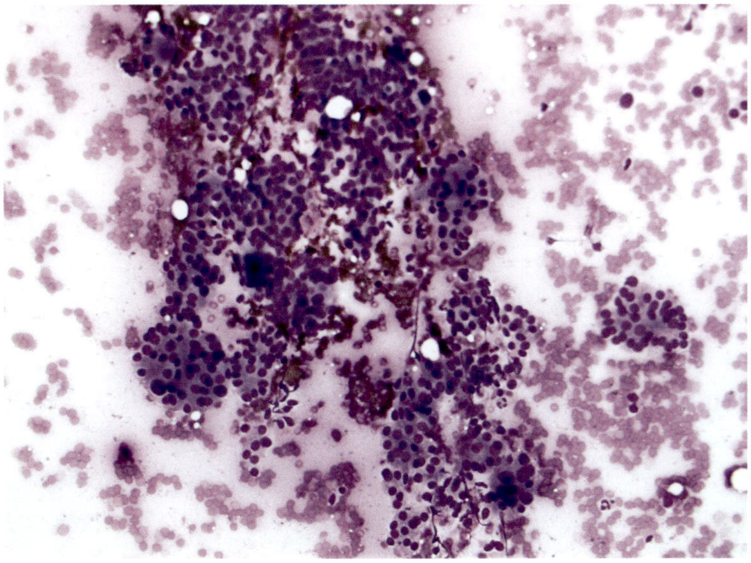

Figure 5.12 — Follicular Neoplasm, FNA. Follicular neoplasms can be very vascular and yield bloody aspirates. In this image, the cells are seen entrapped in blood/fibrin; however the nuclear crowding seen here is real rather than artifactual because the clotting is minimal. These lesions display a significant alteration in follicular cell architecture, characterized by cell crowding, microfollicles, and dispersed isolated cells. (Diff Quik stain)

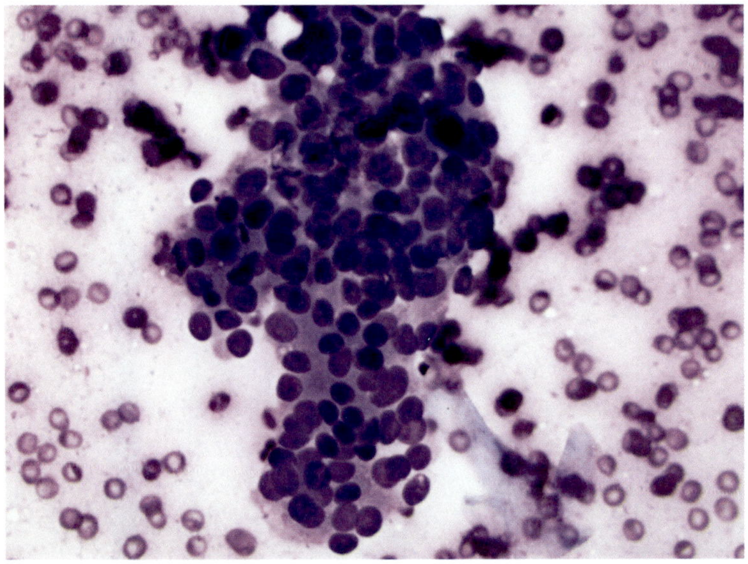

Figure 5.13a — Follicular Neoplasm, FNA. This case displays multiple microfollicles with round nuclei, nuclear crowding, and overlap. Nuclei do not show features worrisome for a follicular variant of papillary thyroid carcinoma (PTC). Literature published prior to TBSRTC show a great variability in the way thyroid aspirates that are suspicious for a follicular neoplasm have been reported. The FNA reporting terminology historically used has ranged from vague and confusing terms like "follicular lesion," "follicular proliferation," and "indeterminate" to the more specific terms like "rule out/suggestive of/suspicious for follicular neoplasm" to the definitive "follicular neoplasm." (Diff Quik)

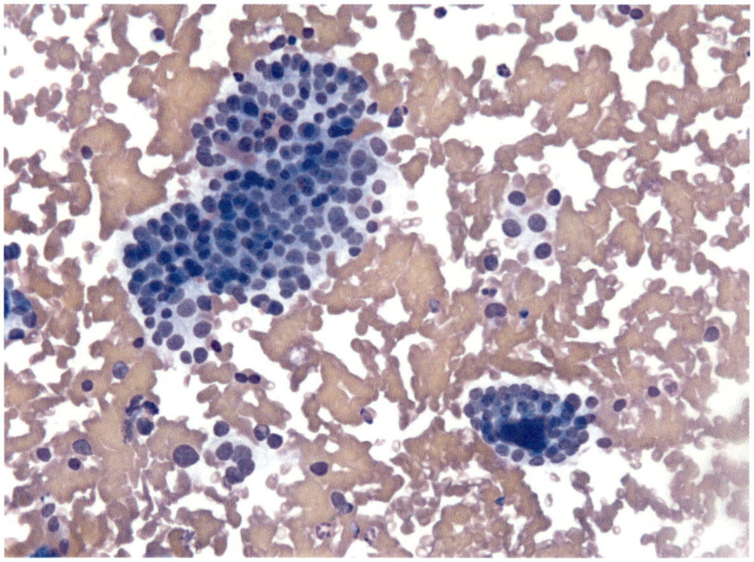

Figure 5.13b — Follicular Neoplasm, FNA. In contrast to the previous example, this follicular neoplasm not only has somewhat cohesive tissue fragments but also numerous isolated single cells. A small amount of colloid is appreciated in the smaller tissue fragment at 4 o'clock. Unless a large amount of dispersed microfollicles are appreciated, the possibility of an adenomatoid nodule is hard to exclude in such cases. (Diff Quik stain)

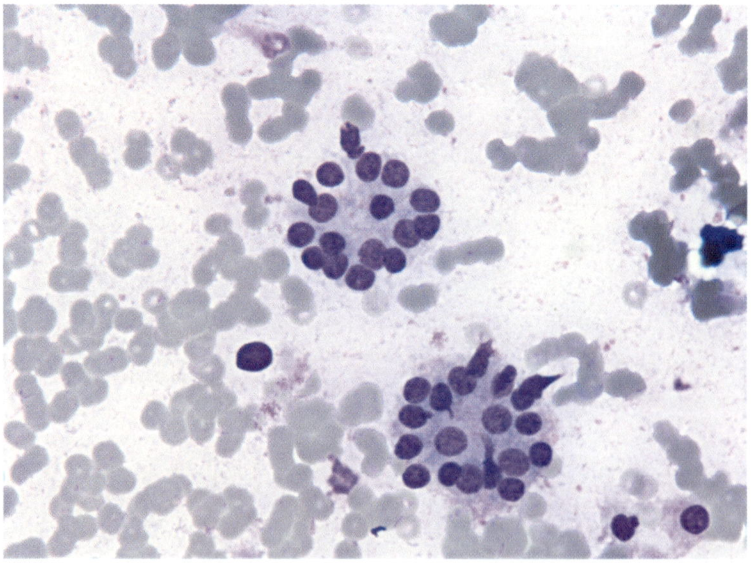

Figure 5.14 — Follicular Neoplasm, FNA. Higher magnification of two microfollicles. Note the uniformity in size and cellular composition. Nuclei are round and colloid is absent. The term "suspicious for a follicular neoplasm" is preferred by most over "follicular neoplasm" for this diagnostic category because a significant proportion of cases (up to 35%) turn out to be adenomatoid nodules rather than follicular neoplasm on follow-up lobectomy. (Diff Quik stain)

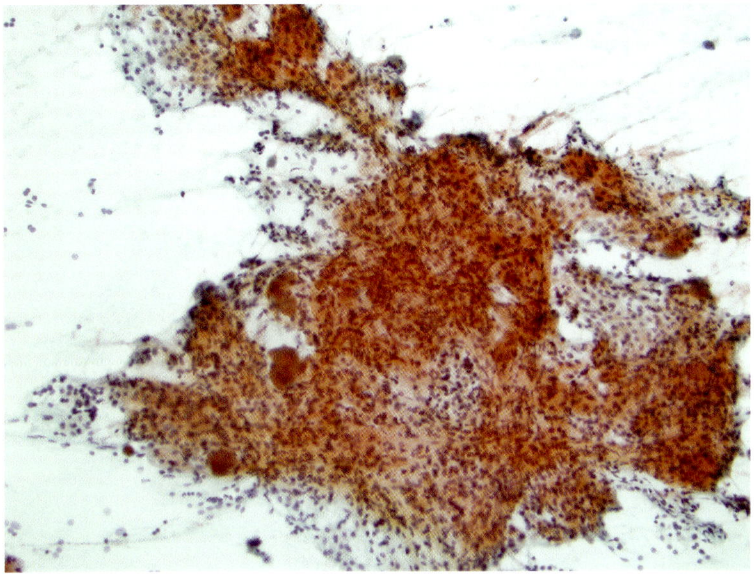

Figure 5.15 — Follicular Neoplasm, FNA. Touch prep with mixed microfollicular/macrofollicular pattern. The cytology was called AUS/FLUS, and the surgical follow-up was follicular adenoma with a mixed microfollicular to normofollicular pattern. Such patterns can be very difficult to classify as hyperplastic or follicular neoplasm and represent the true "grey zone" between these two thyroid lesions. (Papanicolaou stain)

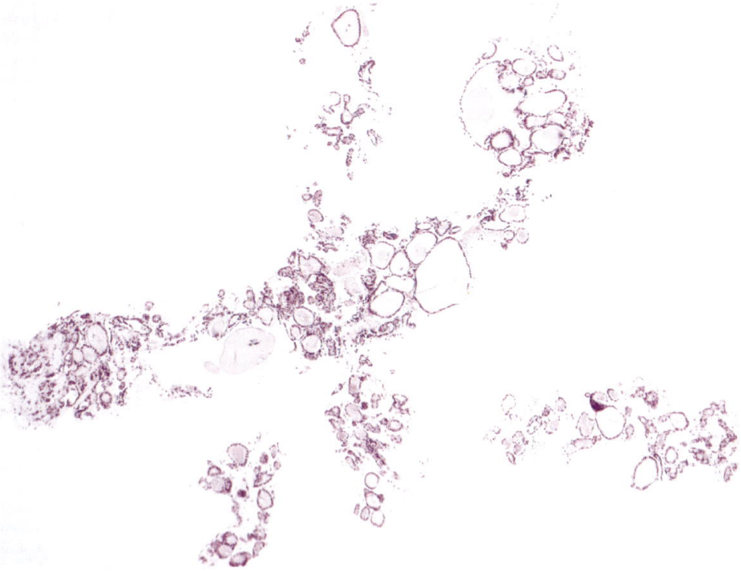

Figure 5.16 — Follicular Neoplasm, Histologic Section. Follicular adenoma. Corresponding core biopsy from touch prep in the previous case showing mixed micro/normo/macrofollicular patterns. It's interesting to note that the majority of follicular neoplasm (FN) cases turn out to be benign—either follicular adenoma or adenomatoid nodule, both of which are more common than follicular carcinoma. Additionally, of those that have a malignant follow-up, a significant proportion are follicular variants of papillary carcinoma. (H&E stain)

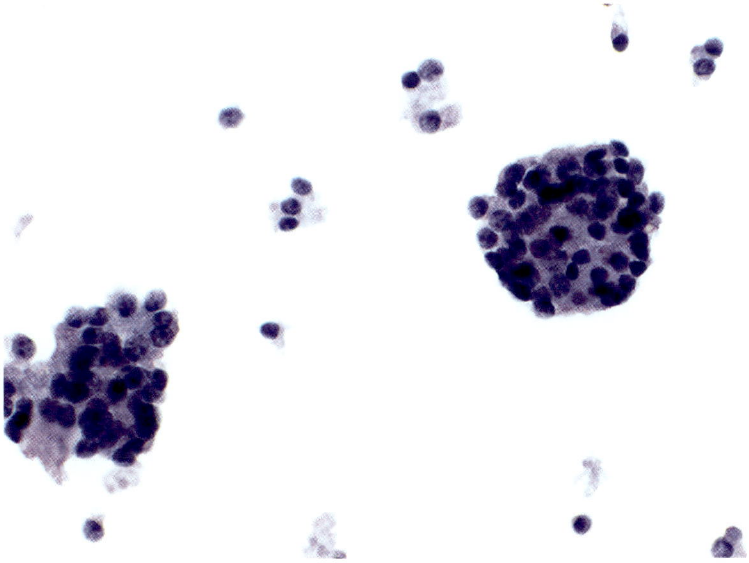

Figure 5.17 — Follicular Neoplasm, FNA. This liquid-based preparation illustrates one intact and one partially intact follicle with few single cells in the background. Due to the technical process involved, there is often a much larger single cell/dishesive pattern on such preparations in cases of follicular neoplasms. Parathyroid lesions should always be entertained in the differential diagnosis in such cases when colloid is totally absent. (Papanicolaou stain)

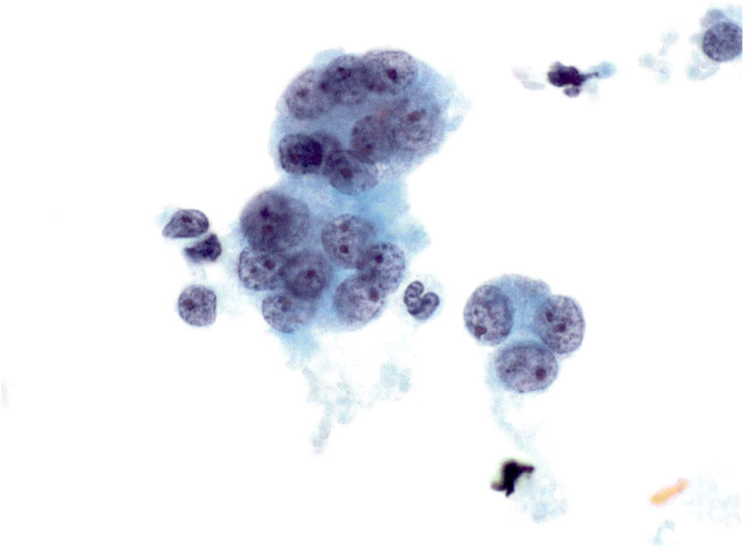

Figure 5.18 — Follicular Neoplasm, FNA. Due to an often pale chromatin of the nuclei seen in liquid-based preparations, the nuclei tend to appear more transparent which brings out the nucleolar prominence in the cells, as nicely displayed in this case. The main purpose of the diagnostic category of "suspicious for a follicular neoplasm" is to identify a thyroid lesion that might be a follicular carcinoma and triage it for surgical lobectomy and a more definitive interpretation. (Papanicolaou stain)

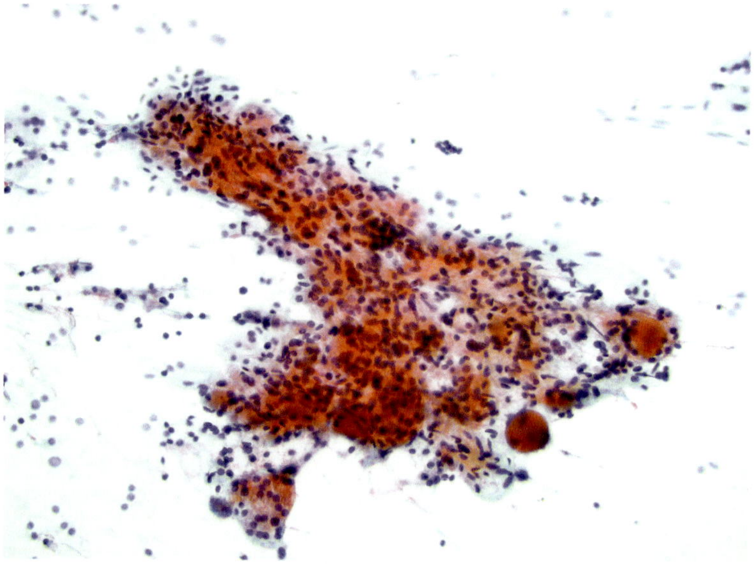

Figure 5.19 — Follicular Neoplasm, FNA. A large partially cohesive tissue fragment containing multiple microfollicles embedded in a loose fibrotic stroma. Some inspissated globules of colloid are also visible. In follicular neoplasms, the neoplastic epithelial cells are normal-sized or enlarged and relatively uniform, with scant or moderate amounts of cytoplasm. Follicular neoplasm may display some nuclear atypia with enlarged, variably sized nuclei and prominent nucleoli. (Papanicolaou stain)

Figure 5.20 — Parathyroid Tissue, FNA. Incidental intrathyroidal parathyroid lesions pose interesting diagnostic issues. FNA of these presumably "thyroid nodules" can lead to misinterpretation of cytomorphological findings because of similarities in cytological features of neoplastic and nonneoplastic parathyroid and thyroid lesions. Cytology in this case shows a microfollicular/crowded cellular pattern. The cells closely resemble thyroid follicular cells. Colloid is absent here but parathyroid secretions can resemble colloid. If parathyroid tissue is not considered in the differential diagnosis, such cases can easily be misdiagnosed as a "follicular neoplasm." Sending the needle rinse for parathyroid hormone (PTH) assay is often helpful in confirming parathyroid tissue, which was done in this case because the patient had hypercalcemia. Subsequent excision confirmed a parathyroid adenoma. (Diff Quik stain)

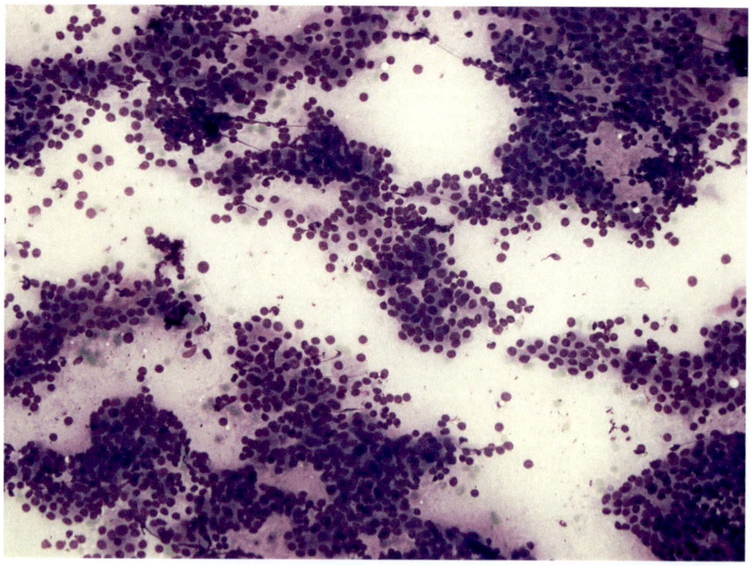

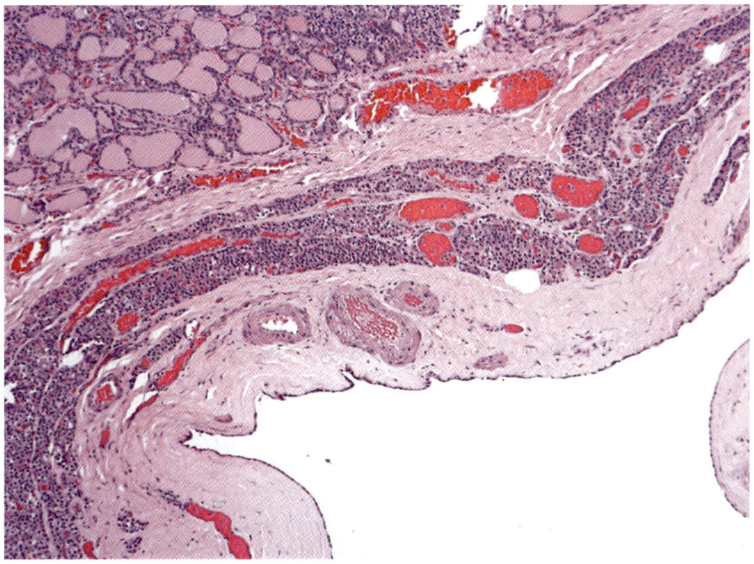

Figure 5.21 — Parathyroid cyst, Histologic Section. Due to the anatomic proximity of the parathyroid glands, a parathyroid cyst can be clinically mistaken for a cyst of the thyroid. The fluid filling the cyst is usually watery and clear to straw-colored. The cysts do not usually extend into the thyroid parenchyma, but tend to be adhered to the surface of the thyroid and separated by partitioning zone of fibrosis. The presence of parathyroid tissue within the cyst wall is very helpful in confirming the parathyroid nature of this cyst. (H&E stain)

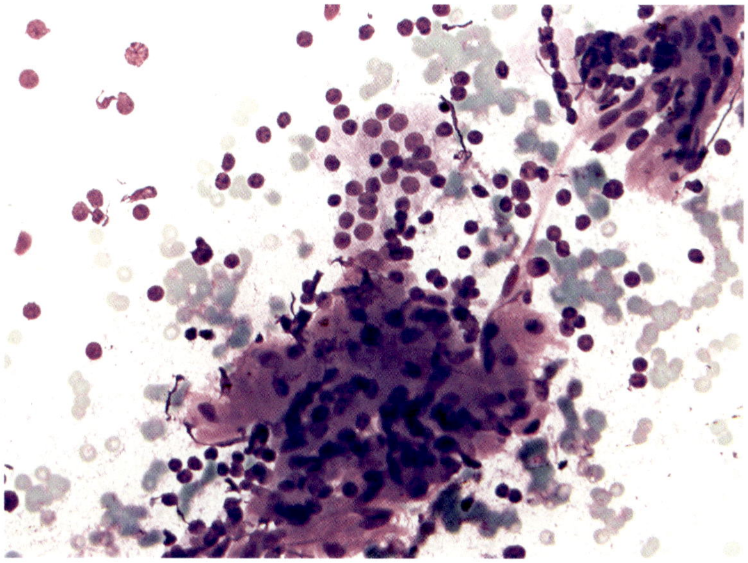

Figure 5.22 — Parathyroid Tissue, FNA. When submitted as a "thyroid FNA" specimen, parathyroid adenomas are often misinterpreted as "follicular neoplasm" due to a significant morphologic overlap between these two groups of lesions. In this case, the cells were thought to have "oncocytic" features on smears. Closer attention to the smear shows prominence of naked nuclei with isolated "endocrine atypia" and endothelial cells/vessels. This case was misdiagnosed as thyroid follicular neoplasm with Hürthle cell change. Subsequent excision showed a parathyroid adenoma. Since parathyroid cells can have oncocytic and clear cell types, the differential diagnosis of parathyroid adenoma should always be considered in cases such as this. (Diff Quik stain)

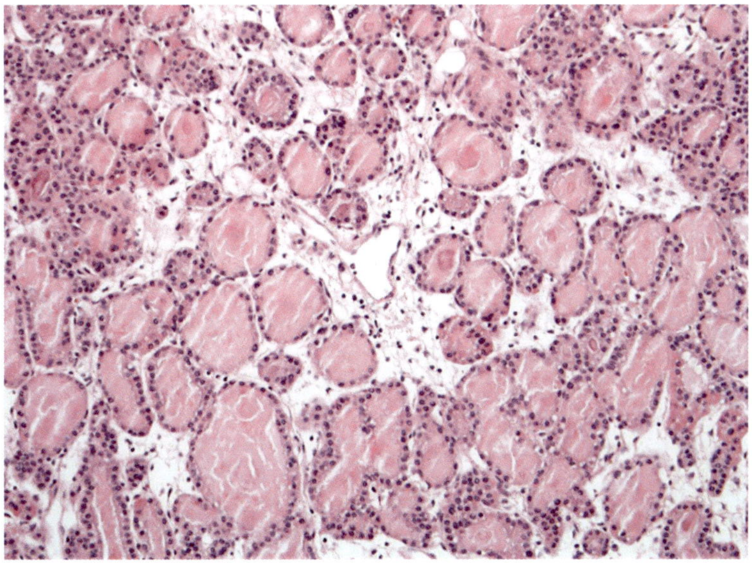

Figure 5.23a — Intrathyroidal Parathyroid Adenoma, Histologic Section. Parathyroid glands sometimes involve the thyroid capsule and occasionally reside within the thyroid parenchyma (intra-thyroidal parathyroid gland). Not surprisingly then, enlarged parathyroid glands can be clinically mistaken for a true thyroid nodule. Moreover, a proliferative parathyroid gland (e.g. hyperplastic parathyroid gland, parathyroid adenoma) can be mistaken for a follicular thyroid neoplasm based on its morphologic features. In the intrathyroidal parathyroid adenoma shown here, the absence of stromal fat and the presence of well formed follicular structures with intraluminal colloid-like material renders its distinction from a thyroid follicular neoplasm extremely difficult on morphologic grounds alone. (H&E stain)

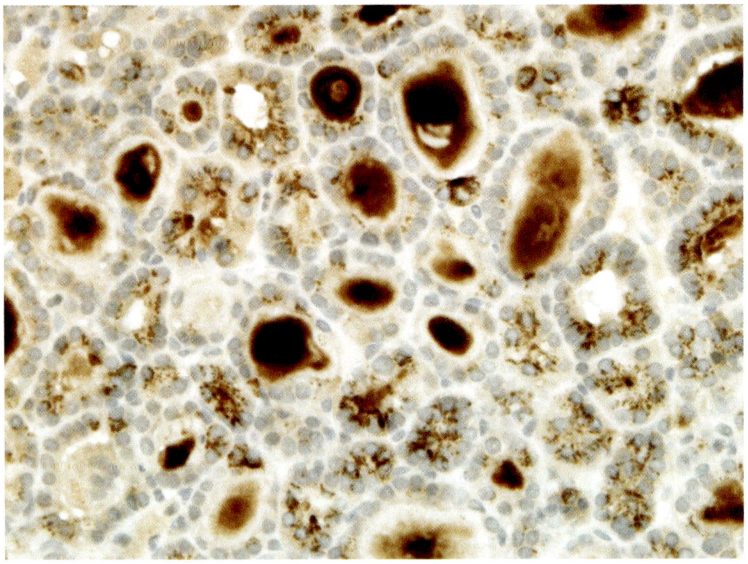

Figure 5.23b — Intrathyroidal Parathyroid Adenoma, Immunohistochemical Staining of Histologic Section. Recognition of the parathyroid nature of this follicular-patterned lesion in the thyroid is assisted by its immunohistochemical staining for parathyroid hormone. (Parathyroid hormone immunostain).

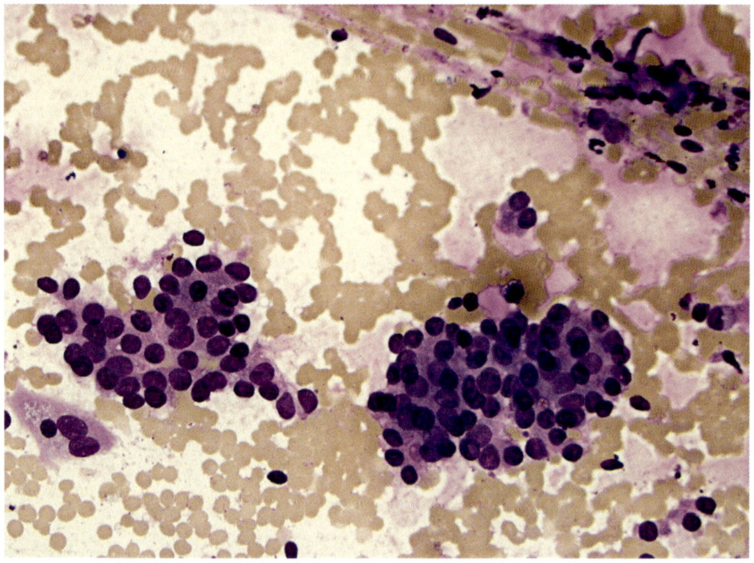

Figure 5.24 — Follicular Neoplasm, FNA. Smear shows microfollicles with enlarged round nuclei and scant colloid. There is nuclear crowding/overlap. It was diagnosed as a follicular neoplasm on cytology; subsequent surgical specimen showed minimally invasive follicular carcinoma. It is virtually impossible to distinguish follicular adenoma from follicular carcinoma on cytology since this depends on assessment of capsular/vascular invasion on the excised specimen. (Diff Quik stain)

Figure 5.25 — Papillary Thyroid Carcinoma, Follicular Variant, FNA. This case depicts hypercellularity with a microfollicular architecture. Nuclei are enlarged with mostly round shapes. Scant colloid is also evident. No nuclear grooves or intranuclear inclusions were noticed and the case was misdiagnosed as "suspicious for a follicular neoplasm." This cytomorphology presents a common problem in thyroid FNA cytology. Approximately 15% to 20% of cases diagnosed as "follicular neoplasm" do turn out to be a follicular variant of papillary carcinoma. (Diff Quik stain)

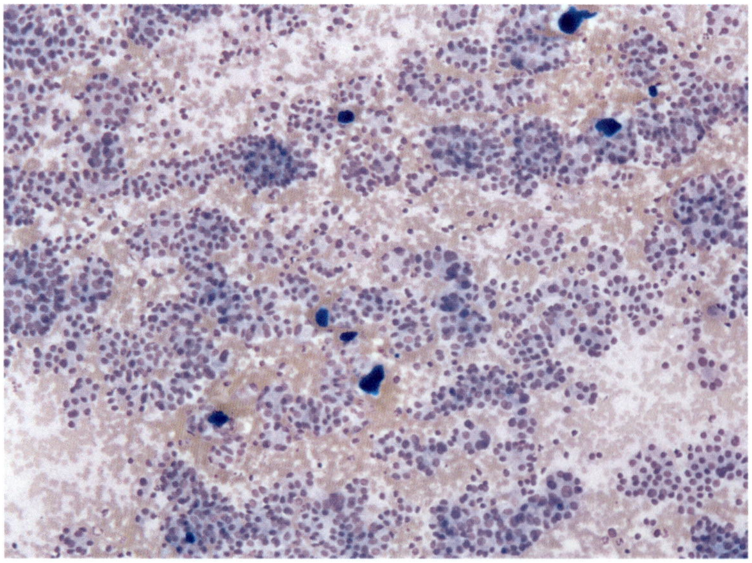

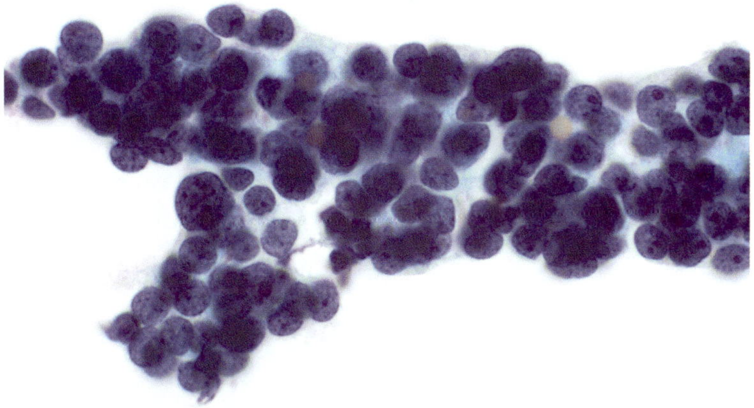

Figure 5.26 — Follicular Neoplasm, FNA. This liquid-based smear shows neoplastic follicular cells with large round and hyperchromatic nuclei in a crowded, trabecular architecture. Small inconspicuous to prominent nucleoli are also evident. Neither a predominantly microfollicular architecture, nor a trabecular pattern can help distinguish an adenoma from a carcinoma and simply represent phenotypic variations that observed in follicular neoplasms. (Papanicolaou stain)

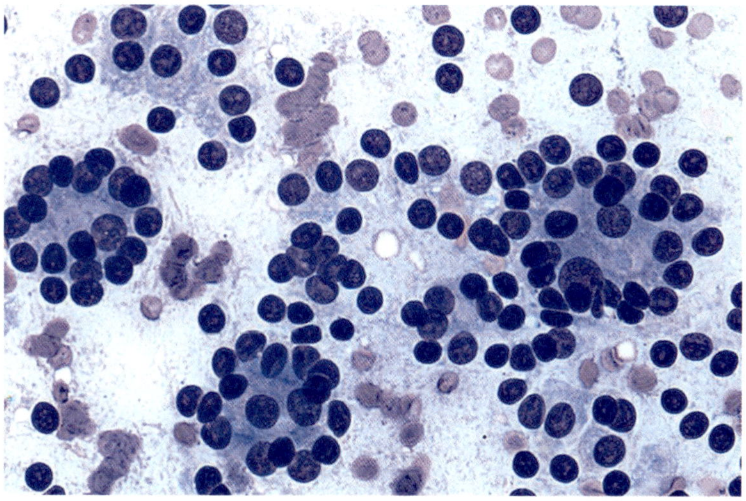

Figure 5.27 — Follicular Neoplasm, FNA. This smear shows multiple well-formed microfollicles. These are complete "rosette-like" or "ring-like" circular structures comprised typically of enlarged follicular cells (typically 12–25 in number). More important than the number of cells forming a microfollicle is the uniformity in their architecture or the so-called "equisize" appearance. Few singly dispersed naked nuclei are also observed in the background. (Diff Quik stain)

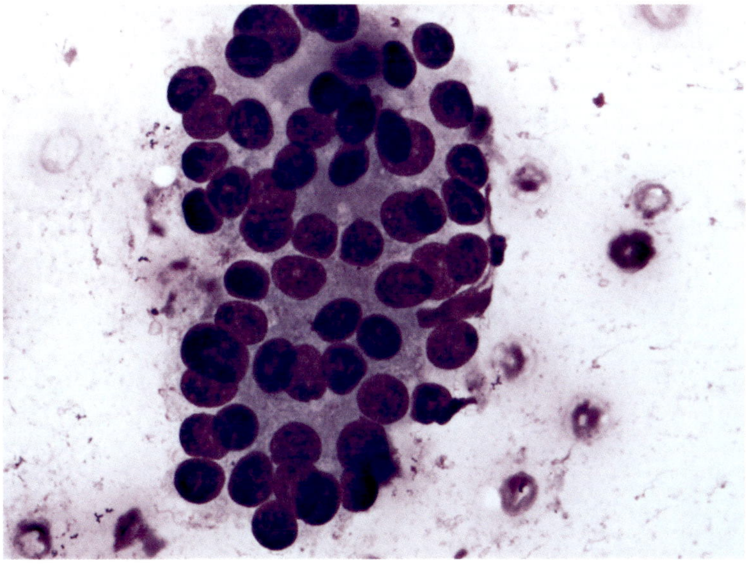

Figure 5.28 — Follicular Neoplasm, FNA. This case displays neoplastic cells with markedly enlarged round nuclei in a follicular growth pattern. Cytoplasm appears granular but lacks the typical appearance of a Hürthle cell. (Papanicolaou stain)

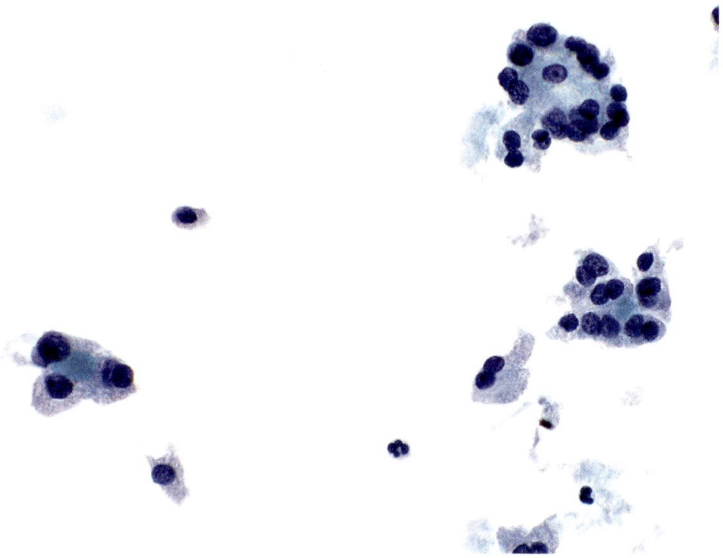

Figure 5.29 — Follicular Neoplasm, FNA. This liquid-based preparation depicts follicular cells with some Hürthle cell features, but they are clearly arranged in microfollicles with colloid droplets visible at the center of the microfollicles at lower left and lower right. The final diagnosis was a follicular adenoma. (Papanicolaou stain)

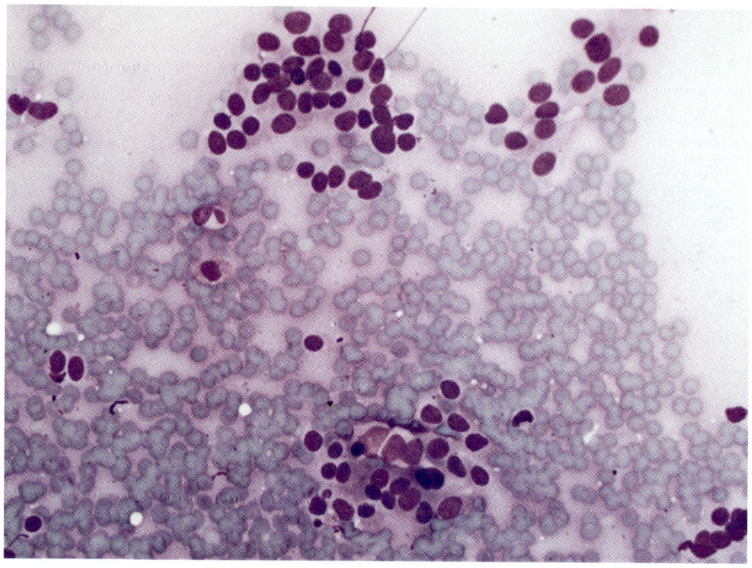

Figure 5.30a — Primary Thyroid Paraganglioma, FNA. This case illustrates a primary thyroid paraganglioma misdiagnosed as follicular neoplasm on cytology. On retrospective review, the smears show that the majority of crowded cells are actually naked nuclei clustering together and possibly representing the sustentacular cells. Primary thyroid paragangliomas are thought to arise from the inferior laryngeal paraganglia, which are sometimes situated within the thyroid capsule. (Diff Quik stain)

Figure 5.30b — Primary Thyroid Paraganglioma, FNA. The tight clustering of the naked nuclei wrongly suggested a microfollicular pattern that led to an erroneous diagnosis of a follicular neoplasm. Colloid was totally absent in this case. Most of the reported cases of primary thyroid paraganglioma occurred in females, with the majority of patients between 40 and 60 years of age. (Diff Quik stain)

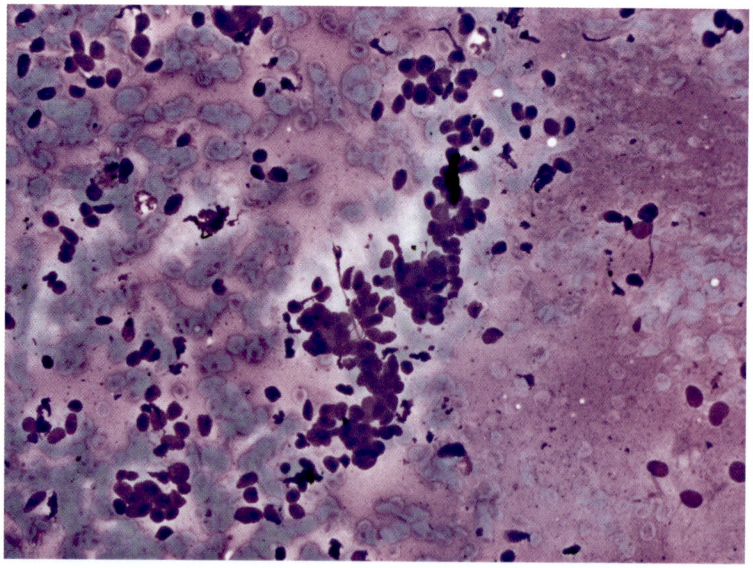

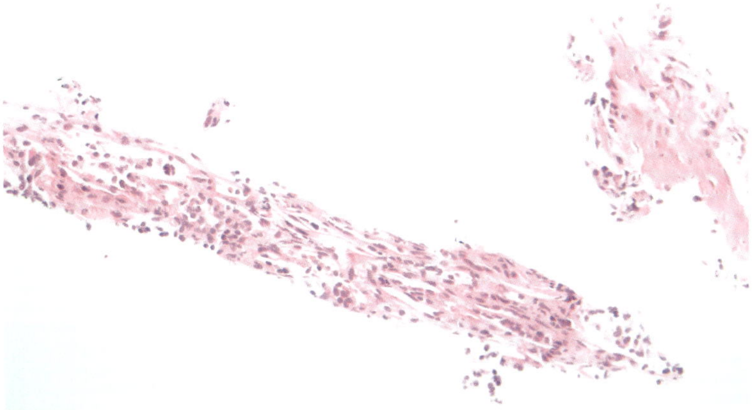

Figure 5.30c — Primary Thyroid Paraganglioma, Histologic Section. Core biopsy taken at a later date displays a predominantly nested "zellballen" pattern with groups of cells surrounded by a vascular stroma. Thyroid paragangliomas are usually asymptomatic, rarely functional, and most often present clinically as a mass in the thyroid/neck. There is no reported association with multiple endocrine neoplasia (MEN) in the literature. (H&E stain)

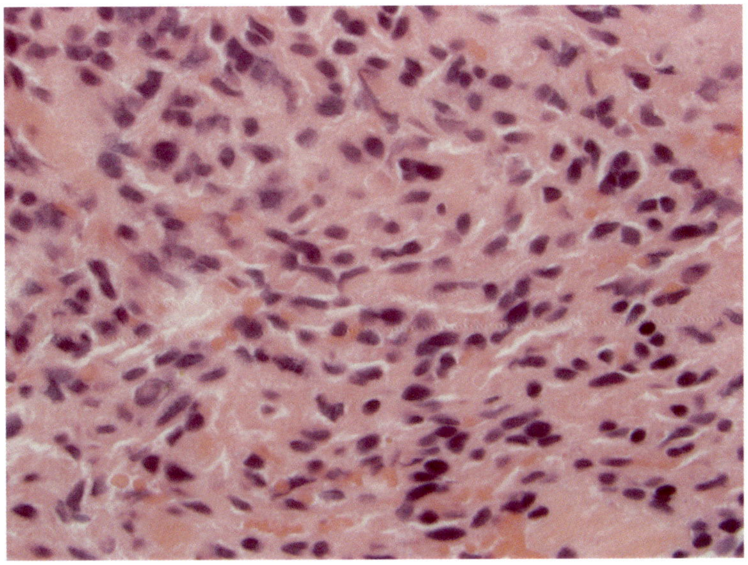

Figure 5.30d — Primary Thyroid Paraganglioma, Histologic Section. On resection, the thyroid tumor shows cells growing in a zellballen pattern and embedded in a fibrous network that is rich with blood vessels. Round tumor cells have amphophilic or acidophilic cytoplasm, and round or ovoid nuclei. Desmoplastic reaction is absent. Total thyroidectomy or lobectomy (for tumors confined to a single thyroid lobe) is the preferred treatment option and is considered to be curative. (H&E stain)

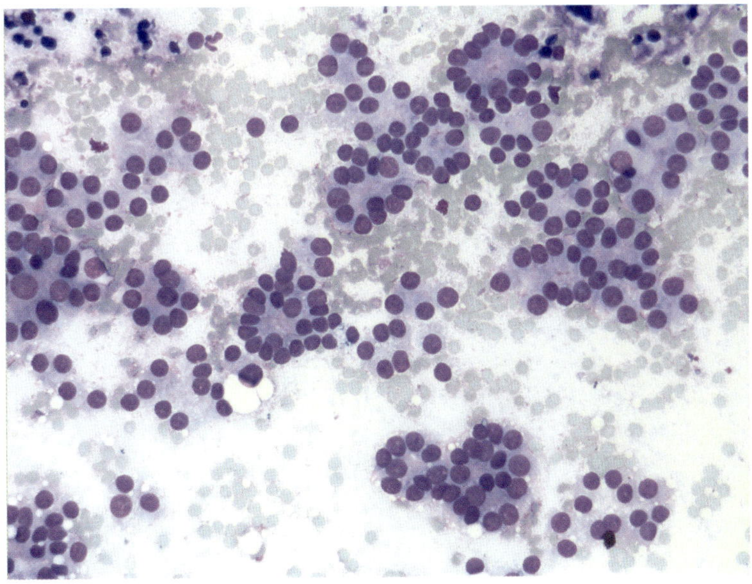

Figure 5.31a — Follicular Neoplasm, FNA. A beautiful illustration of the classic features of a follicular neoplasm—an exclusive microfollicular architecture, enlarged round nuclei, cellular monotony and equisize appearance, and lack of colloid. (Diff Quik stain)

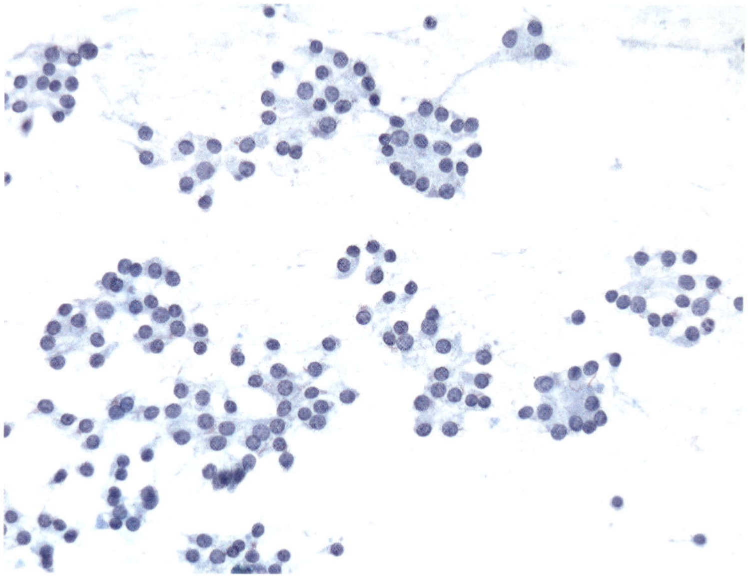

Figure 5.31b — Follicular Neoplasm, FNA. On this alcohol fixed smear, the microfollicles have a more open and loose appearance yet maintain their architectural monotony. (Papanicolaou stain)

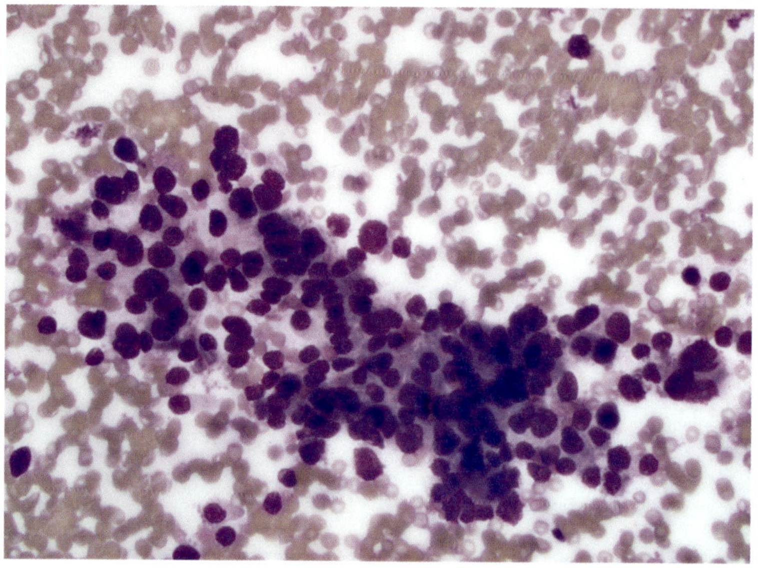

Figure 5.32a — Medullary Thyroid Carcinoma (MTC), FNA. Medullary carcinoma is a great mimicker—often called the "melanoma of the thyroid" because of its highly variable cytologic and histologic patterns. This case showed neoplastic cells with a pattern suggestive of crowded, microfollicles. A useful distinguishing feature here is the variation in cell/nuclear size—this would be unusual for a follicular neoplasm but characteristic for MTC. (Diff Quik stain)

Figure 5.32b — Medullary Thyroid Carcinoma, FNA. Another smear from the previous case. Another area from the case showed a more characteristic dyscohesive pattern with plasmacytoid morphology, much more easily recognizable as MTC. Attention to chromatin pattern of alcohol fixed slides can often help prevent this misinterpretation, especially if the pattern on cytology is entirely or predominantly microfollicular. (Diff Quik stain)

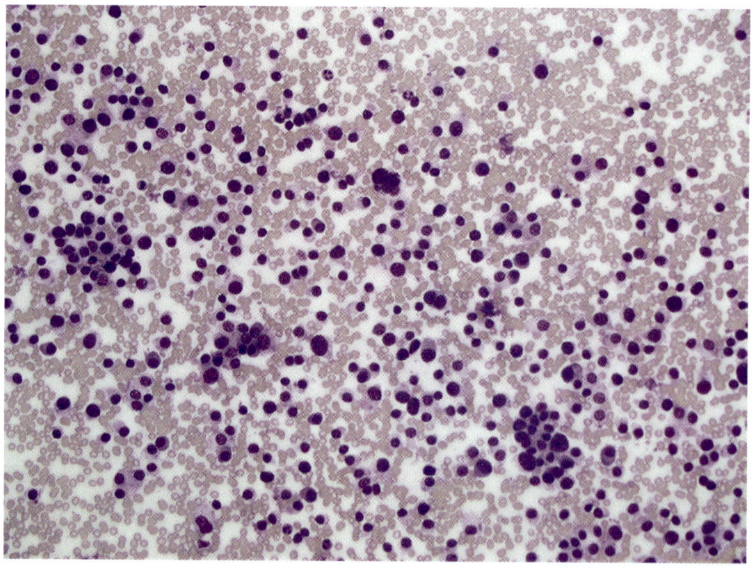

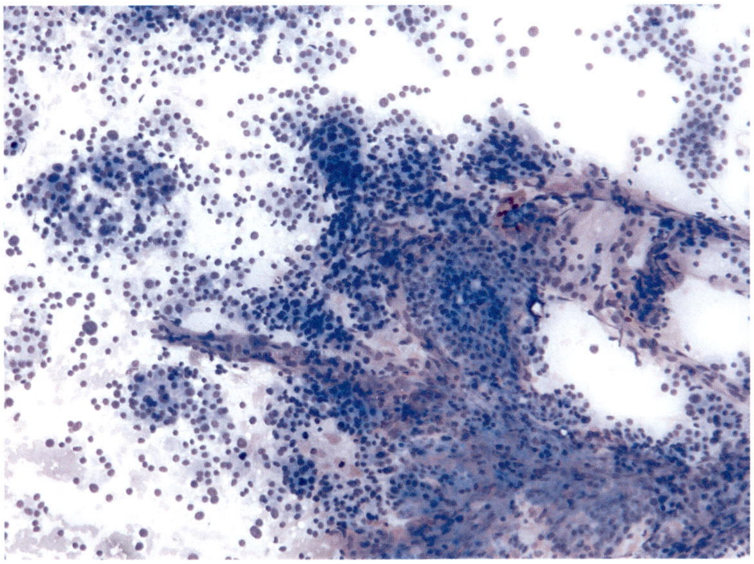

Figure 5.33 — Follicular Neoplasm, FNA. This example of a follicular neoplasm, which turned out to be an adenoma, illustrates significant vascularity often associated with this lesion. Microfollicular architecture is not predominantly present in such cases, however, a trabecular pattern may often be observed. (Diff Quik stain)

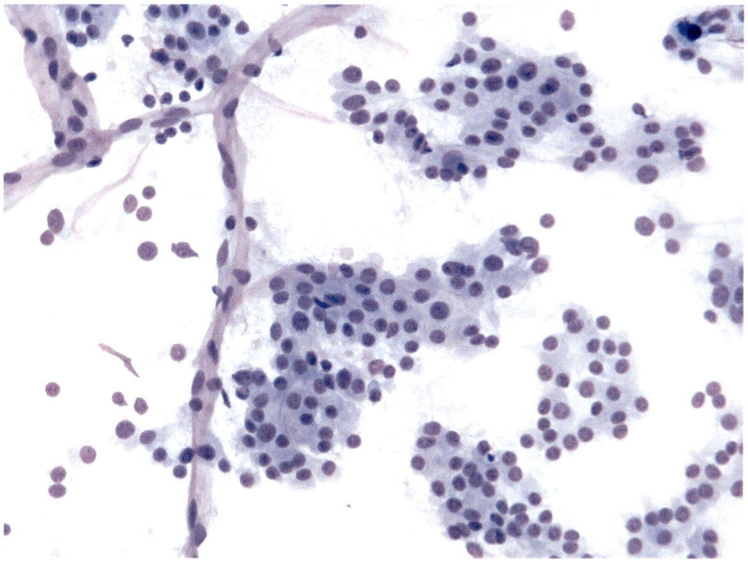

Figure 5.34 — Follicular Neoplasm, FNA. Higher magnification from the previous case shows fine "wire like" arborizing vessels and associated neoplastic follicular cells. Cells have abundant, slightly granular cytoplasm but do not display well-developed Hürthle cell morphology. (Diff Quik stain)

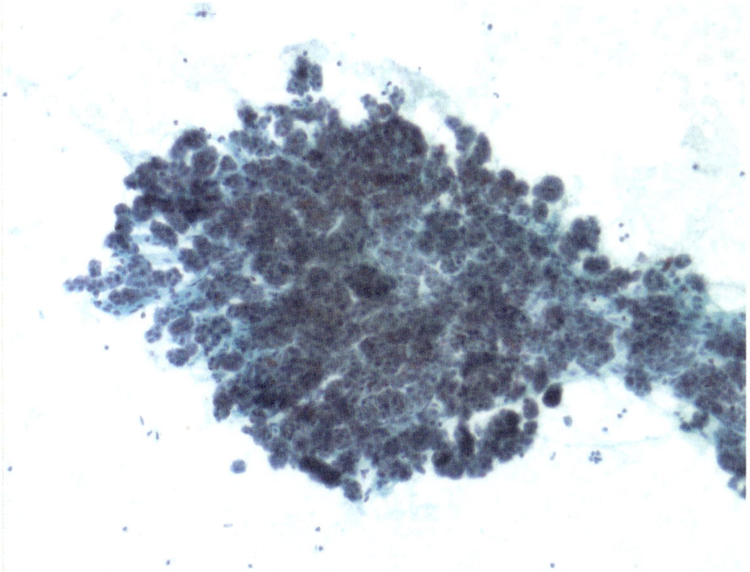

Figure 5.35 — Follicular Neoplasm, FNA. This case, which turned out to be an adenoma, nicely illustrates a crowded fragment of innumerable microfollicles held together with fine stromal fibrous tissue. The appearance almost mimics a tissue core biopsy. Small amount of dot-shaped inspissated colloid is clearly visible in some microfollicles. (Papanicolaou stain)

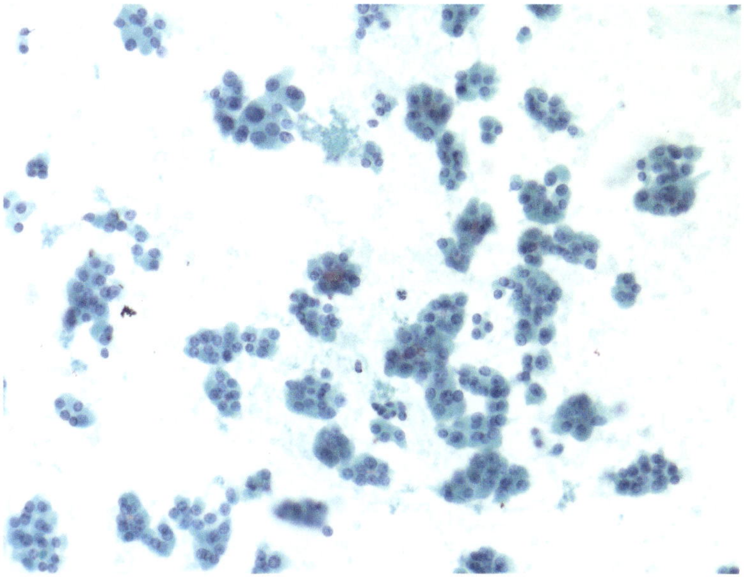

Figure 5.36 — Follicular Neoplasm, FNA. Another example of a follicular neoplasm (an adenoma on follow-up), with numerous uniform "equisize" microfollicles. Nuclei are enlarged but lack prominent nucleoli. Rare follicles have scant inspissated colloid. (Papanicolaou stain)

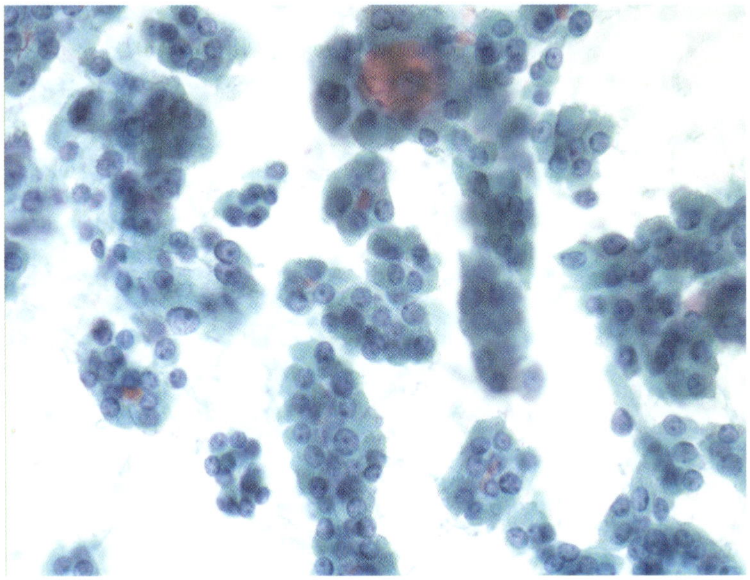

Figure 5.37 — Follicular Neoplasm, FNA. A nice illustration of a mixed, microfollicular and short trabecular pattern is shown here. Nuclei are enlarged with micronucleoli. Some follicles contain intraluminal colloid. Nuclear features of papillary carcinoma are not observed. (Papanicolaou stain)

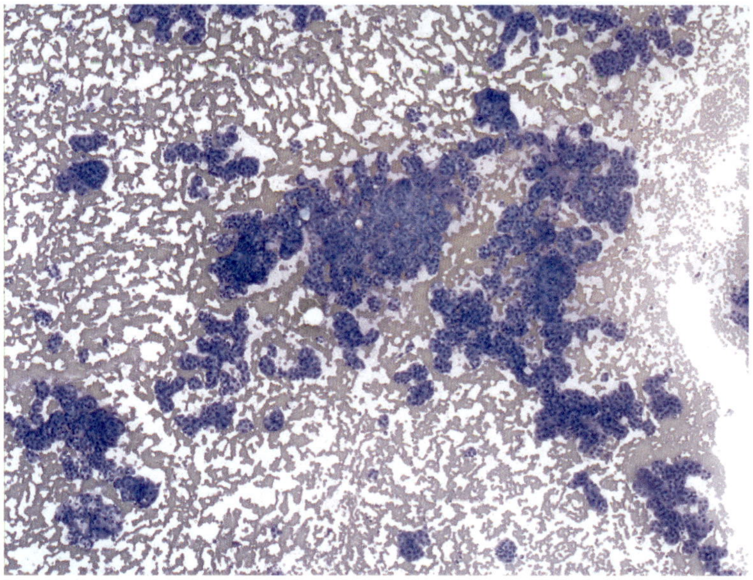

Figure 5.38a — Follicular Neoplasm, FNA. In some cases of follicular neoplasm, the predominant pattern is "trabecular" where the neoplastic cells display branching cord-like formations. Note a total lack of colloid and any other cellular component (usual type of follicular cells, Hürthle cells, etc.). Follow-up revealed a follicular adenoma. (Diff Quik stain)

Figure 5.38b — Follicular Neoplasm, FNA. Higher magnification of the previous case demonstrates cellular monotony forming the trabeculae. Cells have enlarged nuclei and Hürtheloid cytoplasm but lack prominent nucleoli, which are characteristic of a Hürthle cell neoplasm. (Diff Quik stain)

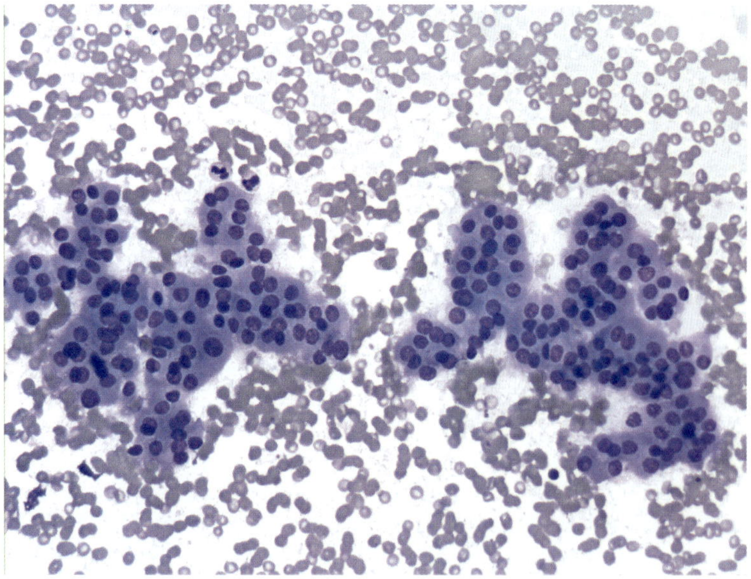

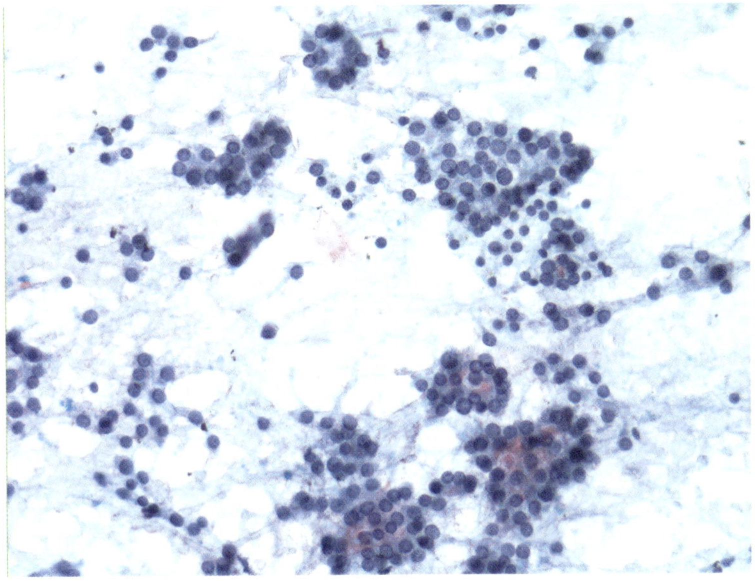

Figure 5.39 — Follicular Neoplasm, FNA. Occasional cases of follicular neoplasm display a loose adherence of neoplastic cells with a large number of singly dispersed naked nuclei. Presence of some colloid (as seen here) helps in the diagnosis of such cases as "thyroid follicular cell" rather than "parathyroid." In the latter case, there is a total lack of colloid and an often vacuolated background. (Papanicolaou stain)

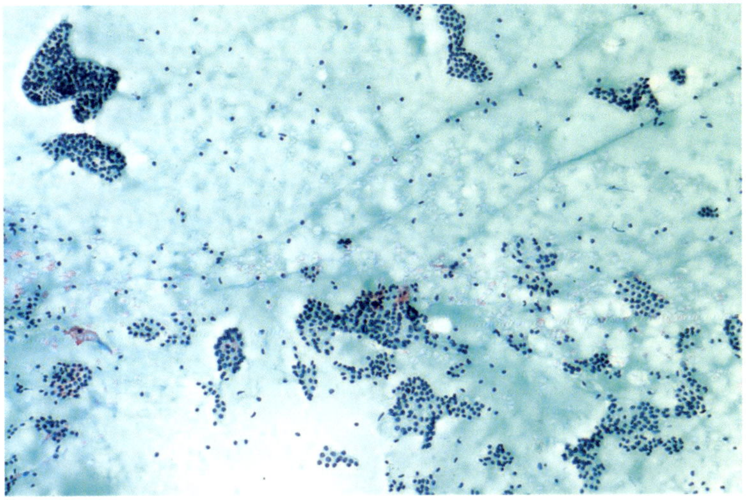

Figure 5.40 — Follicular Neoplasm, FNA. This rather unusual case of follicular neoplasm is colloid-rich (as seen in the smear background) but associated with a predominance of microfollicles. Interestingly, the lobectomy showed follicular carcinoma. A macrofollicular variant of follicular carcinoma has been reported in the literature. (Papanicolaou stain)

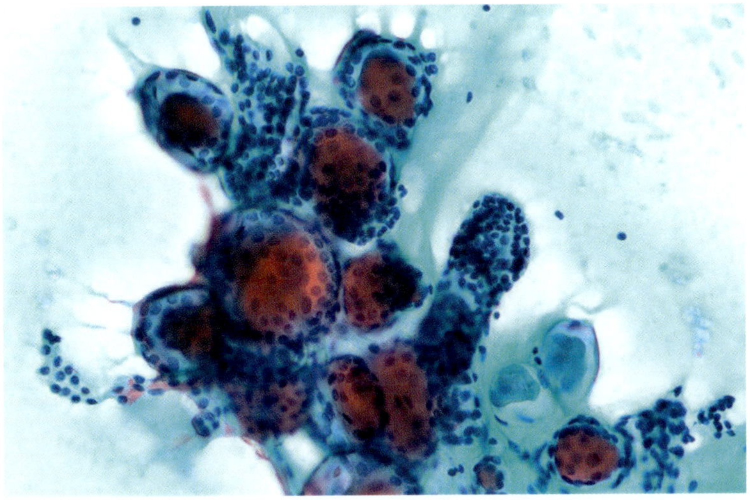

Figure 5.41 — Follicular Neoplasm, FNA. Another unusual case of a follicular neoplasm with abundance of colloid and mixed macro- and microfollicles. Some nuclear enlargement and trabecular architecture is evident. Follow-up revealed a follicular carcinoma. The major differential diagnosis in this case would include the macrofollicular-patterned lesions of the thyroid, the most common of which is an adenomatoid nodule. (Papanicolaou stain)

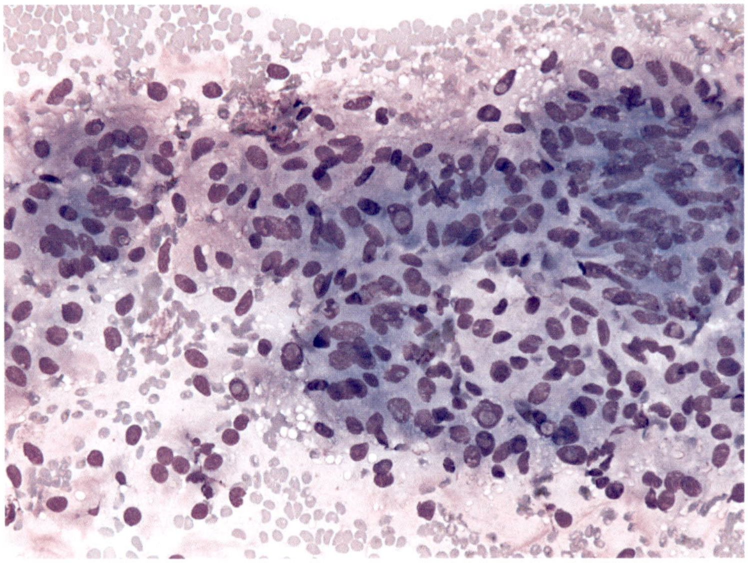

Figure 5.42 — Hyalinizing Trabecular Adenoma, FNA. TBSRTC defines hyalinizing trabecular adenoma (HTA) as "a rare tumor of follicular cell origin characterized by trabecular growth, marked intratrabecular hyalinization, and the nuclear changes of PTC." This hyalinizing trabecular adenoma displays a hypercellular smear comprised of numerous epithelioid and a few spindled cells. No distinct cellular architecture is seen. Few cells have pale metachromatic cytoplasm. Numerous well-formed intranuclear inclusions are present. Colloid is absent. No other nuclear features of papillary carcinoma are present. (Diff Quik stain)

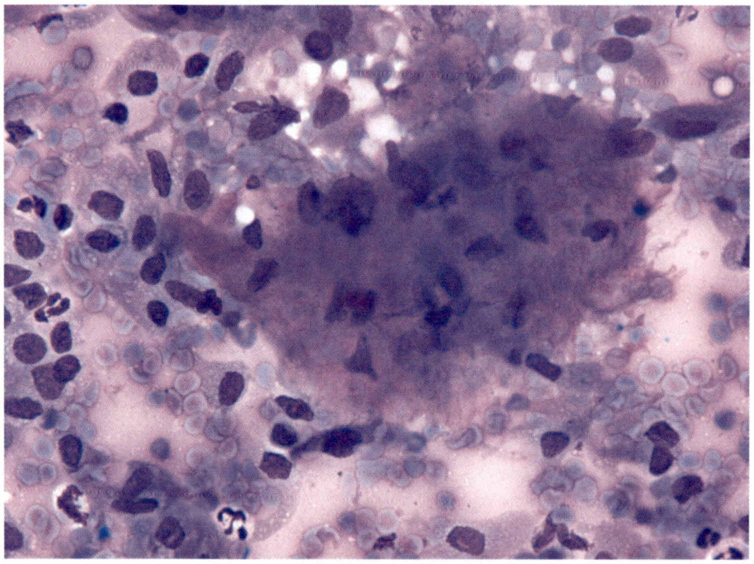

Figure 5.43a — Hyalinizing Trabecular Adenoma, FNA. A few areas contained metachromatic acellular substance, as seen here. Numerous oval to short spindled bare nuclei were seen embedded within this material. This represents hyaline deposits in the stroma of the tumor, which gives this neoplasm its unique name. Occasional psammoma bodies may be present. Grossly, HTA is a well-circumscribed or encapsulated tumor that is usually spherical or oval in shape. It tends to have a solid, bulging appearance on cut section, and ranges in color from yellow to pink, orange, or white. (Diff Quik stain)

Figure 5.43b — Hyalinizing Trabecular Adenoma, FNA. Another case is shown here which contained abundant metachromatic substance associated with numerous ovoid nuclei with intranuclear inclusions. This so-called "hyaline" material morphologically may resemble colloid or amyloid on cytologic smears and hence papillary and medullary carcinoma are the major differential diagnoses of a hyalinizing trabecular adenoma. Some have described cytoplasmic paranuclear yellow bodies, which are considered an uncommon finding. (Diff Quik stain)

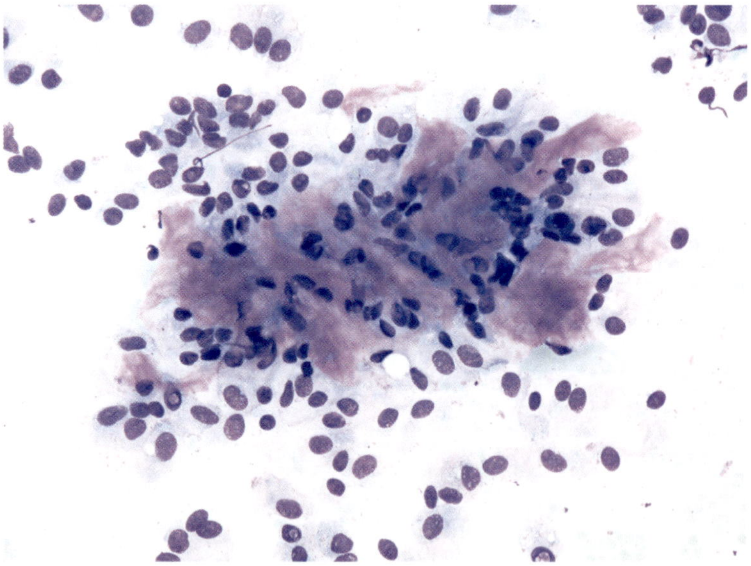

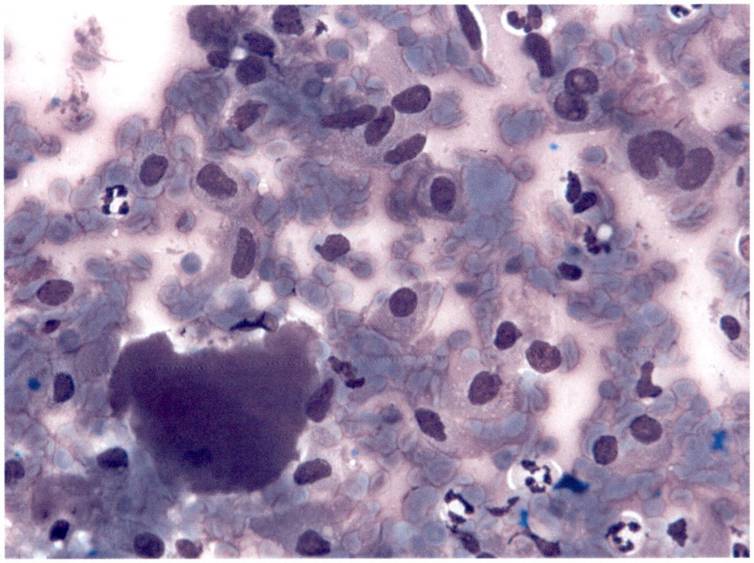

Figure 5.44 — Hyalinizing Trabecular Adenoma, FNA. The majority of these tumors behave in a benign fashion, but malignant HTAs have been reported. A large fragment of amorphous hyaline material is shown here, illustrating the morphological resemblance to colloid or amyloid. It's not surprising that hyalinizing trabecular adenoma is a frequently misdiagnosed entity on FNA cytology due to its rare occurrence and morphologic overlap with both papillary carcinoma and medullary carcinoma. (Diff Quik stain)

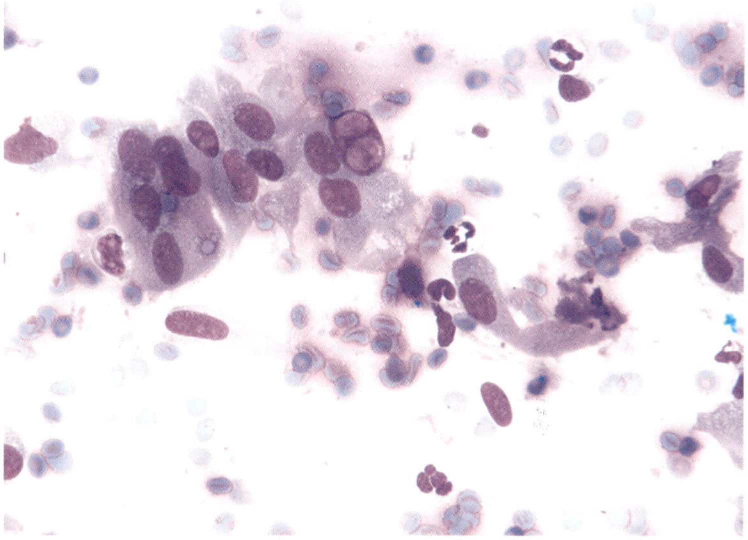

Figure 5.45 — Hyalinizing Trabecular Adenoma, FNA. A loose cluster of neoplastic cells is shown here with epithelioid appearance. Nuclei are round to oval containing multiple intranuclear inclusions. Cytoplasm appears polygonal or more often has a stretched out appearance. Oval nuclear shapes are not unusual. HTA is immunoreactive for thyroglobulin and thyroid transcription factor-1 (TTF-1), reflective of its thyroid follicular cell origin. (Diff Quik stain)

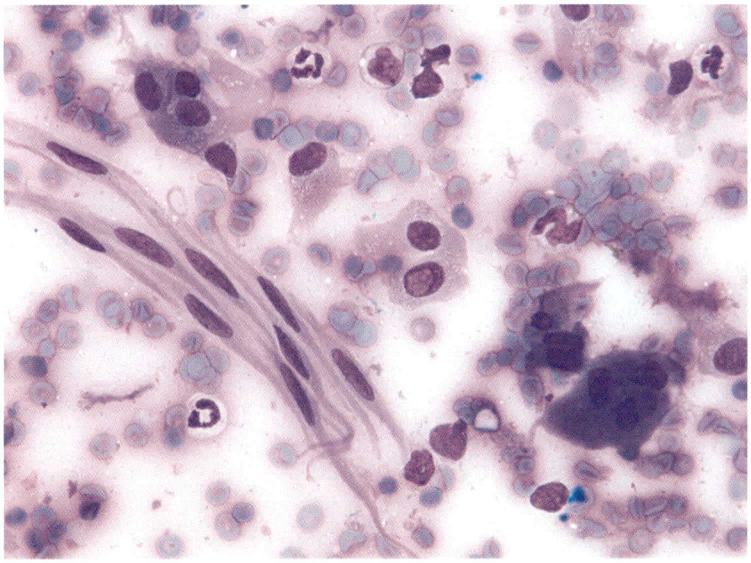

Figure 5.46 — Hyalinizing Trabecular Adenoma, FNA. Occasional cases of this tumor may appear predominantly or exclusively spindled and may resemble mesenchymal neoplasms. In this case, spindle cells with long bipolar cytoplasmic processes are seen juxtaposed with more typical epithelioid cells showing intranuclear inclusions. A multinucleated giant cell is also seen, likely representing a reactive histiocyte. RET/PTC translocations, found in 20% to 40% of sporadic PTC, have been described in some cases of HTA. However, activating BRAF mutations, found in more than 40% to 50% of PTC and believed to be very specific for PTC, have been consistently absent in HTA. (Diff Quik stain)

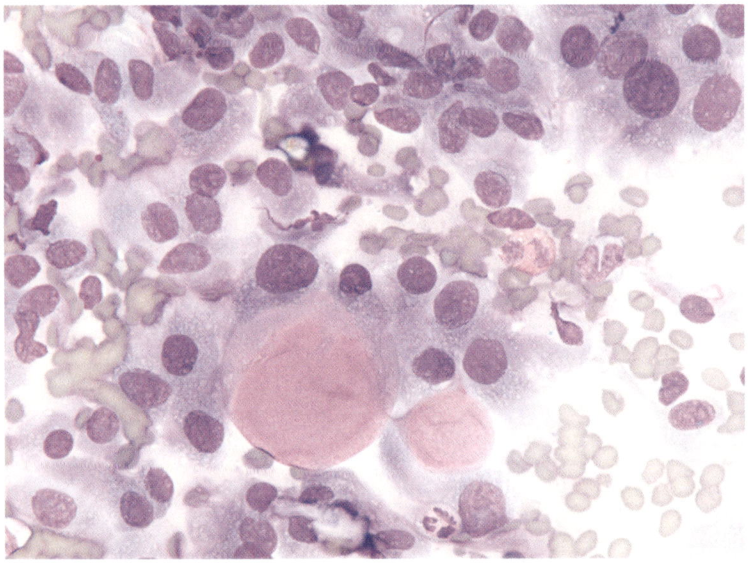

Figure 5.47 — Hyalinizing Trabecular Adenoma, FNA. An unusual appearance of the hyaline substance is seen in a case of hyalinizing trabecular adenoma. The metachromatic material assumes a more globoid appearance resembling "hyaline globules" of an adenoid cystic carcinoma. Notice the rather uniform epithelioid neoplastic cells with abundant finely vacuolated cytoplasm. No intranuclear inclusions were seen in this case, which was initially thought to represent a medullary carcinoma. (Diff Quik stain)

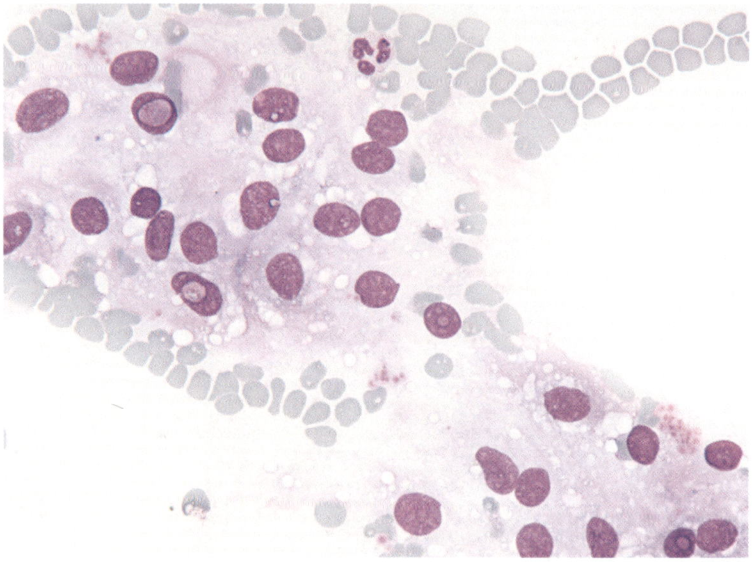

Figure 5.48a — Hyalinizing Trabecular Adenoma, FNA. The cytoplasm in these tumors can display abundant fine to coarse vacuolization resulting in numerous stripped off naked nuclei. Nuclei are uniform, round to oval with well-formed intranuclear inclusions. Nuclear grooves or other features of papillary carcinoma are uncommonly seen. Although a vascular pattern is lacking, the other differential diagnosis here would be a metastatic renal cell carcinoma. (Diff Quik stain)

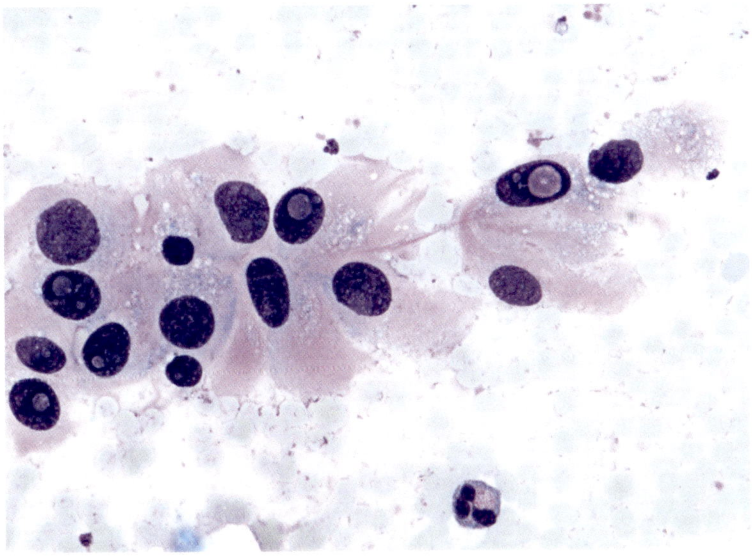

Figure 5.48b — Hyalinizing Trabecular Adenoma, FNA. Higher magnification of another case displays loosely cohesive uniform epithelioid cells with abundant pale metachromatic cytoplasm containing fine granules and vacuolizations. These cells resemble oncocytic differentiation; however, none of the nuclei show macronucleoli. Nuclei depict numerous well-formed inclusions. This case was misdiagnosed on FNA as papillary carcinoma. (Diff Quik stain)

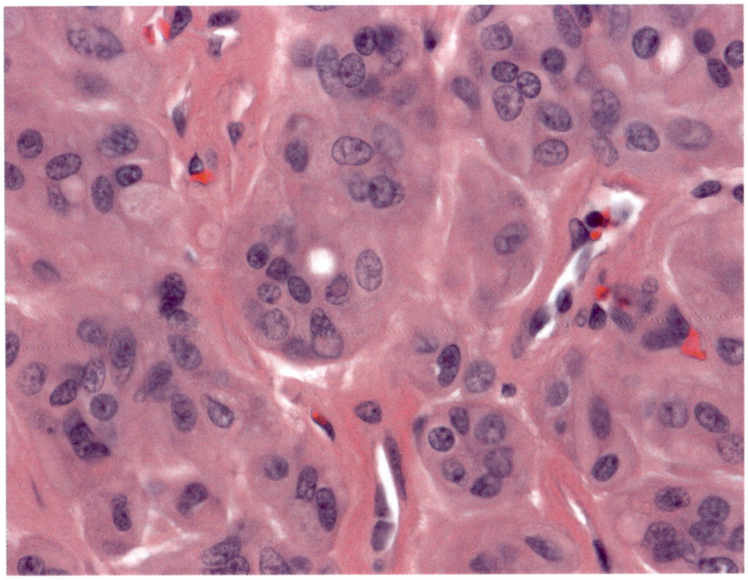

Figure 5.48c — Hyalinizing Trabecular Adenoma, Histologic Section. Higher magnification of the resection specimen from the previous case shows nice cytohistopathologic correlation. Note the neoplastic cells in a nested pattern, intranuclear inclusions and eosinophilic hyaline deposits in the stromal tissues. HTA appears on low power as a well-circumscribed or thinly encapsulated tumor. As the term implies, HTA grows in a trabecular architecture, but can also be focally nested in a zellballen-like pattern reminiscent of paraganglioma (hence the former designation "paraganglioma-like adenoma"). (H&E stain)

6

Hürthle Cell Neoplasm/ Suspicious for a Hürthle Cell Neoplasm

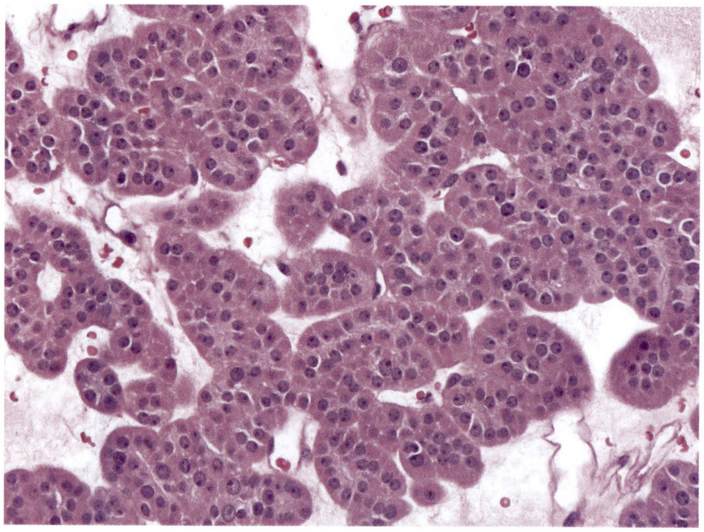

Figure 6.1a — Hürthle Cell Adenoma, Histologic Section. The Hürthle cell adenoma is set apart from the conventional follicular adenoma by the oxyphilic appearance of the cells lining the follicles. The Hürthle cell has a cytoplasm that is abundant, pink, and granular; and a nucleus that is enlarged and vesicular with a prominent central nucleolus. Shown here are nests of Hürthle cells from a Hürthle cell adenoma, but Hürthle cells are also encountered in Hürthle cell carcinomas and in nonneoplastic inflammatory processes, most notably Hashimoto thyroiditis. (H&E stain)

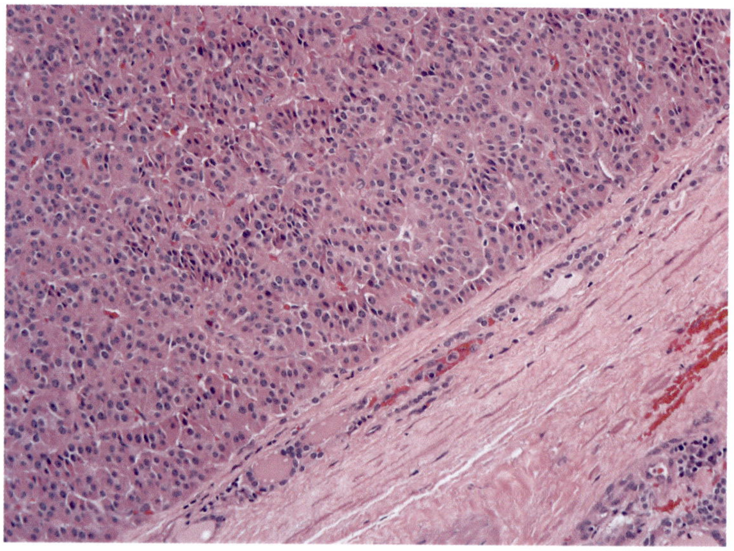

Figure 6.1b — Hürthle Cell Adenoma, Histologic Section. Like conventional follicular adenomas, Hürthle cell adenomas are completely surrounded by a fibrous capsule. The Hürthle cell adenoma may demonstrate a combination of follicular, trabecular and solid patterns of growth. The criteria used to separate Hürthle cell adenomas from Hürthle cell carcinomas are the same as those used for conventional follicular neoplasms, namely the presence of invasive tumor growth. (H&E stain)

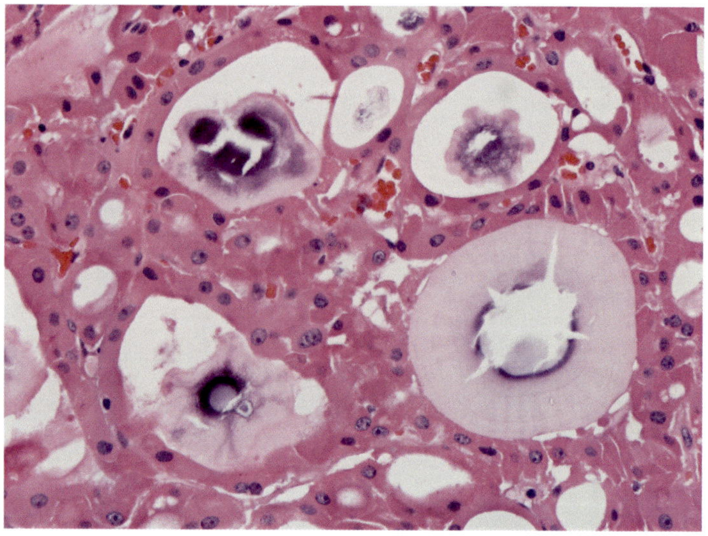

Figure 6.1c — Hürthle Cell Adenoma, Histologic Section. The colloid that fills the follicular spaces sometimes undergoes inspissation and calcification. These intrafollicular concretions are sometimes encountered in Hürthle cell adenomas, and they should not be mistaken for true psammoma bodies of papillary carcinoma. (H&E stain)

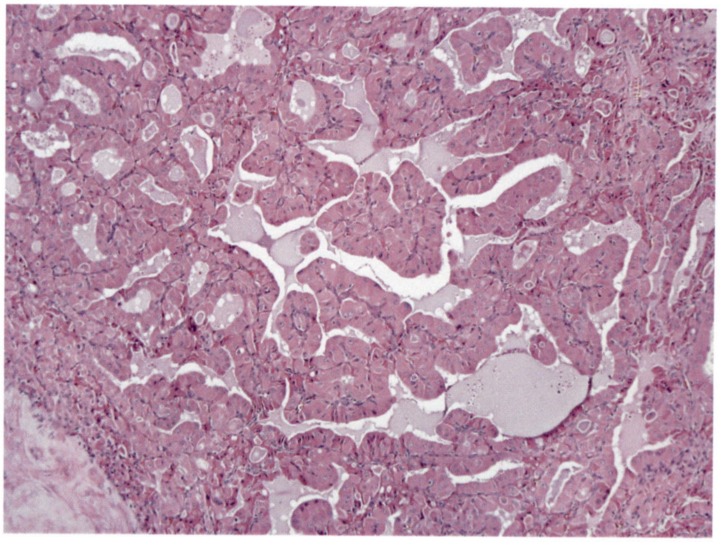

Figure 6.1d — Hürthle Cell Adenoma, Histologic Section. In some Hürthle cell adenomas, sectioning across delicate and elongated interfollicular septae can give rise to pseudopapillary formations. Unlike papillary carcinoma, the cells lining the papillae exhibit eosinophilic granular cytoplasm and vesicular nuclei with prominent nucleoli. (H&E stain)

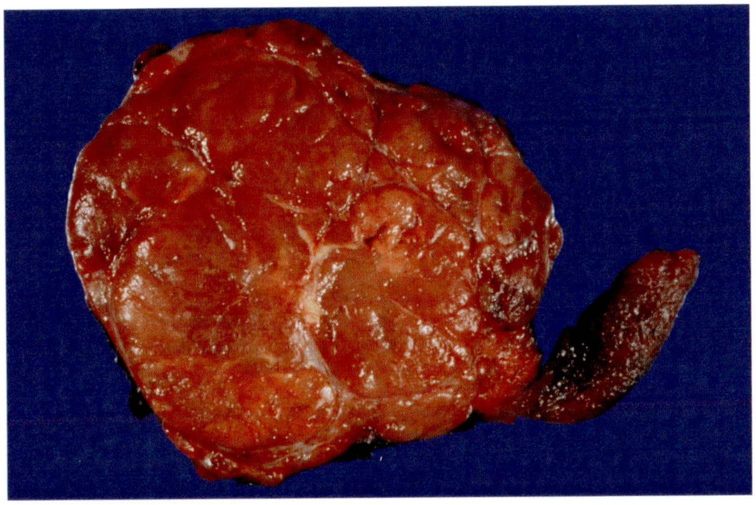

Figure 6.2 — Hürthle Cell Carcinoma, Widely Invasive: Gross Appearance. This lobe of the thyroid is completely effaced by a homogenous solid mass. The tumor capsule is no longer recognizable as it has been completely overridden by the invasive carcinoma. Hürthle cell neoplasms tend to have a mahogany brown color.

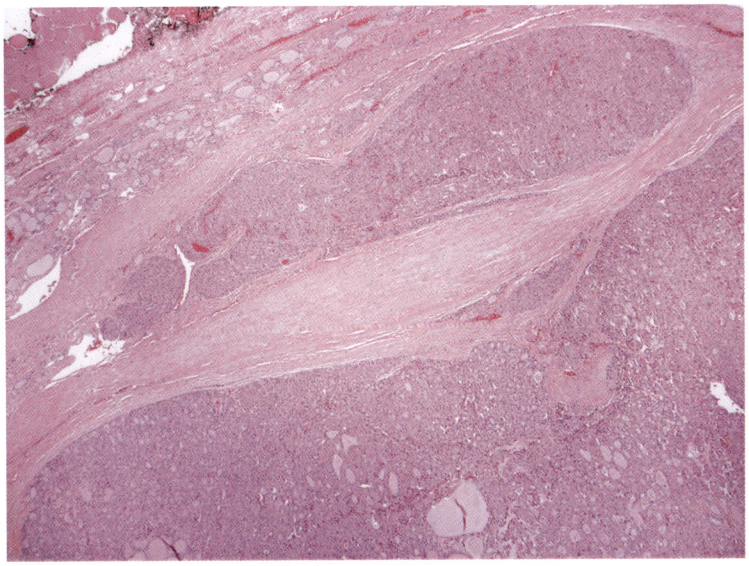

Figure 6.3a — Hürthle Cell Carcinoma, Histologic Section. Like follicular carcinomas, Hürthle cell carcinomas are diagnosed on the basis of invasive tumor growth. Here a tumor nodule invades into the tumor capsule and extends within an intracapsular blood vessel. (H&E stain)

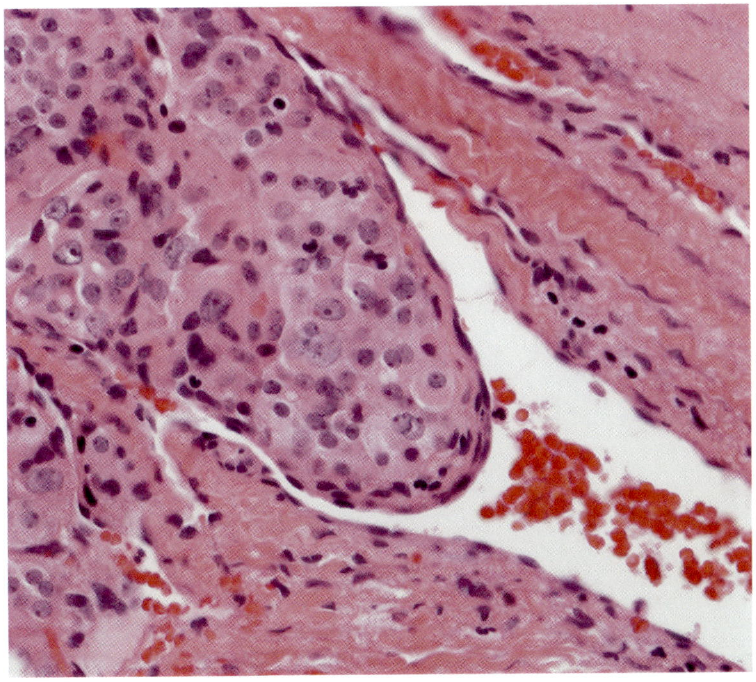

Figure 6.3b — Hürthle Cell Carcinoma, Histologic Section. As Hürthle cell carcinoma propagates within vascular channels, the invasive tumor plugs become lined by a layer of endothelium. (H&E stain)

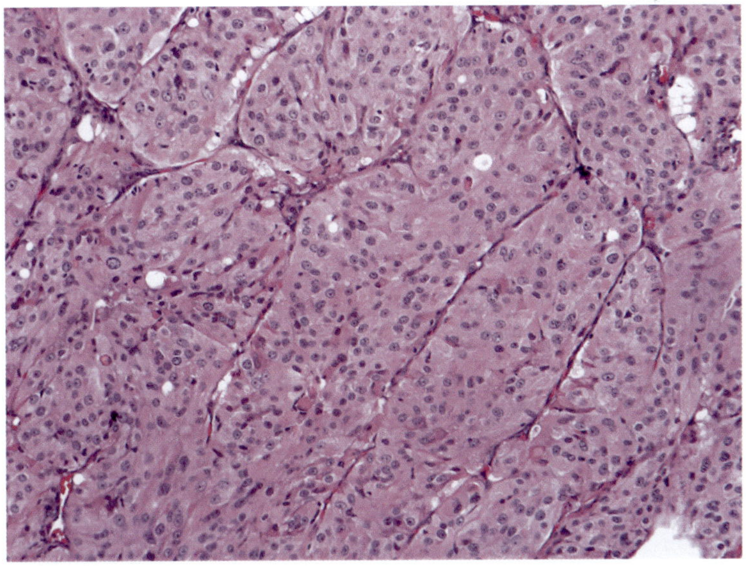

Figure 6.3c — Hürthle Cell Carcinoma, Histologic Section. Most Hürthle cell carcinomas are highly cellular and exhibit a trabecular to solid pattern of growth with varying degrees of cytologic atypia. (H&E stain)

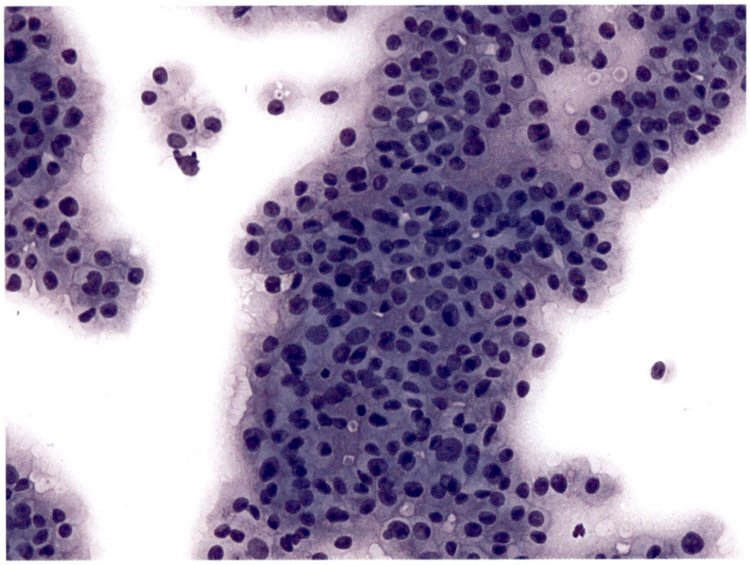

Figure 6.4 — Hürthle Cell Neoplasm, Fine Needle Aspiration (FNA). The Bethesda System for Reporting Thyroid Cytopathology (TBSRTC) defines "suspicious for a Hürthle cell neoplasm" as cellular aspirates that consist exclusively or almost exclusively of Hürthle cells, with minimal to absent colloid, and lacking nuclear features of papillary carcinoma. The Hürthle cells in these aspirates are characterized by abundant homogeneously granular eosinophilic cytoplasm, an enlarged central to eccentrically located round nucleus, and a prominent nucleolus. This case, which turned out to be an adenoma on resection, is characterized by a pure population of Hürthle cells arranged in a loose sheet-like architecture. The neoplastic cells have polygonal outlines, abundant granular cytoplasm, uniform round nuclei displaying often a single prominent nucleolus. No colloid is present in this case. Cytologic distinction between an adenoma and carcinoma (of Hürthle cell type) is not possible on cytologic features only. (Diff Quik stain)

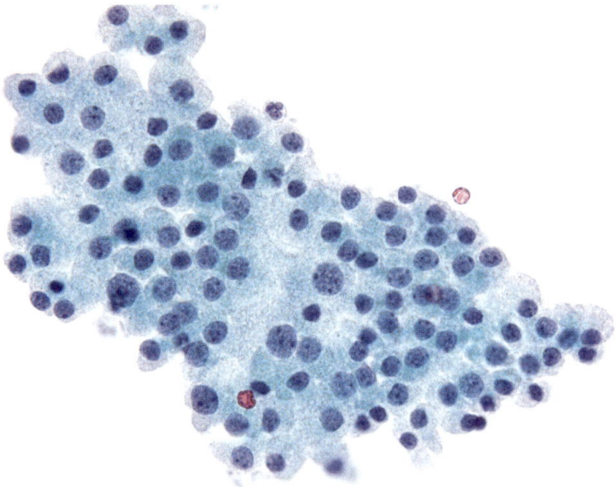

Figure 6.5 — Hürthle Cell Neoplasm, FNA. Hürthle cells can be seen in a thyroid FNA in association with reactive/hyperplastic conditions such as benign nodular hyperplasia, in the setting of chronic lymphocytic thyroiditis as well as in neoplastic conditions such as Hürthle cell adenomas and Hürthle cell carcinomas. This liquid-based preparation displays features similar to those seen in the previous example. However, the background is clean and devoid of blood and debris. The cytoplasmic granularity is enhanced and a fine vacuolization is quite apparent creating a "histiocyte-like" appearance. Chromatin appears slightly more open and coarser compared to direct smears. (Papanicolaou stain)

Figure 6.6 — Hürthle Cell Neoplasm, FNA. This low power image of a liquid-based preparation shows an exclusive Hürthle cell population. Neoplastic cells are arranged in small tissue fragments. Notice the clean background with no colloid, blood, or lymphocytes. The differential diagnosis includes a benign Hürthle cell nodule (an overgrown Hürthle cell in an adenomatoid nodule) and chronic lymphocytic thyroiditis (Hashimoto thyroiditis). However, lack of lymphocytes would make the latter entity, a less likely possibility. (Papanicolaou stain)

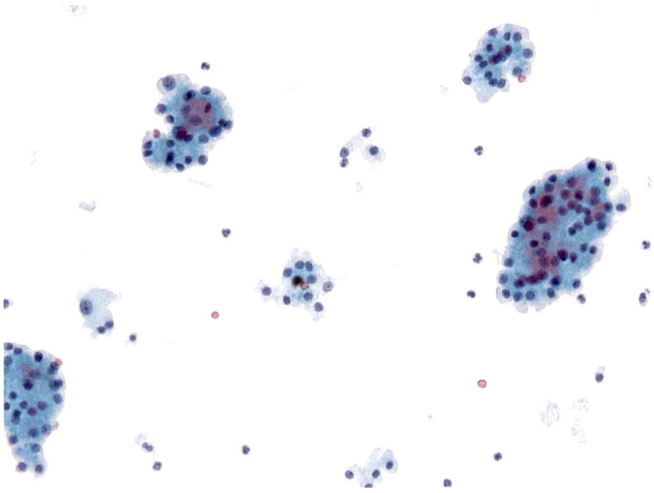

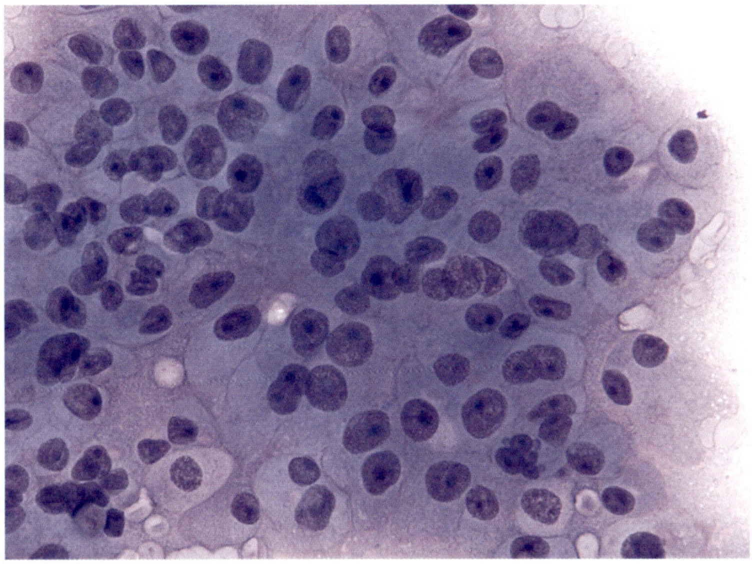

Figure 6.7 — Hürthle Cell Neoplasm, FNA. Higher magnification of this case beautifully illustrates the finer details of Hürthle cells. Notice the relatively large cell size, polygonal cell borders, densely granular and faintly blue cytoplasm, and large nuclei with prominent nucleoli. The aforementioned features simply define "Hürthle" cells. These features are seen in all Hürthle cell lesions such as Hürthle cell neoplasm, Hürthle cell hyperplasia/nodule, and Hürthle cells in Hashimoto thyroiditis. Distinction among these lesions requires a careful evaluation of the presence or absence of the usual-type of follicular epithelium, colloid, and lymphocytes/lymphoid tangles. (Diff Quik stain)

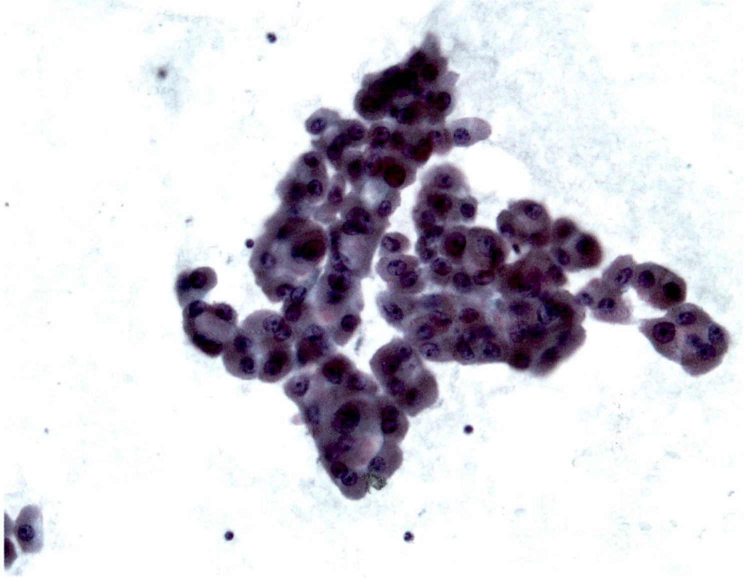

Figure 6.8 — Hürthle Cell Neoplasm, FNA. This alcohol-fixed smear depicts classic features of Hürthle cells, as described in the previous example. Note the heavily granular cytoplasm and macronucleoli, both features enhanced by Papanicolaou staining. The reddish tinge to the cytoplasm is imparted by the slight touch of air-drying artifact as these cells are inherently prone to even the minutest delay in alcohol fixation. The diagnosis of a "Hürthle cell neoplasm" encompasses both Hürthle cell adenoma and carcinoma since the definitive classification rests on the histologic evaluation of the excised mass for invasion. (Papanicolaou stain)

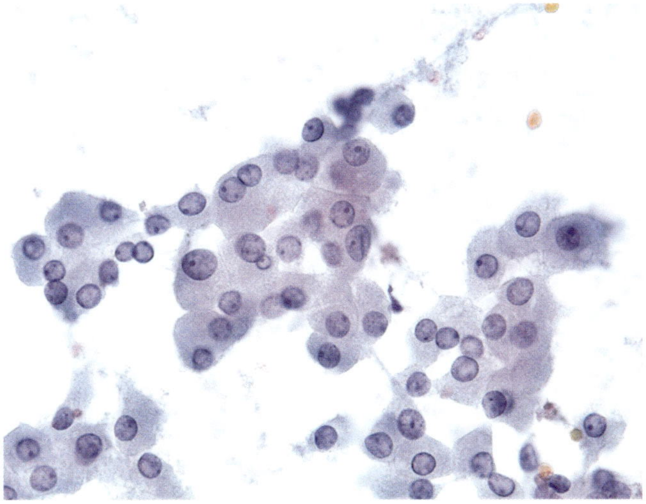

Figure 6.9 — Hürthle Cell Neoplasm, FNA. Higher magnification illustrates the classic features as seen in previous examples. This case does not depict macronucleoli. Presence or absence of prominent nucleoli in Hürthle cell lesions shows poor correlation with the final tissue outcome in these cases. Another feature seen here is frequent binucleation of the neoplastic cells. This feature is not highly specific but seen much more often in Hürthle cell neoplasms than hyperplasia. Once again, the smear does not show colloid and lymphocytes in the background. (Papanicolaou stain)

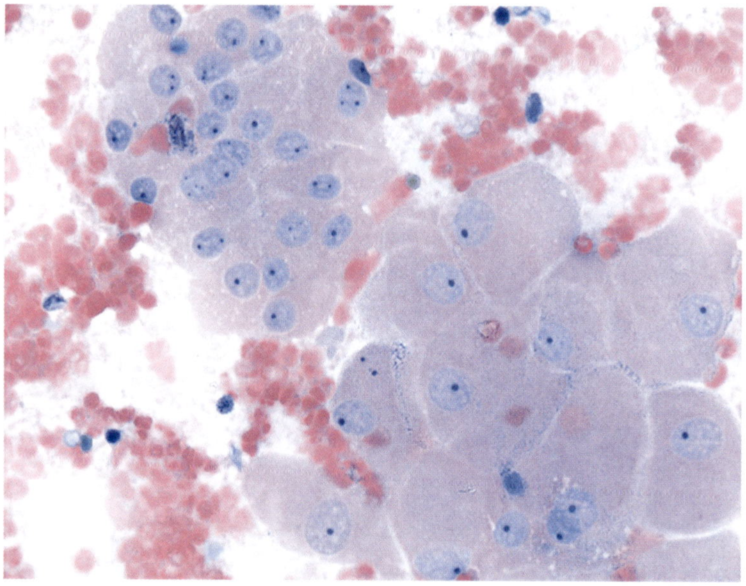

Figure 6.10 — Hürthle Cell Neoplasm, FNA. Large cells with abundant and finely granular cytoplasm are seen. Nuclei are relatively small giving these cells a relatively low N/C ratio. Small nucleoli are present. This case on resection turned out to be an adenoma. FNA cannot distinguish between an adenoma and carcinoma and a cytologic interpretation of "neoplasm" in these cases trigger a lobectomy (hemithyroidectomy). A histopathologic diagnosis of adenoma versus carcinoma dictates whether the patient would need a completion thyroidectomy. (Papanicolaou stain)

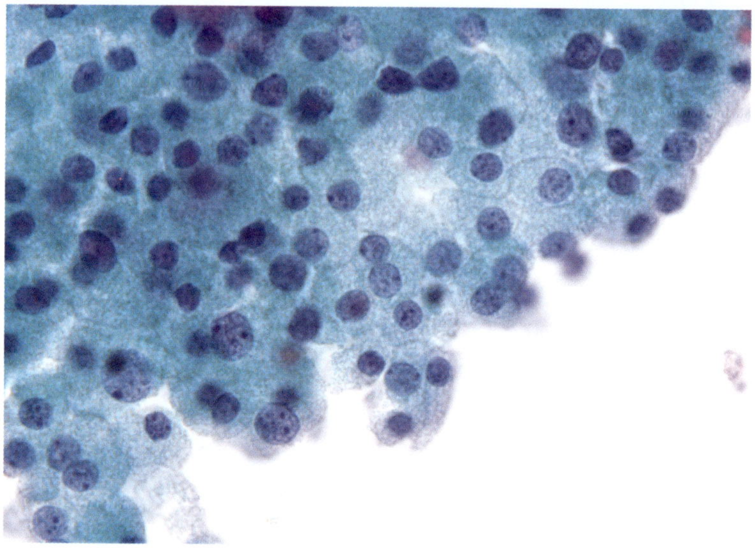

Figure 6.11 — Hürthle Cell Neoplasm, FNA. This liquid-based preparation illustrates the well-defined polygonal cell borders, abundant granular cytoplasm, and coarsely speckled chromatin with nucleoli. Some cells have a clear vacuolated cytoplasm and if such cells are seen singly, they may be misinterpreted as macrophages. (Papanicolaou stain)

Figure 6.12 — Hürthle Cell Neoplasm, FNA. A loose sheet of neoplastic Hürthle cells is shown here. Once again the cytoplasmic borders are well-defined, cytoplasm displays reddish granularity (possibly secondary to subtle air-drying) and nuclei have macronucleoli. In the World Health Organization (WHO) histological classification of thyroid tumors, Hürthle cell adenoma and carcinoma are considered oncocytic variants of follicular adenoma and carcinoma, respectively. However, many studies have shown different underlying genetics for follicular and Hürthle cell tumors. Additionally, since they have such distinctive cytomorphologic features, it is helpful to specify that a sample raises the possibility of a Hürthle cell rather than a follicular neoplasm. This classification also helps fine tune a cytologic differential diagnosis. (Papanicolaou stain)

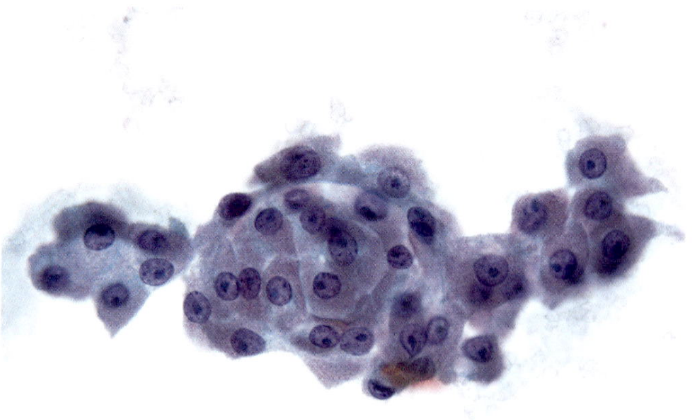

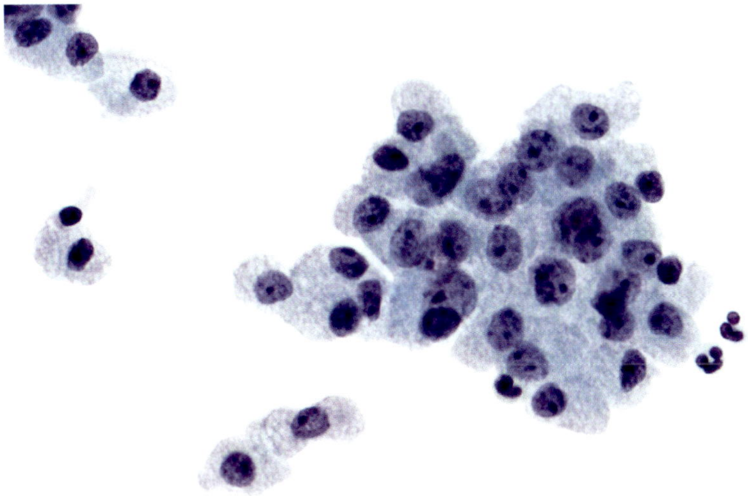

Figure 6.13 — Hürthle Cell Neoplasm, FNA. These Hürthle cells seen on liquid-based preparation can be easily confused with macrophages owing to abundant clear cytoplasm which appears finely vacuolated. However, the nuclear morphology (enlarged nuclei containing macronucleoli) and cellular grouping clearly argues against these being macrophages. The major advantage of using liquid-based cytology are enhancement of cytologic features (both nuclear and cytoplasmic) and better visualization due to a markedly clean slide background devoid of red blood cells. However, since cytomorphology of most thyroid lesions appears different, a reasonable training period is mandatory before switching to liquid-based cytology. (Papanicolaou stain)

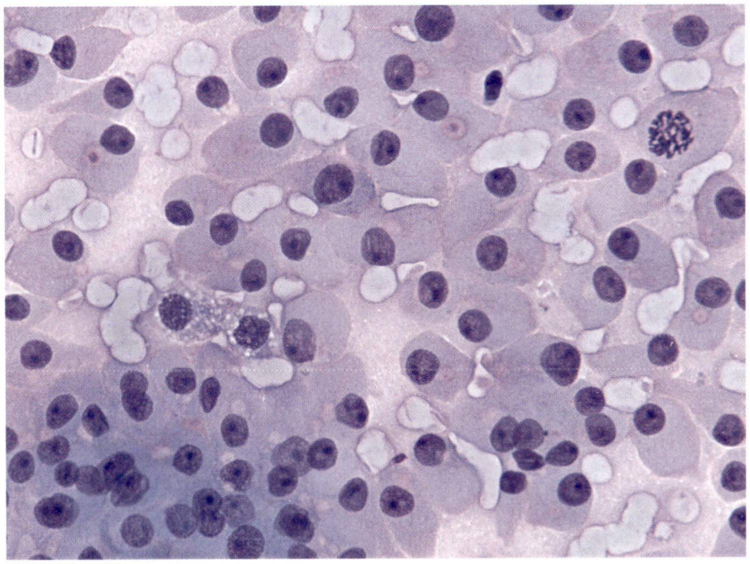

Figure 6.14 — Hürthle Cell Neoplasm, FNA. Mitoses are extremely uncommon in Hürthle cell neoplasms and are often of little or no pathologic significance. These cells are loosely cohesive and display prominent nucleoli. Another eye-catching feature is the presence of occasional intracytoplasmic holes (possibly lumens) containing magenta colored substance, possibly representing colloid-like material. These have often been referred to as "intracytoplasmic colloid inclusions" in the literature and have been reported to be much more common in neoplastic Hürthle cells compared to hyperplastic Hürthle cells. They may often assume a "targetoid" appearance. (Diff Quik stain)

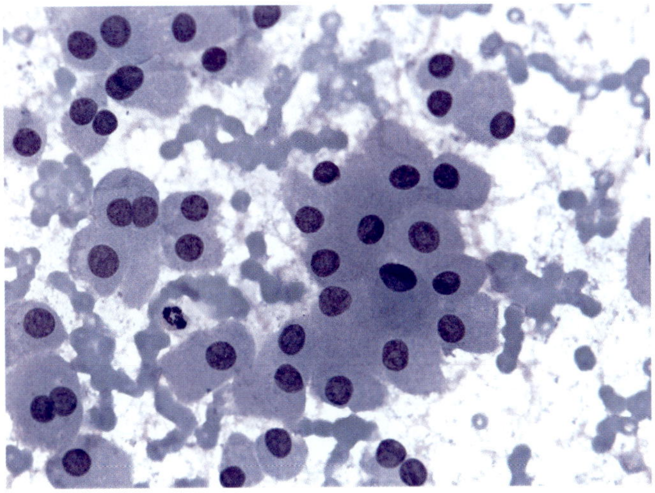

Figure 6.15 — Hürthle Cell Neoplasm, FNA. Neoplastic Hürthle cell displaying classic features as described previously. Note the frequent binucleation. The appearance of these cells can be confused with medullary thyroid carcinoma, which is the major differential diagnosis of Hürthle cell neoplasm. Nuclei in this case are perfectly round excluding the possibility of an oncocytic variant of papillary carcinoma. (Diff Quik stain)

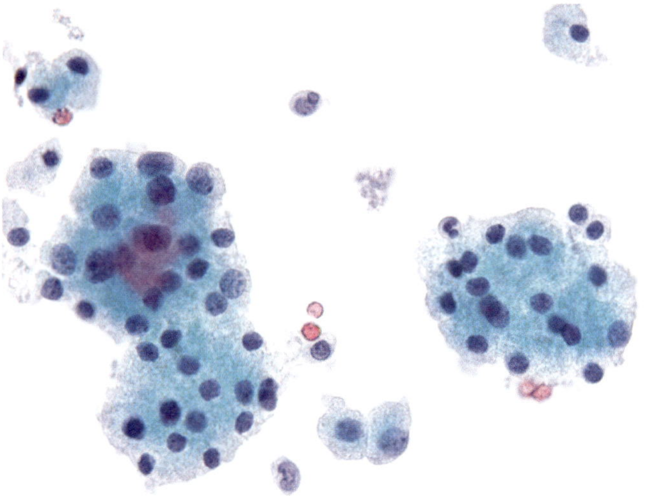

Figure 6.16 — Hürthle Cell Neoplasm, FNA. Another example of Hürthle cell neoplasm on liquid-based preparation. This case turned out to be an adenoma on follow-up resection. Studies have shown that 15% to 45% of Hürthle cell neoplasms turn out to be carcinomas, and the remainder of the neoplasms prove to be adenomas. (Papanicolaou stain)

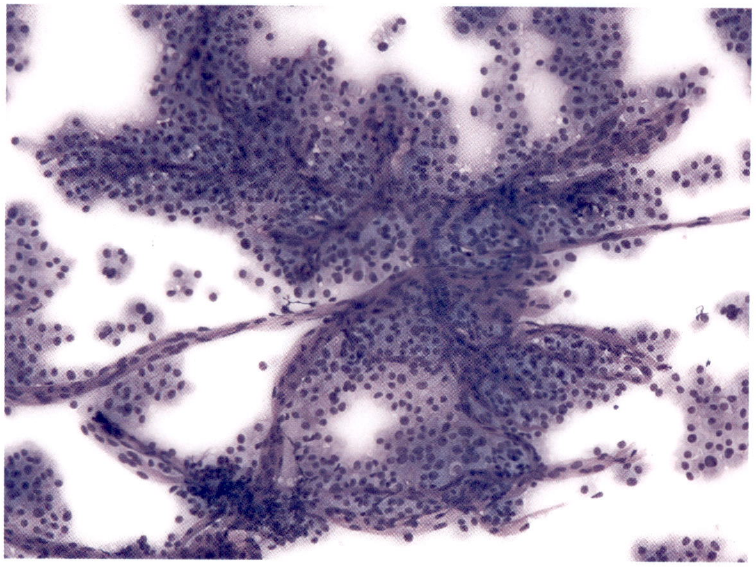

Figure 6.17 — Hürthle Cell Neoplasm, FNA. Traversing capillary vessels are a hallmark of Hürthle cell neoplasms and are rarely seen in a hyperplastic nodule with Hürthle cell change. However, the presence of finely branching capillaries with nests of neoplastic Hürthle cells are not exclusive for carcinoma, as previously believed. This feature can be seen in both, adenomas and carcinomas. However, this particular case on resection did turn out to be a Hürthle cell carcinoma. Presence of this rich arborizing capillary network essentially reflects the vascularity of Hürthle cell neoplasms, a feature often resulting in excessive bleeding on FNA. (Diff Quik stain)

Figure 6.18 — Hürthle Cell Neoplasm, FNA. Another example of a traversing blood vessel is seen in this case, surrounded by abundant Hürthle cells forming loosely cohesive nests. This cytoarchitecture somewhat resembles an FNA appearance of a renal cell carcinoma or a hepatocellular carcinoma. Such perivascular arrangements are unusual for Hürthle cells seen in an adenomatoid nodule or in Hashimoto thyroiditis. Few single cells in the background display binucleation. (Diff Quik stain)

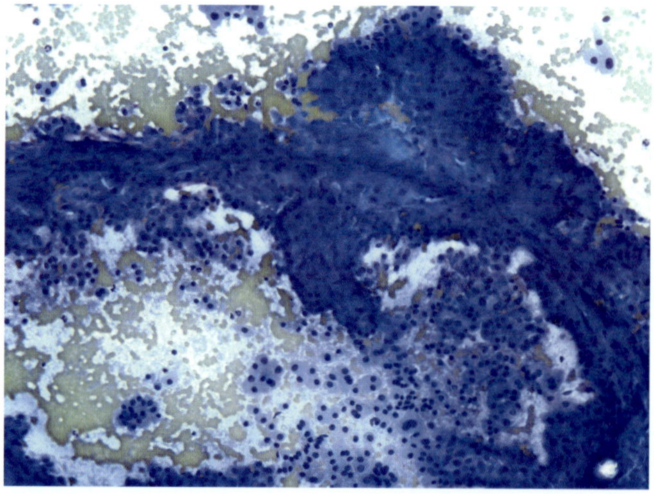

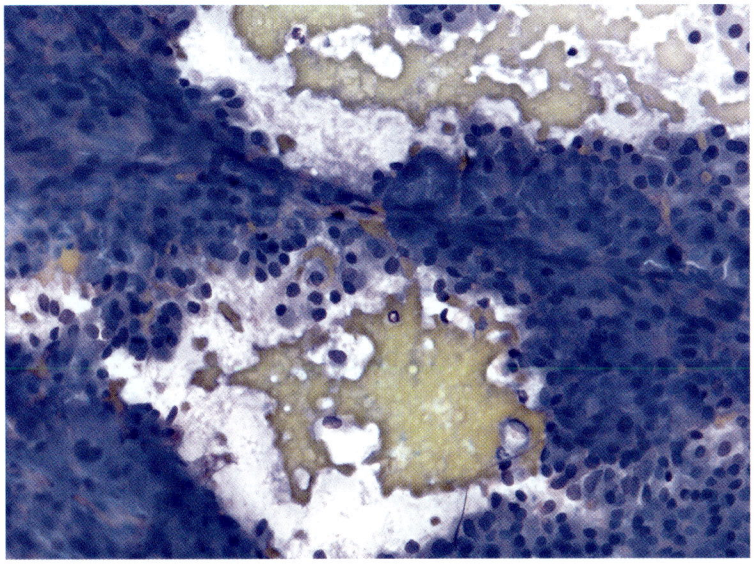

Figure 6.19 — Hürthle Cell Neoplasm, FNA. Higher magnification in this case beautifully illustrates the fine wire-like capillary vessel and associated loose nests of neoplastic Hürthle cells. Although medullary carcinoma is in the differential, such perivascular formations are rarely seen in the latter tumor. (Diff Quik stain)

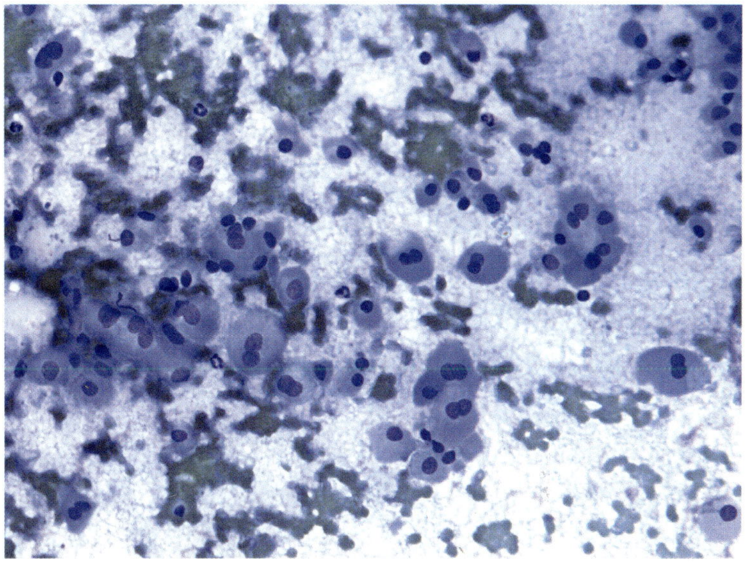

Figure 6.20 — Hürthle Cell Neoplasm, FNA. Binucleation with figure "8" nuclei is an often underreported feature of Hürthle cell neoplasms. However, it's not entirely specific and is occasionally (and focally) seen in hyperplastic Hürthle cells. Once again, the closest differential diagnosis here would be a medullary carcinoma. It's often easy to correlate the cytomorphologic findings with the patient's peripheral blood calcitonin level. (Diff Quik stain)

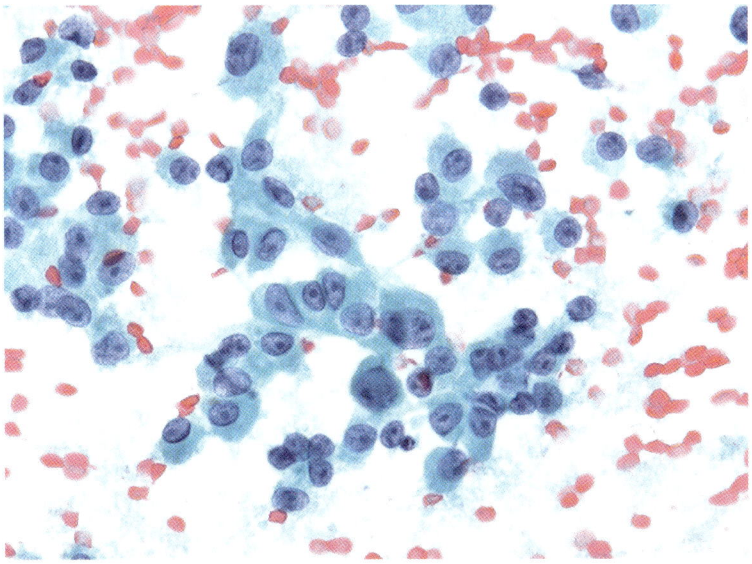

Figure 6.21 — Hürthle Cell Neoplasm, FNA. This case turned out to be a Hürthle cell carcinoma on follow-up. However, presence of macronucleoli is poorly associated with malignancy in Hürthle cell lesions. N/C ratios are significantly increased in this case and some cells display eccentrically placed nuclei which is an unusual feature for a Hürthle cell neoplasm and is often associated with medullary thyroid carcinoma. (Papanicolaou stain)

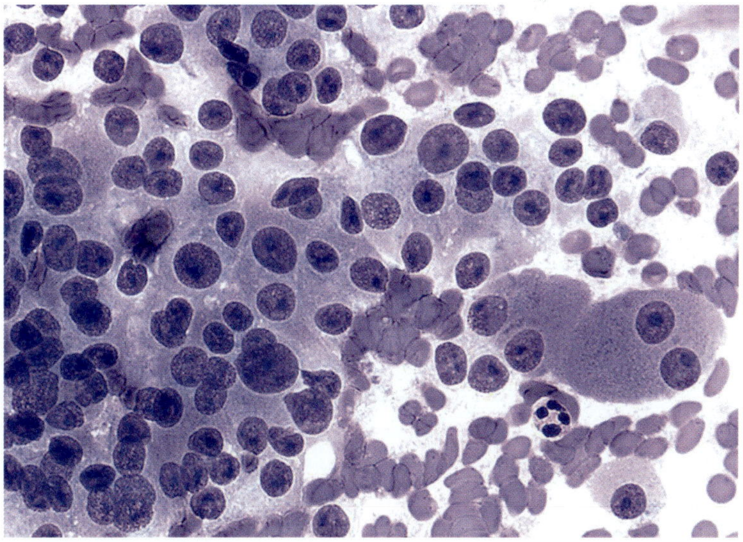

Figure 6.22 — Hürthle Cell Neoplasm, FNA. Helpful diagnostic features of a Hürthle cell neoplasm are seen here such as prominent binucleation in most cells, large nuclei, and macronucleoli. Cytoplasm shows dense granularity. (Diff Quik stain)

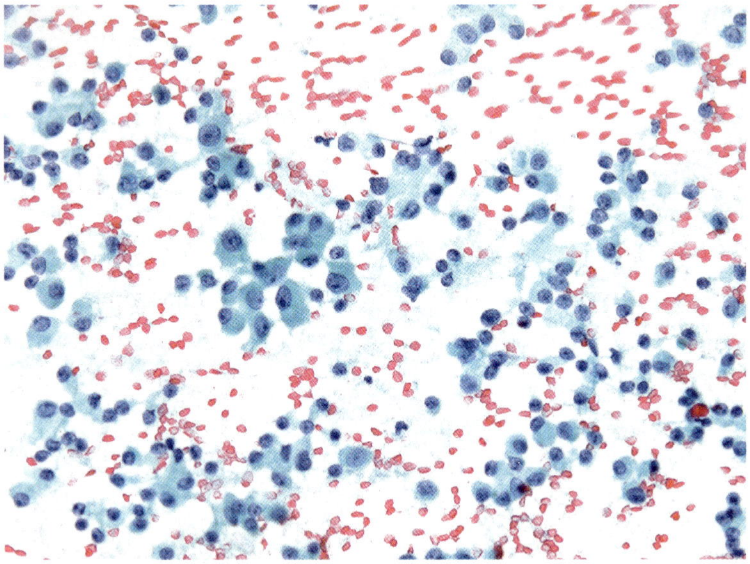

Figure 6.23 — Hürthle Cell Neoplasm, FNA. This case of a Hürthle cell neoplasm was initially confused with medullary thyroid carcinoma owing to a uniform population of mostly dispersed cells and eccentric nuclei (plasmacytoid cells). However, presence of prominent nucleoli is an unusual feature for medullary carcinoma. (Papanicolaou stain)

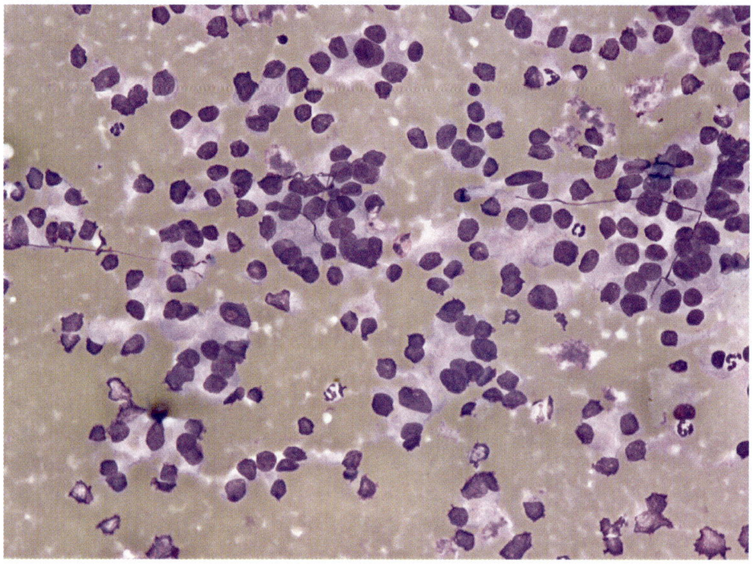

Figure 6.24 — Hürthle Cell Neoplasm, FNA. Often the dense cytoplasmic granularity renders Hürthle cells to cytoplasmic disruption secondary to vigorous smearing resulting in a large population of bare nuclei, as seen in this case. This often adds to diagnostic confusion with both medullary carcinoma and less often with a parathyroid lesion. (Diff Quik stain)

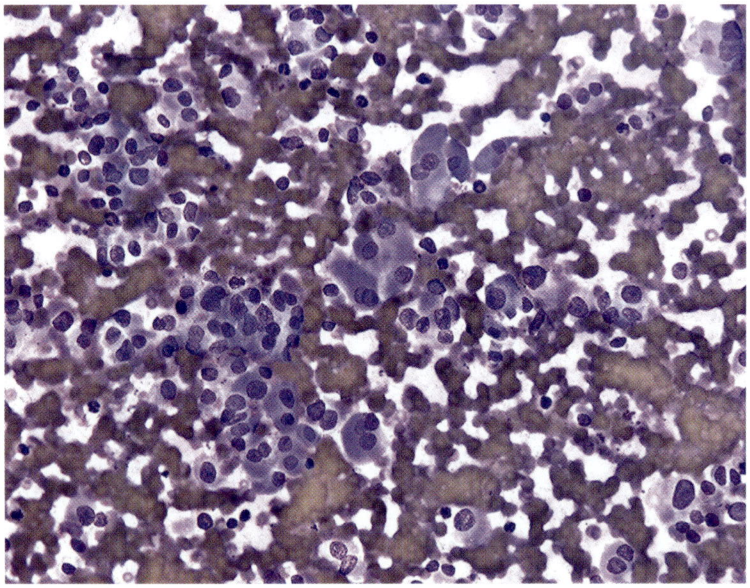

Figure 6.25 — Hürthle Cell Neoplasm, FNA. Another example of a Hürthle cell neoplasm which was initially confused with a medullary thyroid carcinoma due to prominent plasmacytoid morphology of the neoplastic cells. Presence of macronucleoli would be unusual for medullary carcinoma. On follow-up resection, this case turned out to be a widely invasive Hürthle cell carcinoma. (Diff Quik stain)

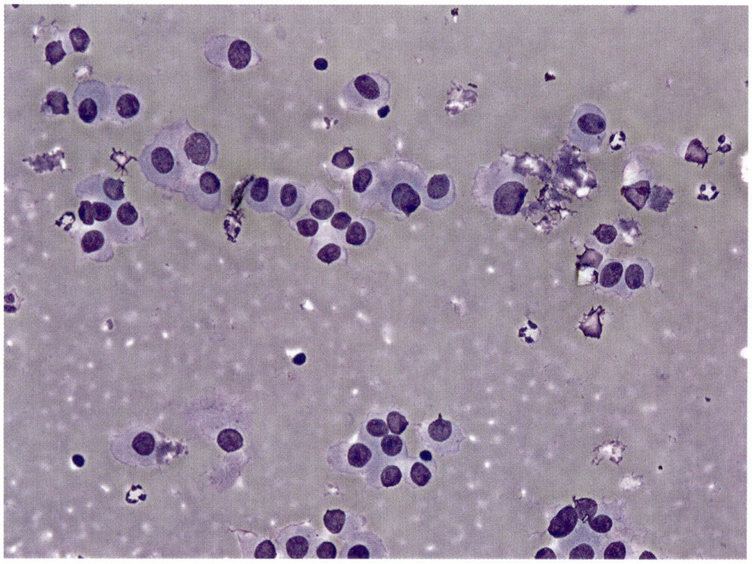

Figure 6.26 — Hürthle Cell Neoplasm, FNA. Medullary thyroid carcinoma remains one of the most important differential diagnoses of a Hürthle cell neoplasm. The dispersed cell population, cellular monotony, and eccentric nuclear placement in this Hürthle cell neoplasm was originally misinterpreted as medullary carcinoma. (Diff Quik stain)

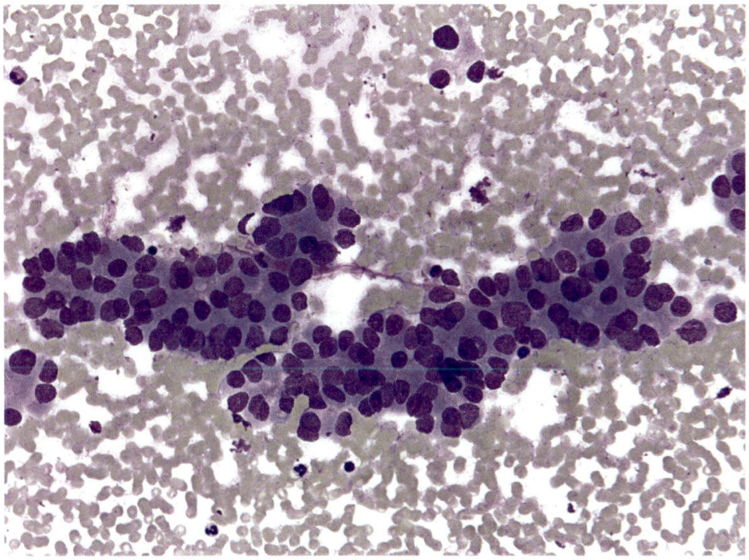

Figure 6.27 — Hürthle Cell Neoplasm, FNA. An unusual trabecular pattern is depicted in this image. Nuclei are round to oval with suggestion of palisading. Classic Hürthle cell features are lacking and differential diagnosis would include an oncocytic variant of papillary thyroid carcinoma. Intranuclear inclusions are almost never seen in Hürthle cell neoplasm. (Diff Quik stain)

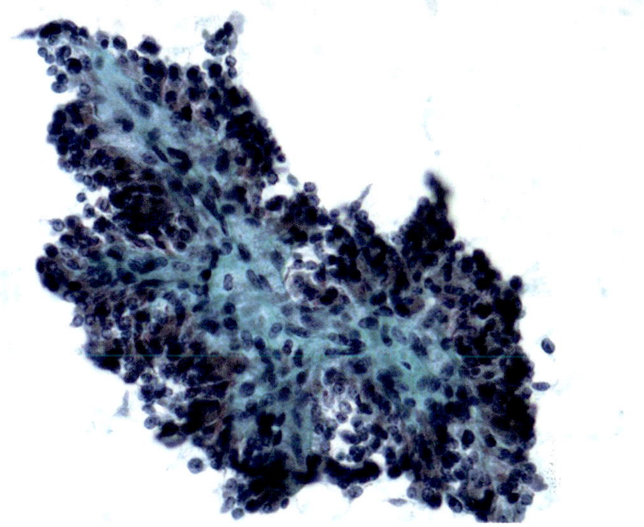

Figure 6.28 — Hürthle Cell Neoplasm, FNA. Presence of vascular proliferation in Hürthle cell neoplasms when surrounded by neoplastic cells may create a papillary-like appearance, as beautifully illustrated in this example. This case turned out to be a Hürthle cell carcinoma on resection. Hürthle cell features are mostly lacking in this particular case, which created diagnostic confusion. However, the nuclei are perfectly round arguing against a papillary carcinoma. (Papanicolaou stain)

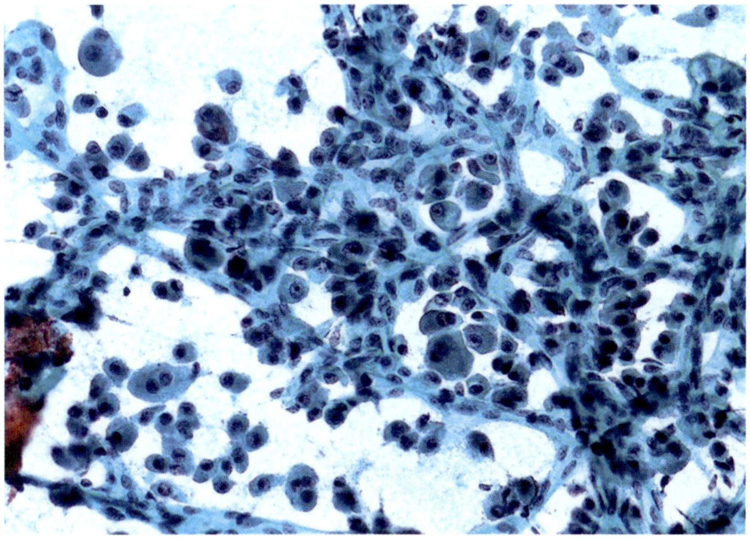

Figure 6.29 — Hürthle Cell Neoplasm, FNA. A rich network of fine arborizing capillaries is depicted in this case surrounded by mostly single cells with well-developed Hürthle cell features. Cytoplasm is densely granular and nuclei show macronucleoli. Follow-up revealed Hürthle cell carcinoma. (Papanicolaou stain)

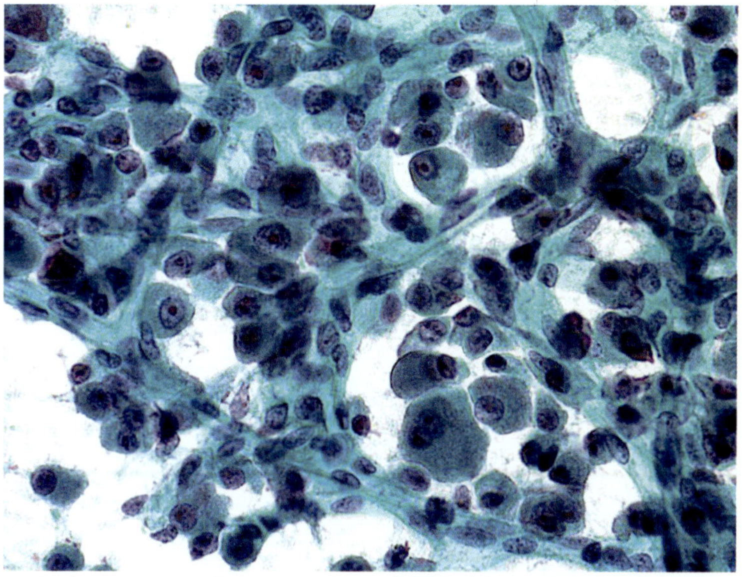

Figure 6.30 — Hürthle Cell Neoplasm, FNA. Higher magnification of the previous case displays the intimate relationship of the neoplastic Hürthle cells to vascular endothelium. Additionally, the cells display binucleation and macronucleoli. None of these morphologic features have good positive predictive value for a carcinoma diagnosis in such cases. (Papanicolaou stain)

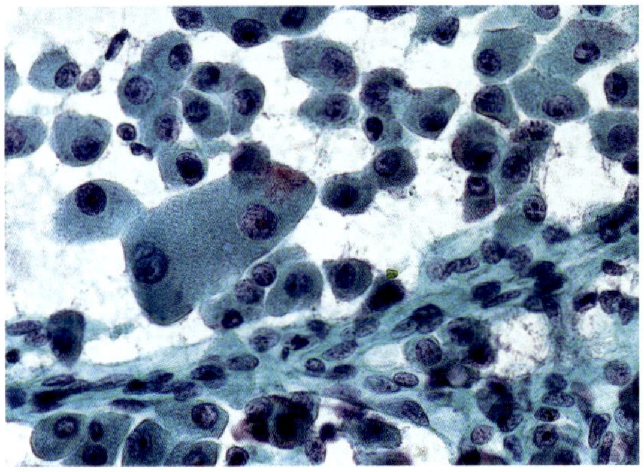

Figure 6.31 — Hürthle Cell Neoplasm, FNA. Another view of the same tumor displays a traversing vessel and extensive pleomorphism of the neoplastic cells, which also contain eosinophilic macronucleoli. Studies have shown that presence of significant nuclear enlargement and a large nodule size are more common in neoplasms than benign hyperplasia of Hürthle cells. Others have concluded that statistically significant cytologic features that favor carcinoma over benign lesions (adenoma and hyperplasia) include small cell dysplasia, large cell dysplasia, nuclear crowding, and cellular dyshesion. Most experts, however, strongly recommend against attempting to distinguish Hürthle cell adenoma from carcinoma on FNA. (Papanicolaou stain)

7

Suspicious for Malignancy

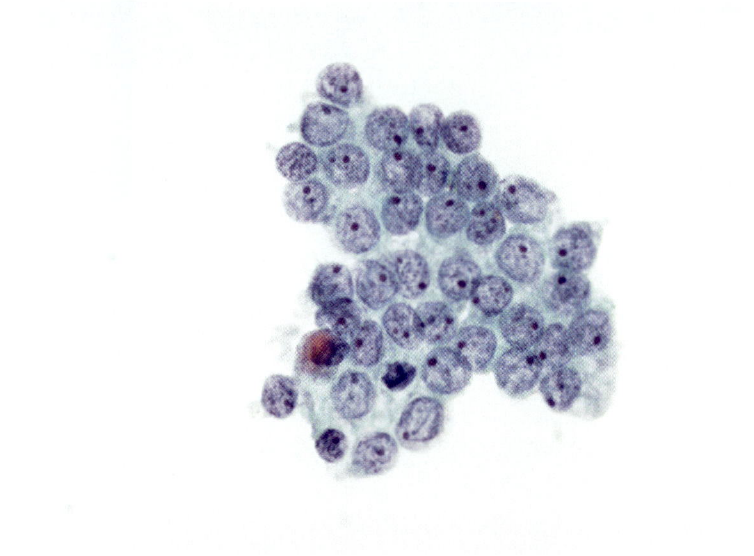

Figure 7.1 — Suspicious for Malignancy, Fine Needle Aspiration (FNA). Suspicious for papillary carcinoma. The suspicious for malignancy category encompasses aspirates that elicit a high level of concern for malignancy but are less than definitive. Such aspirates are qualitatively and/or quantitatively insufficient to completely fulfill diagnostic criteria for the entity in question. The positive predictive value for this category is typically in the 60% to 75% range. Aspirates are most frequently suspicious for papillary carcinoma. In this cellular specimen, nuclei are enlarged, with powdery chromatin, rounded nuclear contours, infrequent nuclear grooves, and small distinct nucleoli. Nuclear molding and intranuclear pseudoinclusions are absent. (Liquid based preparation, Papanicolaou stain)

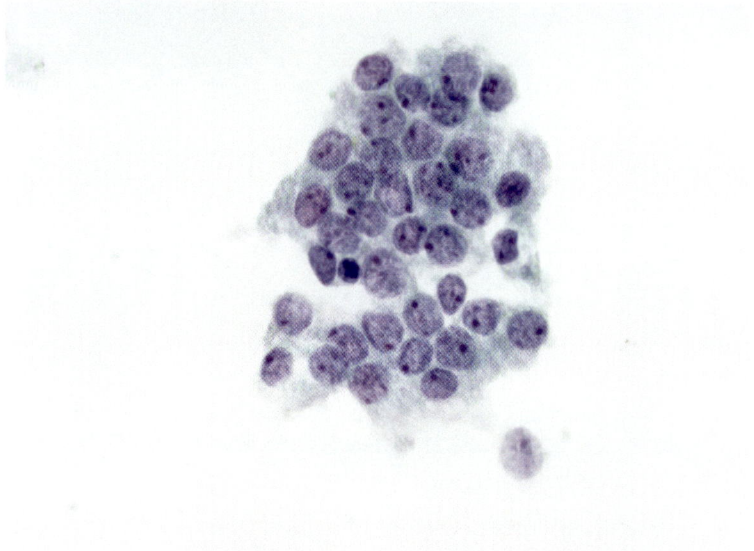

Figure 7.2 — Suspicious for Malignancy, FNA. Suspicious for papillary carcinoma. In comparison to Figure 7.1, the cytologic features are similar with enlarged nuclei, pale chromatin, and only slight nuclear contour irregularities. In contrast to the prior aspirate, this specimen was sparsely cellular. This specimen proved to be a follicular adenoma, while the diagnosis in Figure 7.1 was papillary carcinoma. (Liquid based preparation, Papanicolaou stain)

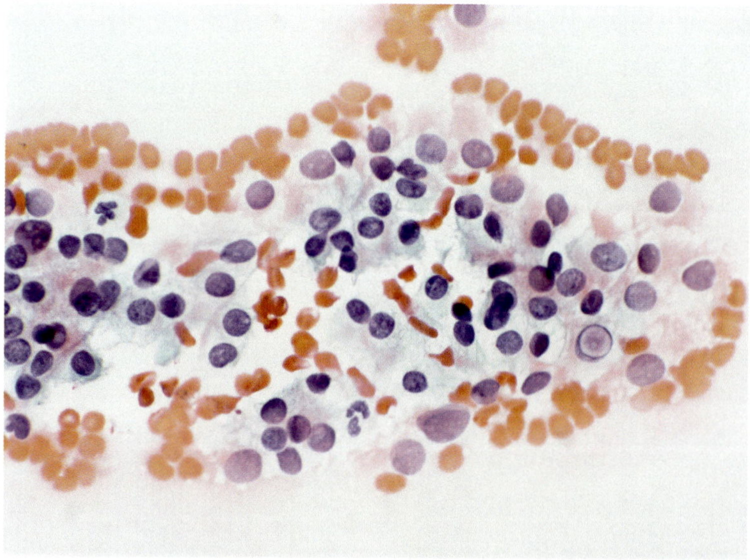

Figure 7.3 — Suspicious for Malignancy, FNA. Suspicious for papillary carcinoma. In this example, the suspicious cells exhibit air-drying artifact. Nevertheless, a well-defined intranuclear pseudoinclusion is present (lower right of group) and there is the suggestion of pseudoinclusions in other nuclei. Papillary carcinoma was confirmed histologically. (Papanicolaou stain)

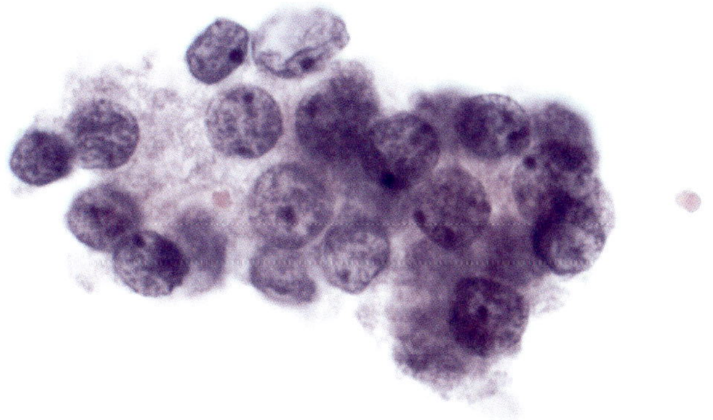

Figure 7.4 — Suspicious for Malignancy, FNA. Suspicious for papillary carcinoma. Nuclei are enlarged and overlapping with pale chromatin. Most nuclei have regular nuclear contours; however, a nucleus at the upper portion of the group is quite irregular with a prominent nuclear groove. There is also the suggestion of two microfollicles abutting one another. This case was a follicular variant of papillary carcinoma on resection. Follicular variants often have more subtle cytologic features of papillary carcinoma that result in a suspicious rather than malignant cytologic diagnosis. (Liquid based preparation, Papanicolaou stain)

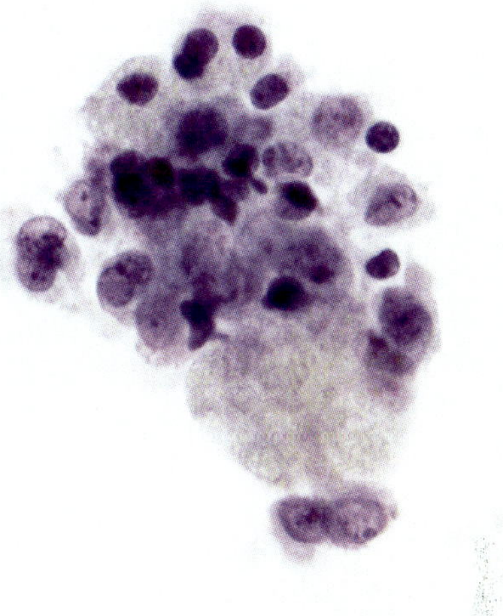

Figure 7.5 — Suspicious for Malignancy, FNA. Suspicious for cystic papillary carcinoma. This case is comprised mostly of hemosiderin-laden macrophages. Only rare follicular cells with enlarged pale nuclei and slightly irregular nuclear contours are identified. Cystic degeneration is a common pitfall in the diagnosis of papillary carcinoma. However, the worrisome cells in this case are rare and not well visualized. A diagnosis of atypical cells of undetermined significance may be more appropriate. See Figure 7.6 for corresponding histology. (Liquid based preparation, Papanicolaou stain)

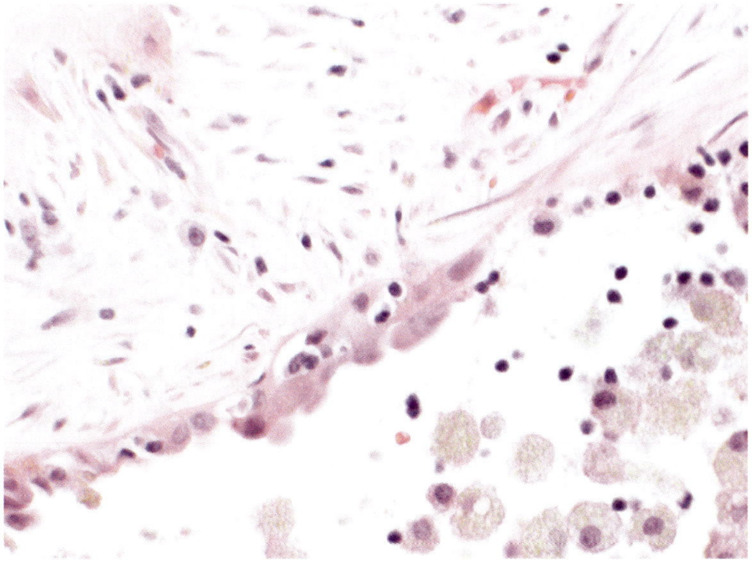

Figure 7.6 — Suspicious for Malignancy, FNA. Suspicious for cystic papillary carcinoma, benign cyst on resection. The corresponding histology to Figure 7.5 is of a benign hyperplastic nodule with extensive cystic degeneration. In addition to numerous hemosiderin-laden macrophages within the cyst, reactive cyst lining cells with enlarged pale nuclei are present in the cyst wall. These cells correlate with the cytologic cells of concern, but are not diagnostic of papillary carcinoma. (H&E stain)

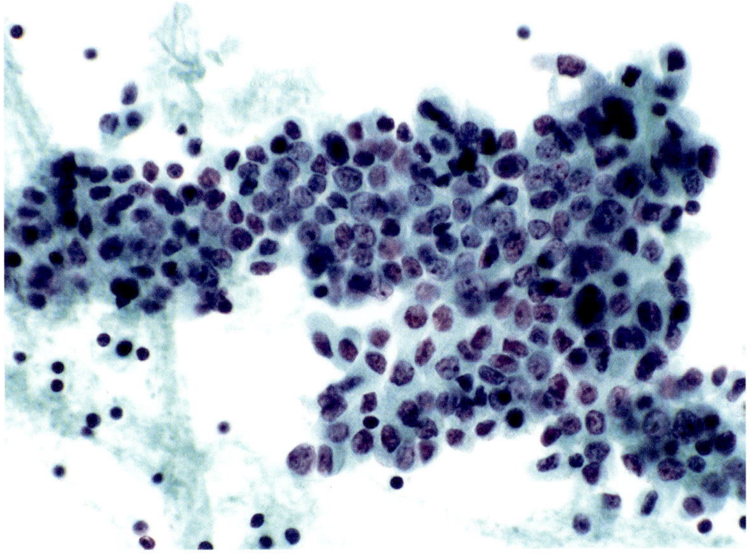

Figure 7.7 — Suspicious for Malignancy, FNA. Suspicious for papillary carcinoma in Hashimoto thyroiditis. In some instances, other features of the aspirate raise concern for alternative diagnoses. Nuclear changes in Hashimoto thyroiditis overlap changes of papillary carcinoma warranting caution in rendering a malignant diagnosis if the cytologic features are not definitive. In this aspirate with characteristic features of Hashimoto thyroiditis elsewhere, occasional lymphoid cells can be appreciated in the background of this image. The follicular cells present exhibit many cytologic features of papillary carcinoma with enlarged, pale nuclei having irregular nuclear contours and focal nuclear molding. The presence of Hashimoto thyroiditis created slight uncertainty resulting in a suspicious diagnosis. Papillary carcinoma was confirmed at surgery. (Liquid based preparation, Papanicolaou stain)

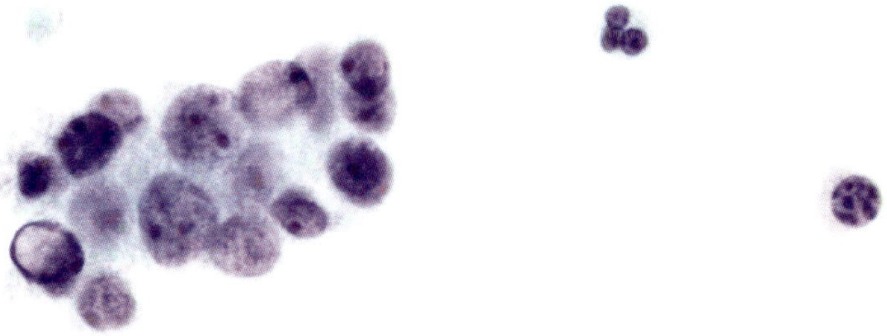

Figure 7.8 — Suspicious for Malignancy, FNA. Suspicious for papillary carcinoma in Hashimoto thyroiditis. This case from a patient with Hashimoto thyroiditis also exhibits features concerning for papillary carcinoma. Among the enlarged, overlapping nuclei with pale chromatin is a single nucleus with an apparent intranuclear pseudoinclusion (far left). However, this nucleus appears degenerated and the cell is largely devoid of cytoplasm. Papillary carcinoma was identified on the resected specimen. (Liquid based preparation, Papanicolaou stain)

Figure 7.9a — Suspicious for Malignancy, FNA. Suspicious for papillary carcinoma in Hashimoto thyroiditis. Cytologic changes in Hürthle cells are potentially confounding in Hashimoto thyroiditis. This group of oncocytic cells from a case of Hashimoto thyroiditis has cytologic features that are highly suspicious for papillary carcinoma including pronounced nuclear contour irregularities and multiple nuclei with intranuclear pseudoinclusions. An oncocytic variant of papillary carcinoma in a background compatible with Hashimoto thyroiditis was diagnosed histologically. (Liquid based preparation, Papanicolaou stain)

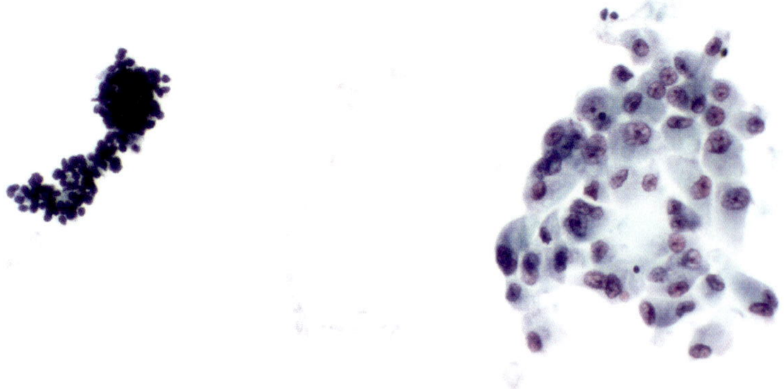

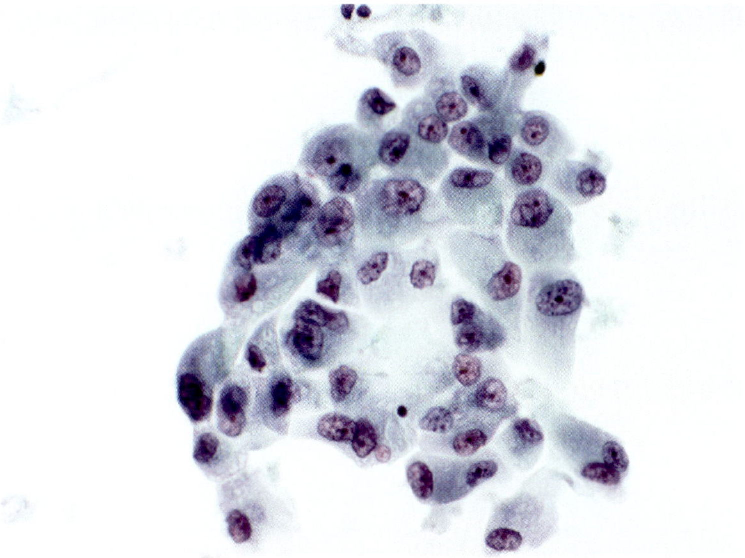

Figure 7.9b — Suspicious for Malignancy, FNA. Higher magnification of the previous case shows oval-shaped nuclei with markedly convoluted nuclear contours and grooves. (Liquid based preparation, Papanicolaou stain)

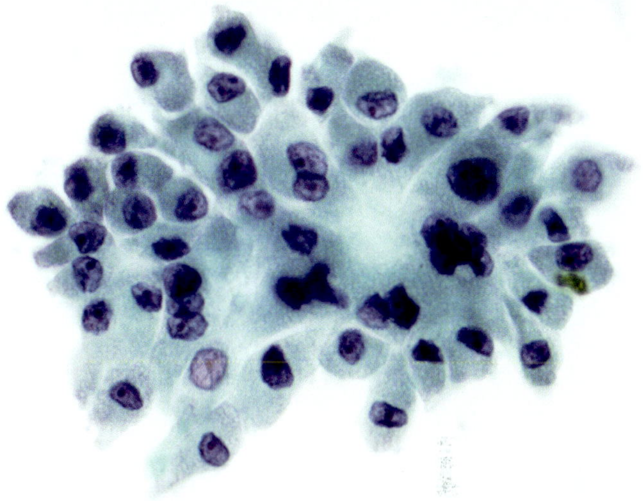

Figure 7.10 — Suspicious for Malignancy, FNA. Suspicious for papillary carcinoma, oncocytic variant. Unusual variants of tumors can create diagnostic uncertainty with features that overlap other entities. These cells, similar in appearance to those in the case shown in Figure 7.9b, have abundant granular cytoplasm suggesting the diagnostic of a Hürthle cell neoplasm. However, the nuclei with pale chromatin and occasional grooves are suspicious for papillary carcinoma. The corresponding histology is shown in Figure 7.11. (Liquid based preparation, Papanicolaou stain)

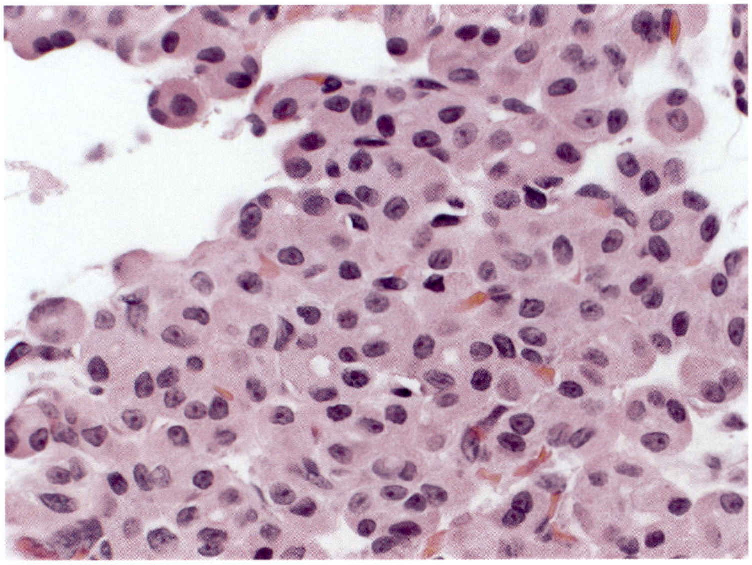

Figure 7.11 — Suspicious for Malignancy, FNA. Papillary carcinoma, oncocytic variant. The surgical specimen of the nodule aspirated in Figure 7.10 confirms the diagnosis of the oncocytic variant of papillary carcinoma. The cells have abundant granular eosinophilic cytoplasm, but unlike a Hürthle neoplasm, there are characteristic cytologic features of papillary carcinoma. Nuclei have fine chromatin with frequent nuclear grooves and pronounced nuclear contour irregularities. (H&E stain)

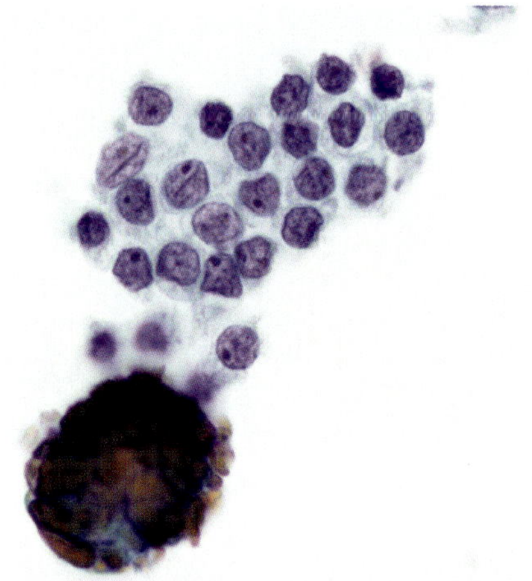

Figure 7.12 — Suspicious for Malignancy, FNA. Suspicious for papillary carcinoma, macrofollicular variant. This field is representative of the findings throughout this hypercellular specimen. Abundant colloid is present and numerous macrofollicular sheets of follicular cells are also seen. While these findings would typically signify a benign thyroid nodule, the nuclei are suspicious for papillary carcinoma including fine pale chromatin, focal nuclear molding, and prominent nuclear grooves. The surgical specimen is shown in Figure 7.13. (Liquid based preparation, Papanicolaou stain)

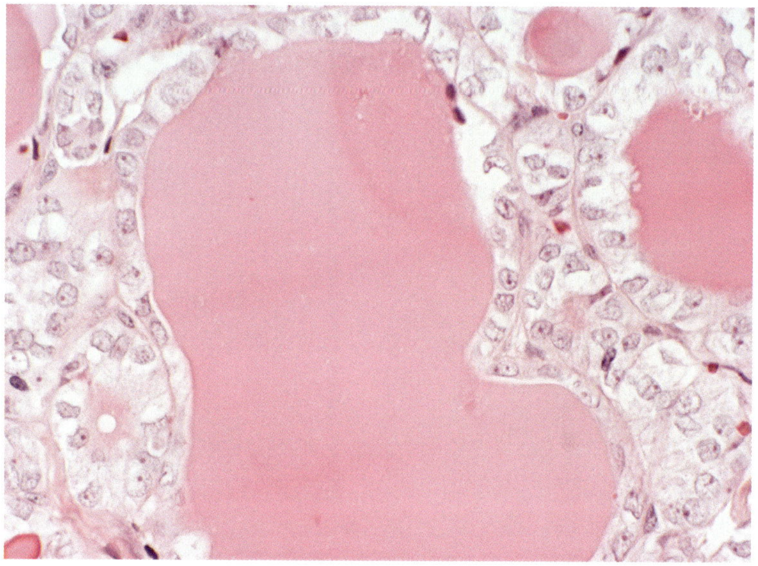

Figure 7.13 — Suspicious for Malignancy, FNA. Surgical resection from the previous case. (H&E stain)

Figure 7.14 — Suspicious for Malignancy, FNA. Suspicious for papillary carcinoma (hyalinizing trabecular tumor). The suspicious cells in this case are few in number as the aspirate was sparsely cellular overall. However, the nuclei are enlarged, chromatin is powdery, and intranuclear pseudoinclusions are readily identified. The excised mass was a hyalinizing trabecular tumor (shown in Figure 7.15). These tumors are notoriously difficult to distinguish from papillary carcinoma and are typically called either suspicious for papillary carcinoma or malignant on FNA. (Liquid based preparation, Papanicolaou stain)

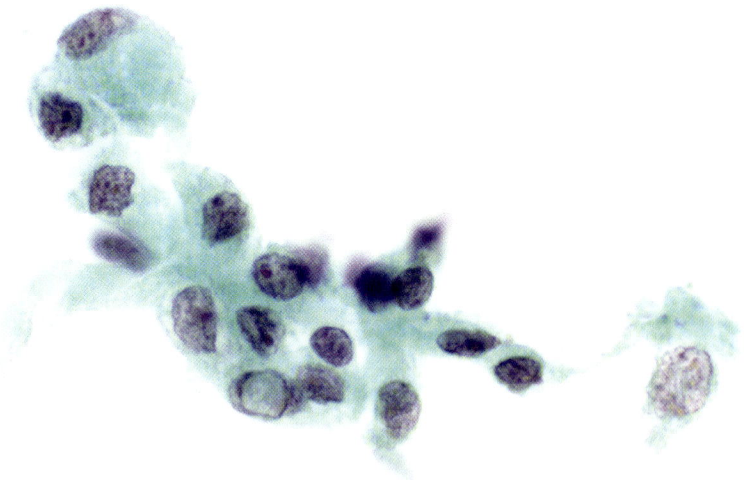

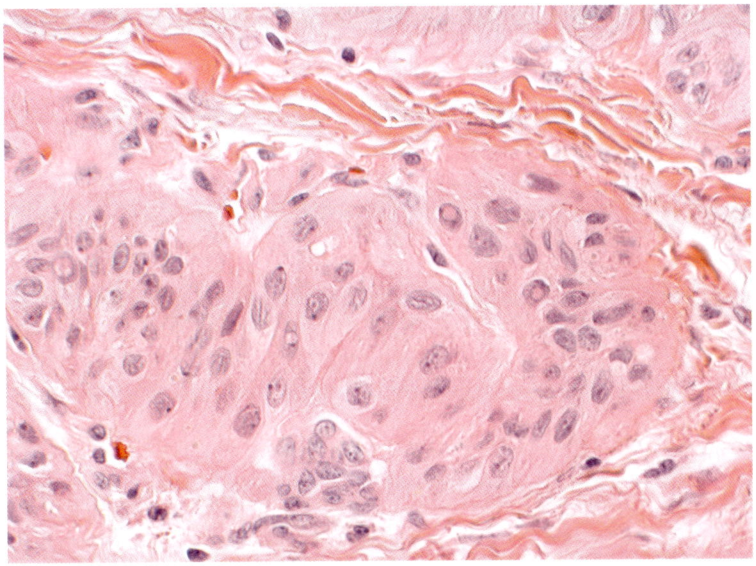

Figure 7.15 — Suspicious for Malignancy, FNA. Hyalinizing trabecular tumor. The corresponding excision specimen from Figure 7.14 demonstrates the appearance of a hyalinizing trabecular tumor. The elongated neoplastic follicular cells grow in a nested pattern separated by fibrous septae. Nuclei are oval with pale chromatin, prominent nuclear grooves, and frequent intranuclear pseudoinclusions. Hyalinizing trabecular tumor is a controversial entity thought by some to be related to papillary carcinoma. Although most behave in a benign fashion, uncommon malignant behavior has been described. (H&E stain)

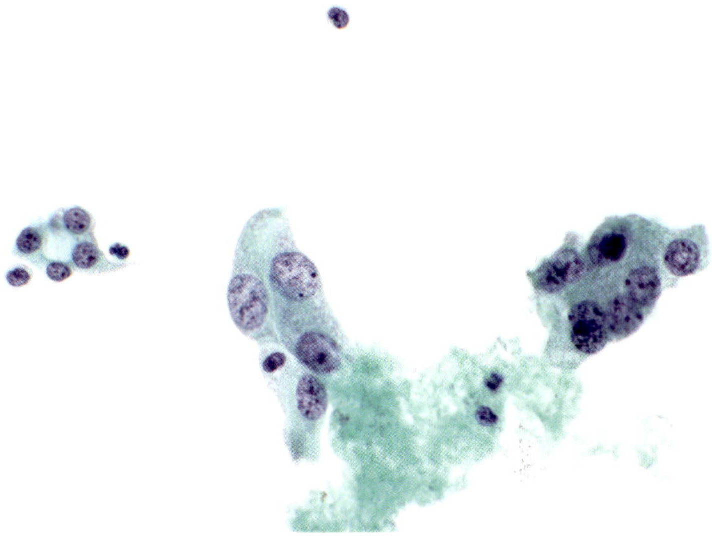

Figure 7.16 — Suspicious for Malignancy, FNA. This aspirate is difficult to classify precisely. Cytoplasm of some cells is oncocytic. Nuclei vary considerably in size with some having pale chromatin, although most cells have rounded nuclear contours. Possible diagnoses include a Hürthle cell neoplasm and papillary carcinoma (possibly an oncocytic variant). The latter diagnosis was slightly favored prospectively. The thyroidectomy specimen is shown in Figure 7.17. (Liquid based preparation, Papanicolaou stain)

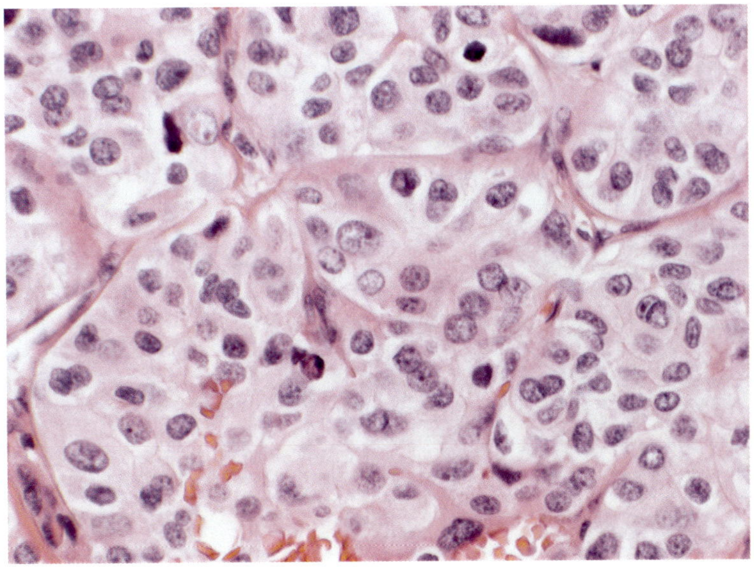

Figure 7.17 — Suspicious for Malignancy, FNA. Poorly differentiated (insular) carcinoma. The case shown here and in Figure 7.16 further demonstrates the difficulty in recognizing less common entities. On histology, the tumor grows in a nested pattern with a representative mitotic figure and apoptotic body shown in this field. Poorly differentiated thyroid carcinoma is challenging to recognize in most cytologic preparations. When present, high nuclear to cytoplasmic ratios, apoptosis, mitoses, and necrosis are helpful findings. Frequently, however, these tumors are difficult to distinguish from well-differentiated follicular neoplasms. (H&E stain)

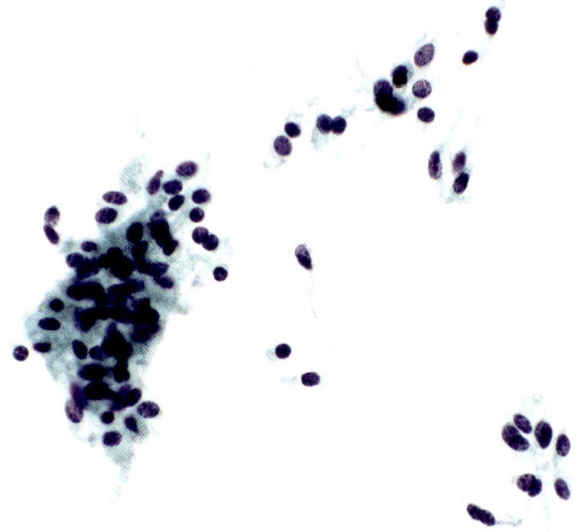

Figure 7.18 — Suspicious for Malignancy, FNA. Suspicious for medullary carcinoma. Medullary carcinoma is readily detected in thyroid FNA. Issues of quantity and/or quality of the cells may preclude definitive diagnosis as does an unusual appearance of the cells. This case shows typical features of a spindle cell variant of medullary carcinoma. This hypercellular specimen exhibits loose clusters and single cells with long cytoplasmic processes. Nuclei are round to oval with uniform, hyperchromatic, and speckled chromatin. Amyloid is not identified. In this case, confirmatory immunocytochemical stains were attempted, but actually introduced doubt regarding the diagnosis. Both thyroglobulin and calcitonin stains were equivocal and carcinoembryonic antigen (CEA), which is positive in most medullary carcinomas, was negative. Consequently, a suspicious diagnosis was rendered with a recommendation to assess the serum calcitonin to confirm the diagnosis. The excised tumor is shown in Figure 7.19. (Liquid based preparation, Papanicolaou stain)

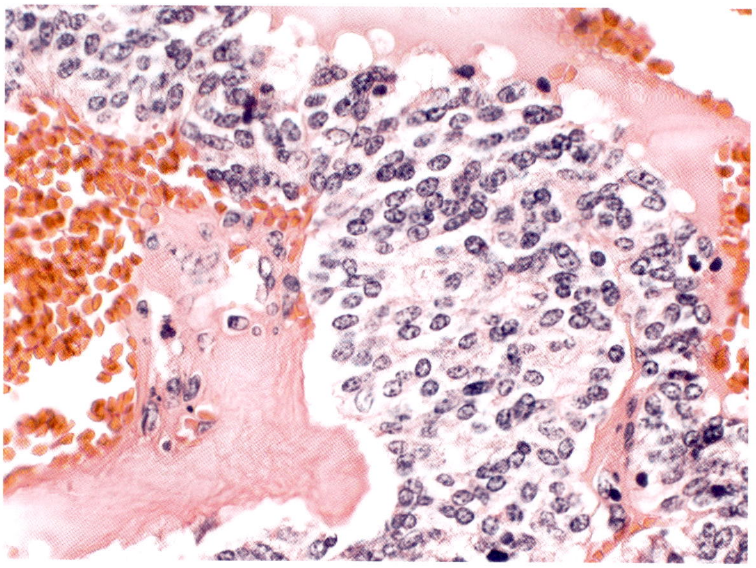

Figure 7.19 — Suspicious for Malignancy, FNA. Medullary carcinoma. The tumor aspirated in Figure 7.18 shows the characteristic neuroendocrine features of a medullary carcinoma with coarse granular chromatin. Amyloid is also present. (H&E stain)

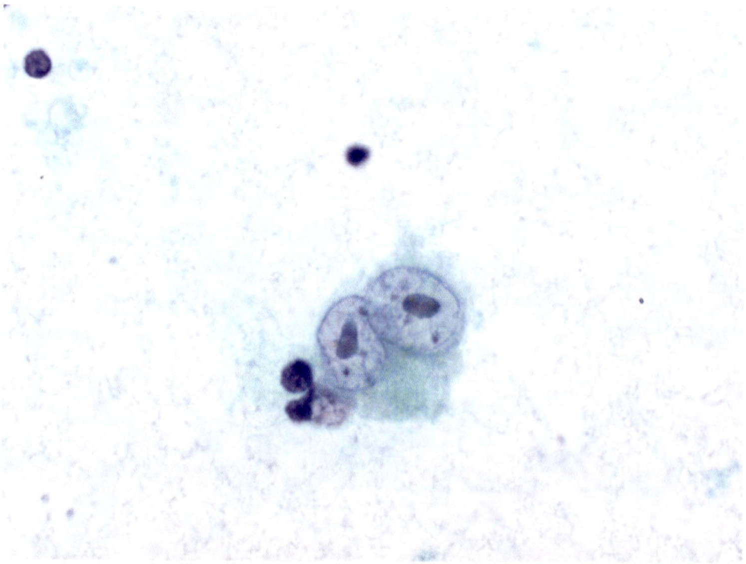

Figure 7.20 — Suspicious for Malignancy, FNA. Suspicious for Hodgkin lymphoma. A suspicious for lymphoma diagnosis is appropriate when cell preservation or quantity is an issue in the presence of a suspected clonal population of lymphoid cells. Fragile cells of diffuse large B cell lymphoma may preclude definitive diagnosis morphologically and can also be problematic when performing confirmatory immunophenotyping by flow cytometry. The polymorphous nature of aspirates of extranodal marginal zone lymphomas of mucosa associated lymphoid tissue (MALT) type will require confirmatory marker studies for a malignant diagnosis. Otherwise, a suspicious or even atypical diagnosis is more appropriate. This image shows the only Reed-Sternberg cell identified in this paucicellular aspirate. Accordingly, a diagnosis of suspicious for Hodgkin disease was rendered and subsequently confirmed on biopsy. (Filter preparation, Papanicolaou stain)

8

Papillary Thyroid Carcinoma and Variants

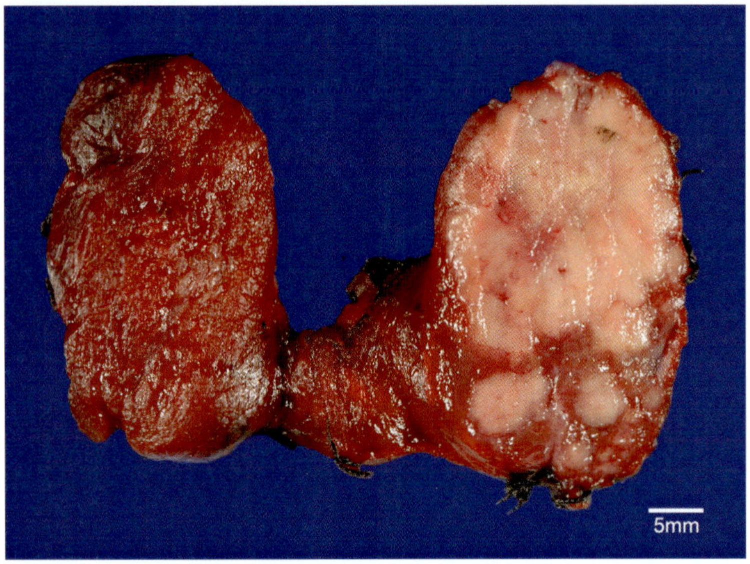

Figure 8.1 — Papillary Carcinoma, Gross Appearance. The gross appearance of papillary carcinoma can vary considerably depending on the presence and degree of fibrosis, encapsulation, and cystic change. The typical papillary carcinoma has a cut surface that is whitish tan, fleshy, and firm. The papillary architecture seen microscopically can sometimes be appreciated grossly as a fine granularity of the cut surface. The invasive edge of conventional papillary carcinomas may be highly infiltrative or well demarcated, but it usually lacks the uniform encapsulation of follicular neoplasms. Papillary carcinoma is often a multifocal process. Accordingly, the thyroid parenchyma of both lobes should be carefully inspected for additional tumor nodules. In this case, the right lobe harbors multiple tumor foci.

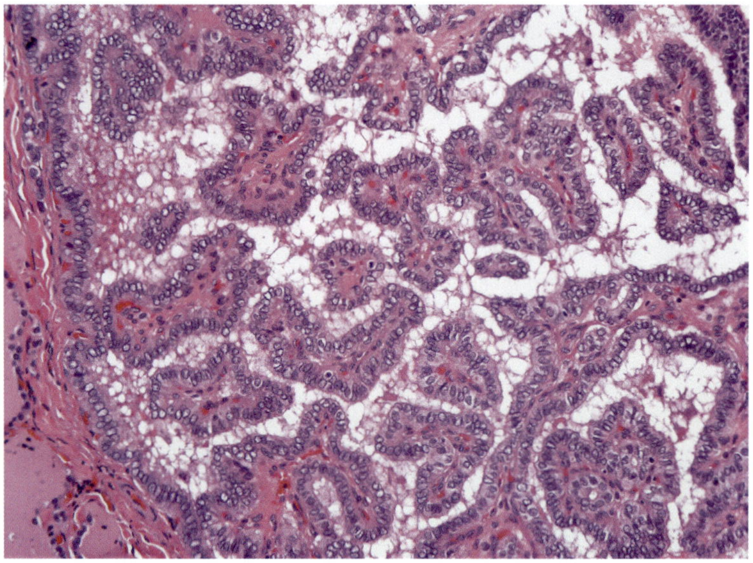

Figure 8.2a — Papillary Carcinoma, Classic Type, Histologic Section. Classic papillary carcinomas exhibit a papillary architecture where central fibrovascular cores support an atypical epithelial proliferation. Compared to benign papillary hyperplasia encountered in Graves disease and multinodular adenomatoid hyperplasia, the papillae in papillary carcinoma are much longer and convoluted with complex tertiary branching. More importantly, the follicular epithelium lining the papillae exhibits cytologic atypia including nuclear enlargement with chromatin pallor. (H&E stain)

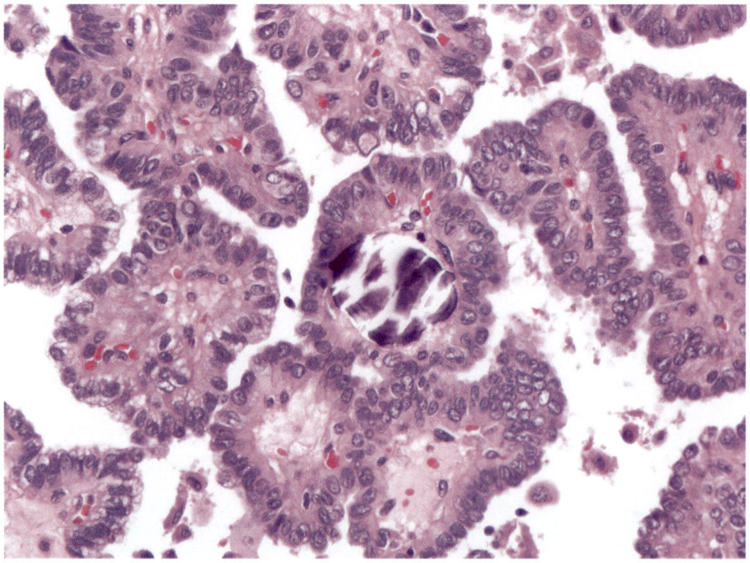

Figure 8.2b — Papillary Carcinoma, Classic Type, Histologic Section. Some papillary carcinomas show a type of tumoral calcification known as psammomatous calcification. Psammoma bodies are seen as round purple laminated concretions that show shatter artifact in nondecalcified tissue sections. They typically occur in the tips of the papillae, but they may be encountered as isolated bodies within the interstitium of the nonneoplastic thyroid parenchyma and even within cervical lymph nodes. Their presence in these sites strongly infers the presence of a papillary carcinoma in the ipsilateral thyroid lobe. Note the cytologic atypia of the cells lining the papillae including the presence of pseudoinclusions in some of the nuclei. (H&E stain)

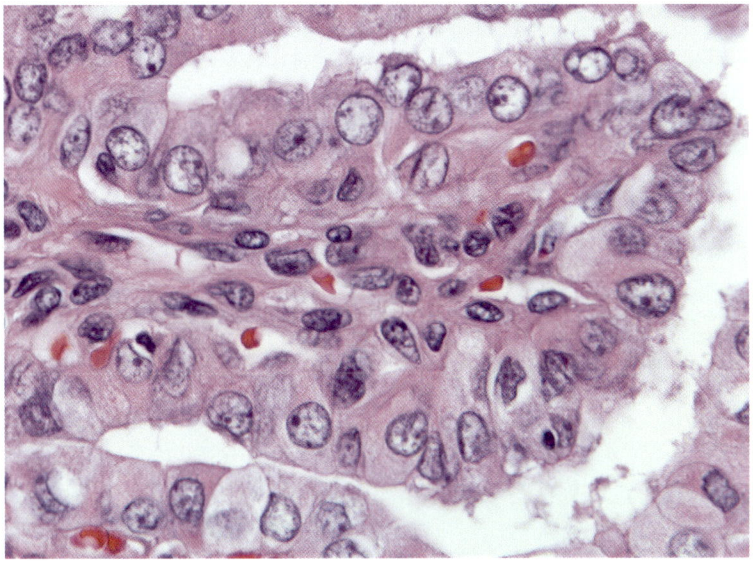

Figure 8.2c — Papillary Carcinoma, Classic Type, Histologic Section. The hallmark diagnostic feature of papillary carcinoma is its atypical nuclear morphology. In well fixed tissue sections, the nuclei tend to be enlarged and elongated. The chromatin has a propensity to condense along the nuclear membrane resulting in a sharply etched nuclear outline with an optically clear center. The nuclear contours may be indented giving rise to irregular nuclear shapes. The tumor cells lining the papillae lack uniform spacing and polarity. Instead, they are crowded and haphazardly aligned. (H&E stain)

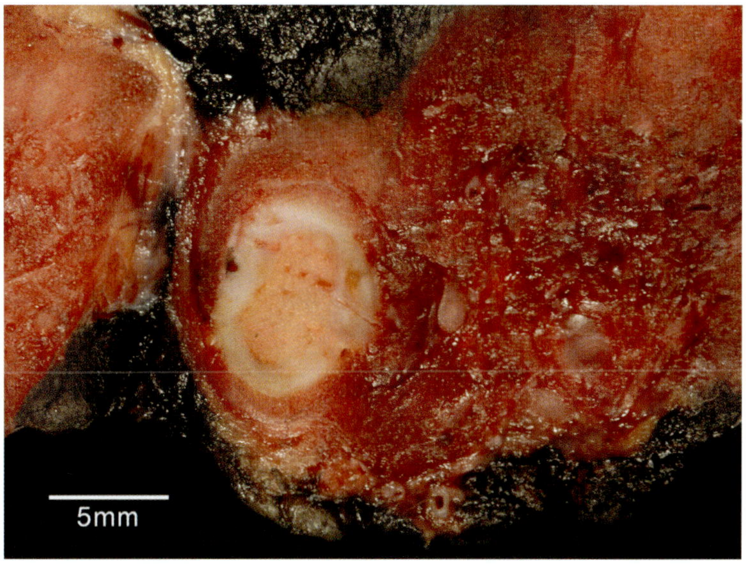

Figure 8.3 — Papillary Microcarcinoma, Gross Appearance. Papillary microcarcinoma is technically defined as a papillary carcinoma that measures less than 1.0 cm. Papillary microcarcinomas are often firm and sclerotic, but the degree of fibrosis is highly variable. They may be either encapsulated or unencapsulated. At times they may be palpable and even accessible to fine needle aspiration (FNA), but most are incidentally discovered during macroscopic and microscopic examination.

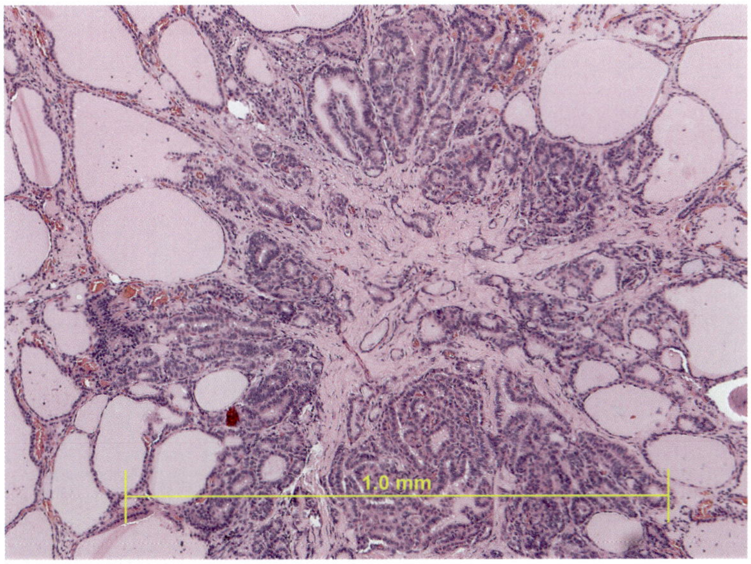

Figure 8.4 — Papillary Microcarcinoma, Histologic Section. In its most classic form, papillary microcarcinomas radiate outward from a stellate central scar to permeate the surrounding thyroid parenchyma in an infiltrative fashion. They may show any combination of papillary and follicular growth. Not all papillary microcarcinomas, however, are sclerotic and infiltrative. At the other end of the morphologic spectrum, papillary microcarcinomas may exhibit a pure follicular growth pattern, lack any fibrosis, and be entirely surrounded by a fibrous capsule. (H&E stain)

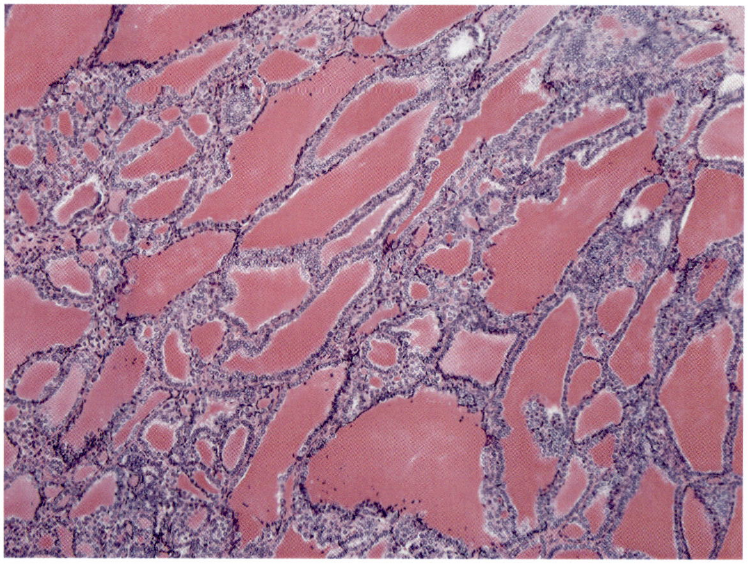

Figure 8.5a — Follicular Variant of Papillary Carcinoma, Histologic Section. The follicular variant of papillary carcinoma is notable for the conspicuous absence of papillary fronds. Instead, this variant demonstrates a pure follicular pattern of growth. When well formed papillary fronds are present, they are a very focal finding. The follicles often occur as elongated tubular structures that are filled with darkly stained eosinophilic colloid. Although well formed papillary fronds are not readily observed, buds of tumor epithelium often project into the luminal spaces in a way that resembles an attempt at primitive frond formation. Psammoma bodies may occasionally be observed, but not with the frequency with which they are seen in conventional papillary carcinoma. In the absence of psammoma bodies and papillary architecture, the diagnosis of a follicular variant of papillary carcinoma rests on its atypical cellular features. (H&E stain)

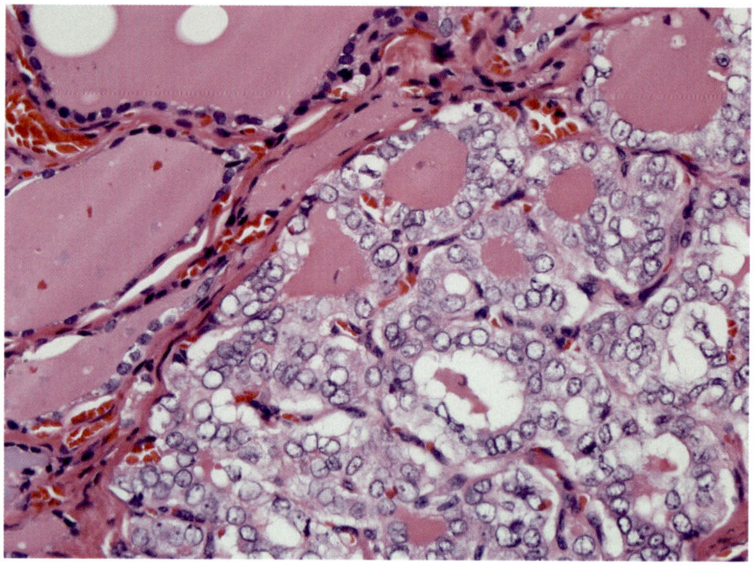

Figure 8.5b — Follicular Variant of Papillary Carcinoma, Histologic Section. The follicles are filled with a darkly stained pink colloid. Absorption of colloid gives rise to a scalloped zone of clearing at the interface of the colloid and the lining epithelium. Although not highly specific, intrafollicular multinucleated giant cells are frequently noted in the follicular variant of papillary carcinoma. The diagnosis of this form of papillary carcinoma mostly rests on recognition of the cellular features of papillary carcinoma. The tumor cells forming the follicles exhibit all of the same atypical features as those lining the papilla of conventional papillary carcinoma. These features include nuclear enlargement, nuclear overlapping, chromatin clearing, nuclear grooves, and nuclear pseudoinclusions. (H&E stain)

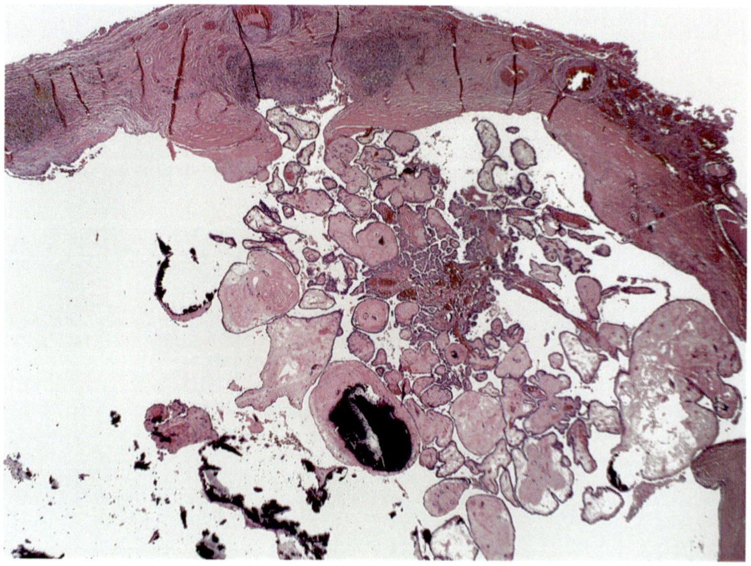

Figure 8.6 — Encapsulated Variant of Papillary Carcinoma, Histologic Section. Most papillary carcinomas show some degree of infiltration. In the encapsulated variant, however, the papillary carcinoma is completely separated from the surrounding thyroid tissue by a fibrous wall. Central cystic degeneration is a common finding in the encapsulated variant. (H&E stain)

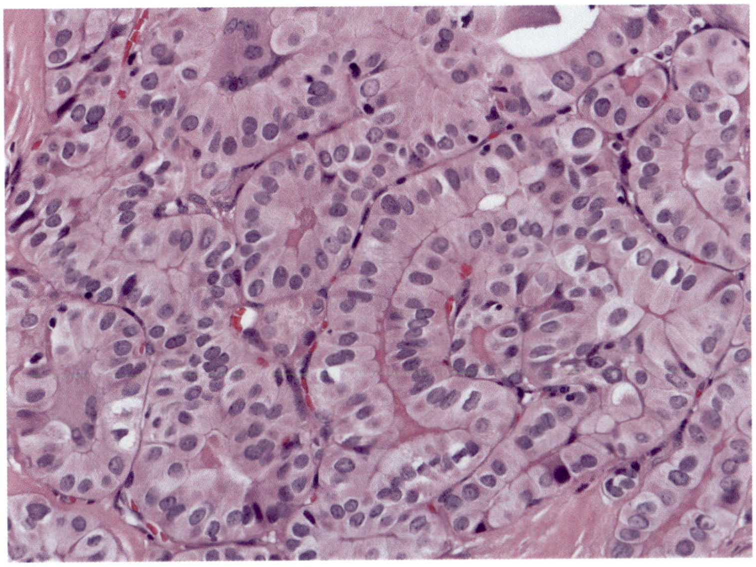

Figure 8.7 — Tall Cell Variant of Papillary Carcinoma, Histologic Section. Relative to conventional papillary carcinoma, the tall cell variant is clinically more aggressive. Extension beyond the thyroid with infiltration of local structures is a common occurrence in this subtype of papillary carcinoma. Its hallmark morphologic feature is the loftiness of the tumor cells. By definition, the height of the tumor cell is at least two to three times its width. In addition to its height, the cytoplasm is very eosinophilic. Indeed, this variant is often included in the differential diagnosis of other pink cell tumors such as Hürthle cell neoplasms. Unlike Hürthle cell neoplasms, the cytoplasm of this variant of papillary carcinoma lacks the prominent granularity of true oncocytic change. Nuclear elongation, longitudinal nuclear grooves, and nuclear pseudoinclusions are particularly well developed in the tall cell variant. The nuclei tend to be uniformly aligned along the basal aspect of the tumor cells. This variant exhibits much less cellular crowding, nuclear overlapping, and dyspolarity than conventional papillary carcinoma. (H&E stain)

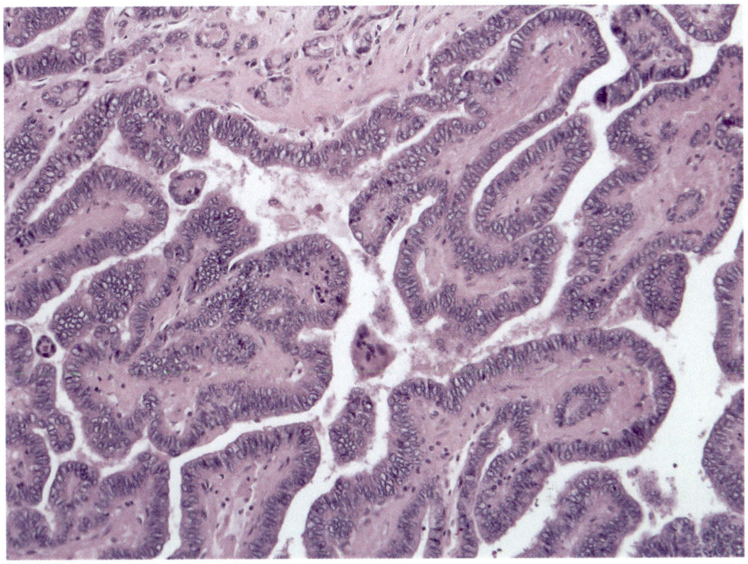

Figure 8.8a — Columnar Cell Variant of Papillary Carcinoma, Histologic Section. The columnar variant represents another aggressive form of papillary carcinoma. Papillary formations are well developed and often take on a villous-like quality. It is sometimes confused with the tall cell variant as both forms are made up of tumor cells with tall cytoplasm. (H&E stain)

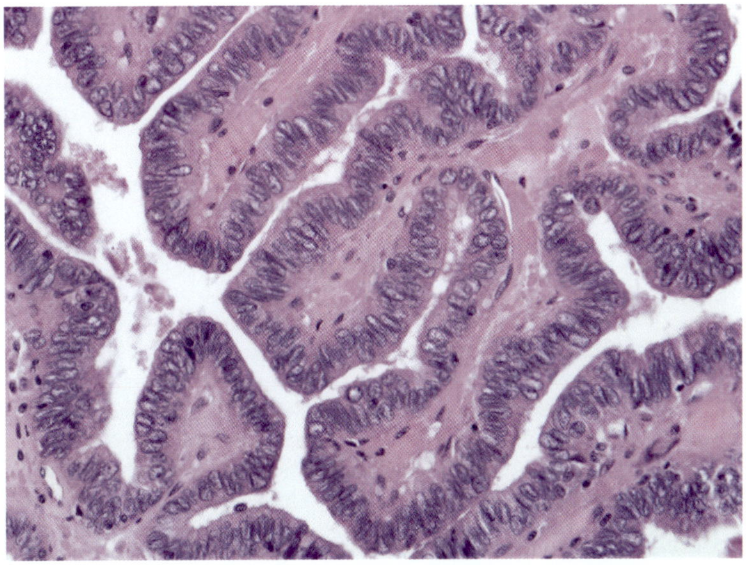

Figure 8.8b — Columnar Cell Variant of Papillary Carcinoma, Histologic Section. In contrast to the tall cell variant with its eosinophilic cytoplasm and uniformly aligned nuclei, the columnar cell variant does not exhibit cytoplasmic eosinophilia, and its nuclei are crowded, overlapping, and stratified in a picket fence-like array. The columnar variant of papillary carcinoma is highly reminiscent of adenocarcinoma of colorectal and endometrial origin. Accordingly, the differential diagnosis of the columnar cell variant includes metastatic carcinoma from one of these extrathyroidal sites. Immunohistochemistry can be useful in resolving this differential diagnosis as the columnar variant of papillary thyroid carcinoma retains its immunoreactivity for thyroglobulin and TTF-1. (H&E stain)

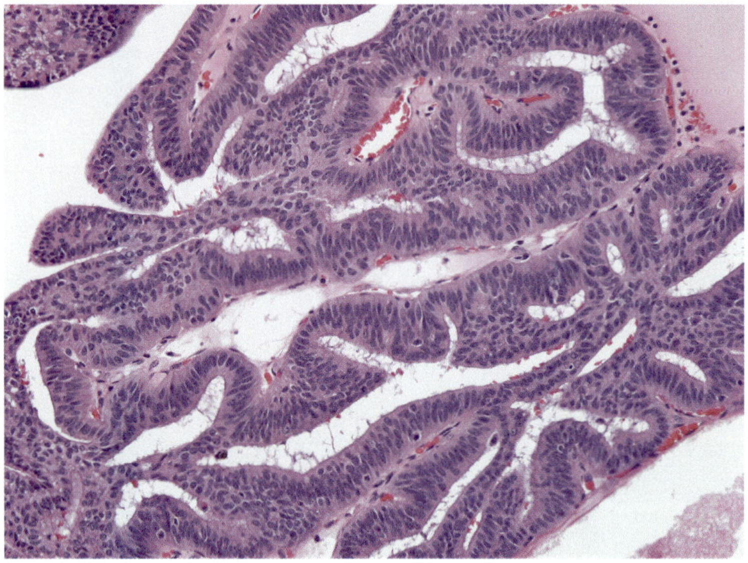

Figure 8.9a — Cribriform-Morular Variant of Papillary Carcinoma, Histologic Section. The cribriform-morular variant of papillary carcinoma typically exhibits an admixture of cribriform, follicular, papillary, trabecular, and solid patterns of growth with morular formations. The descriptor "cribriform" refers to those areas where the tumor cells form anastamosing bars and arches in the absence of an intervening fibrovascular stroma. The cells lining the cribriform structures are sometimes tall and hyperchromatic with nuclear crowding and stratification. Although confusion with the columnar variant is a concern, the cribriform variant is morphologically more diverse (eg, cribriform and morular components), and it typically lacks the tumor necrosis and high grade cytologic features of the columnar variant. The distinction is important as the cribriform-morular variant lacks the aggressive clinical behavior of the columnar variant. (H&E stain)

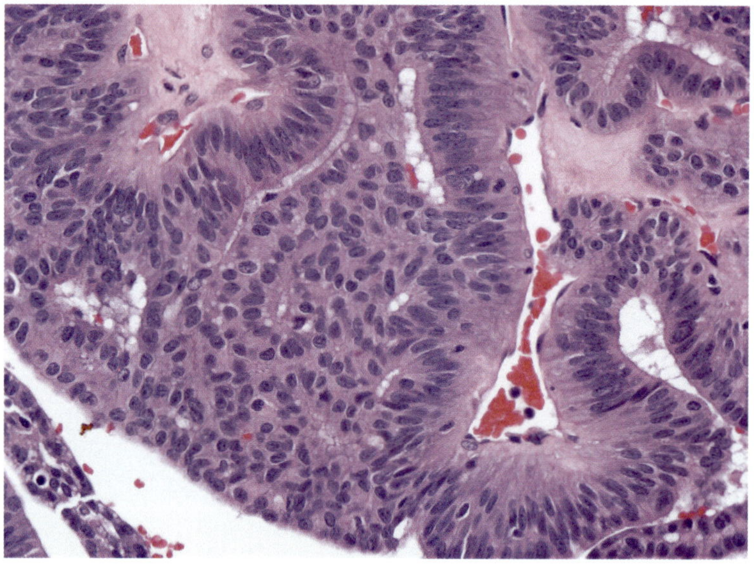

Figure 8.9b — Cribriform-Morular Variant of Papillary Carcinoma, Histologic Section. The term "morular" refers to the presence of solid nests of slightly spindled tumor cells in a whorled arrangement. (H&E stain)

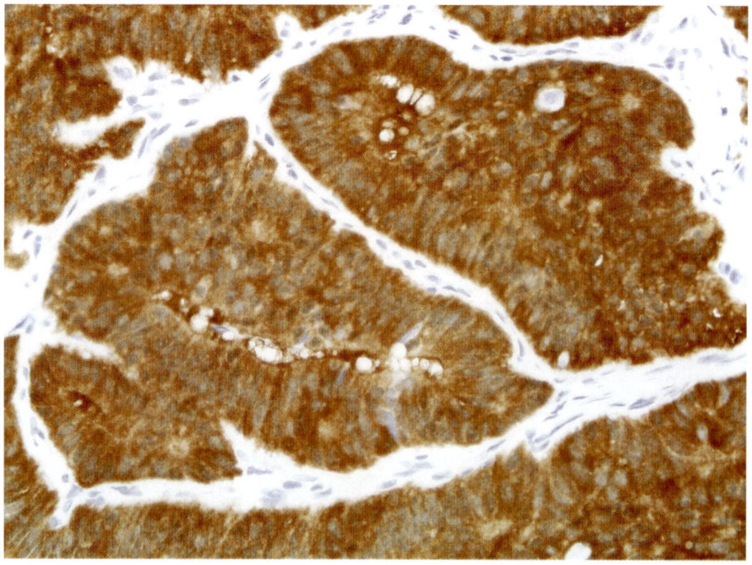

Figure 8.9c — Cribriform-Morular Variant of Papillary Carcinoma (Beta-Catenin Staining), Histologic Section. Although the cribriform-morular variant can occur sporadically, it is also the form of thyroid carcinoma that is encountered in patients who carry a germ line mutation of the adenomatous polyposis coli (APC) gene. Accordingly, this variant is important for the pathologist to recognize as it may represent an extracolonic manifestation of familial adenomatous polyposis. Recognition may be aided by the immunohistochemistry. The cribriform-morular variant often exhibits abnormal nuclear and cytoplasmic accumulation of the beta-catenin gene product. (Immunostain)

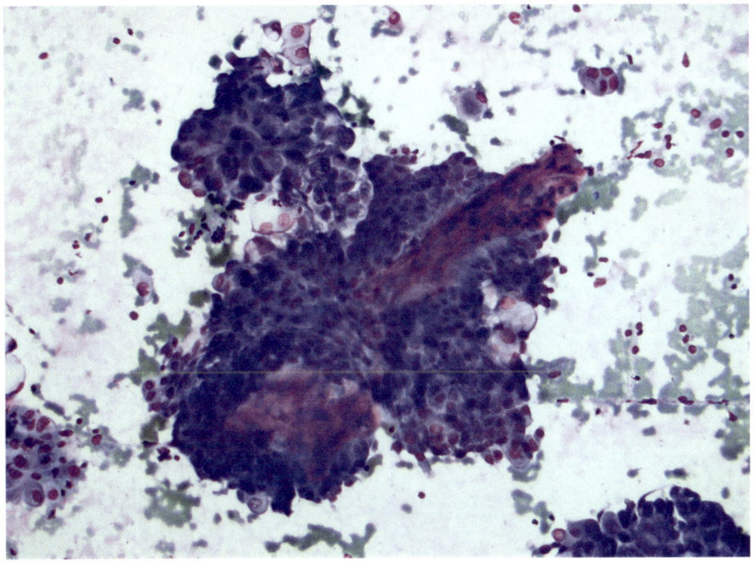

Figure 8.10a — Papillary Thyroid Carcinoma, FNA. Papillary thyroid carcinoma (PTC) can present on FNA smears in wide variety of architectural patterns. Seeing true papillae with fibrovascular cores, as in this image is not the most common pattern; and papillary architecture is not a major diagnostic criterion for PTC. Other patterns include macrofollicles or sheets and microfollicles. Identification of architecture is a first step; evaluation of nuclear features is critical for the ultimate diagnosis of PTC. Papillary thyroid carcinoma is the most common malignant neoplasm of the thyroid, accounting for approximately 80% of all cancers at this site. (Diff Quik stain)

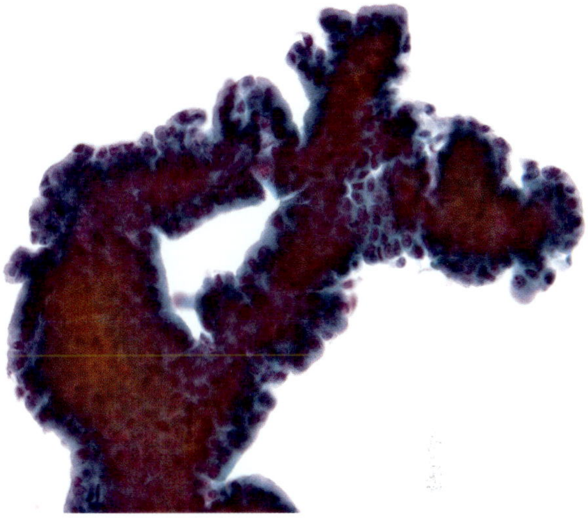

Figure 8.10b — Papillary Thyroid Carcinoma, FNA. The Bethesda System for Reporting Thyroid Cytopathology (TBSRTC) defines PTC as "a malignant epithelial tumor derived from thyroid follicular epithelium and displays characteristic nuclear alterations." Papillary architecture may be present but is not required for the diagnosis. A well-developed true papillary architecture is shown here. The central portion (stained darker) contains slender fibrovascular cores. Notice focal palisading of the neoplastic cells at the edge of the branching papillary fronds. (Liquid-based preparation, Papanicolaou stain)

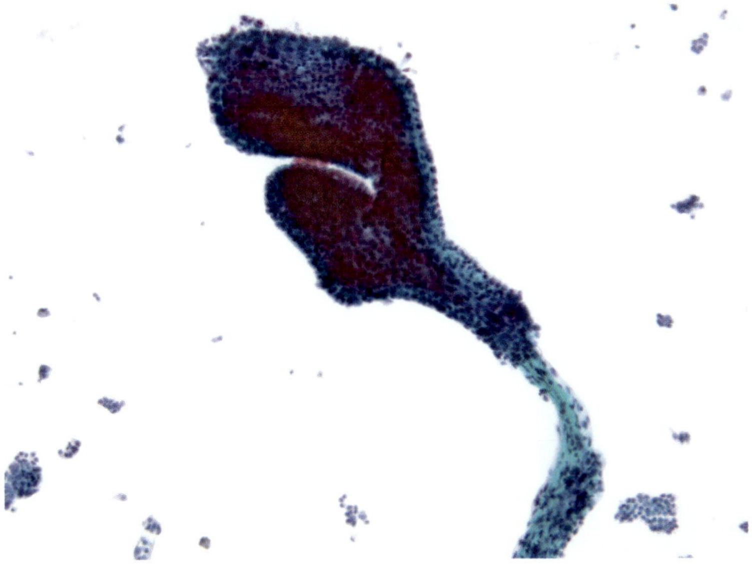

Figure 8.10c — Papillary Thyroid Carcinoma, FNA. This case beautifully demonstrates the classic papillary pattern of PTC. Papillary architecture (with true fibrovascular cores), although quite specific for PTC, is only seen in a minority of cases (15%–20%). More often, PTC demonstrates flat monolayered sheets or papillary-like architecture (without fibrovascular cores). Notice the long and slender piercing capillary vessel surrounded by scant fibrous stroma at the inferior aspect of the epithelial fragment. (Liquid-based preparation, Papanicolaou stain)

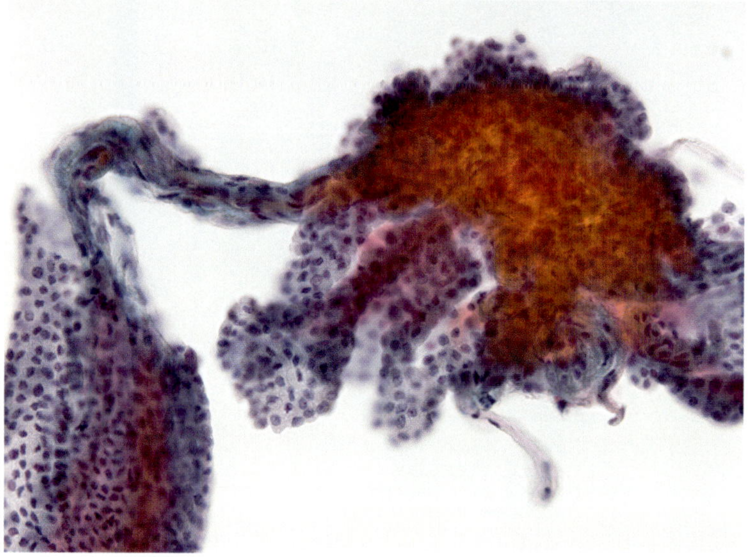

Figure 8.10d — Papillary Thyroid Carcinoma, FNA. Another example illustrating the basic architecture of a true papillary tumor fragment, that is, nests of epithelial cells with classic nuclear features of PTC, surrounding fine capillaries with associated scant fibrous stroma. Presence of fibrovascular cores distinguish true papillary from papillary-like tissue fragments. Papillary-like architecture is less specific and is seen in many benign and neoplastic lesions of the thyroid. (Liquid-based preparation, Papanicolaou stain)

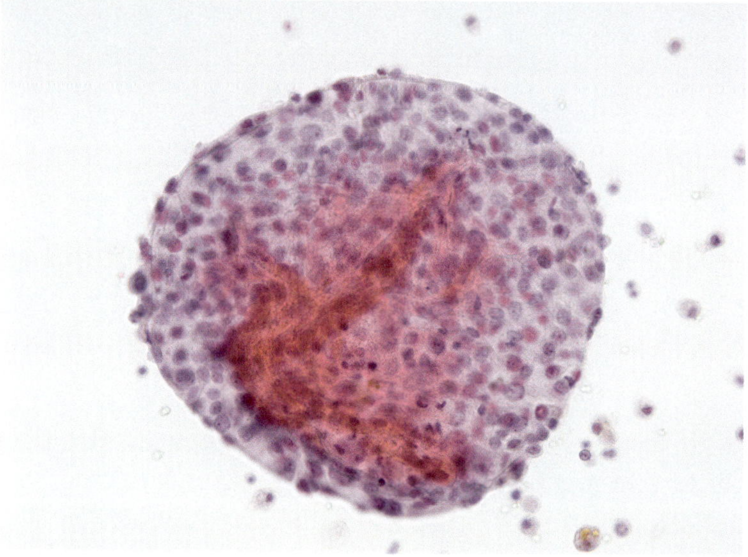

Figure 8.10e — Papillary Thyroid Carcinoma, FNA. Liquid-based preparations offer a great appreciation of PTC cytomorphology. They bring out the cellular details and architectural characteristics in a relatively clean slide background. This image shows a beautiful illustration of papillary formation (likely representing tip of the papillary frond). Notice the fine branching vessel surrounded by malignant epithelial cells. (Liquid-based preparation, Papanicolaou stain)

Figure 8.11a — Papillary Thyroid Carcinoma, FNA. This example illustrates hypercellular smear with numerous fine piercing capillaries (center of the field) forming cores of the papillary formations. Risk factors for PTC include external radiation to the neck during childhood, ionizing radiation, genetic factors, and nodular hyperplasia. PTC occurs in all age groups, including children, with a peak incidence in the third to fourth decades, and the male/female ratio is 1:3. (Diff Quik stain)

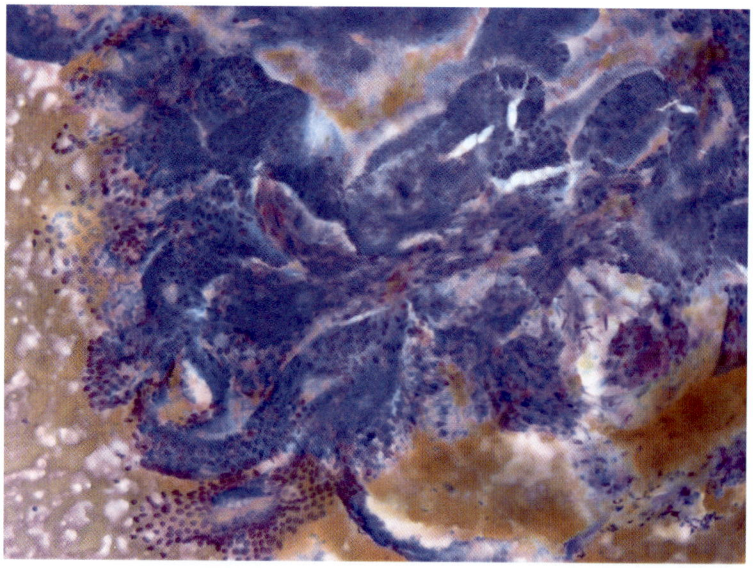

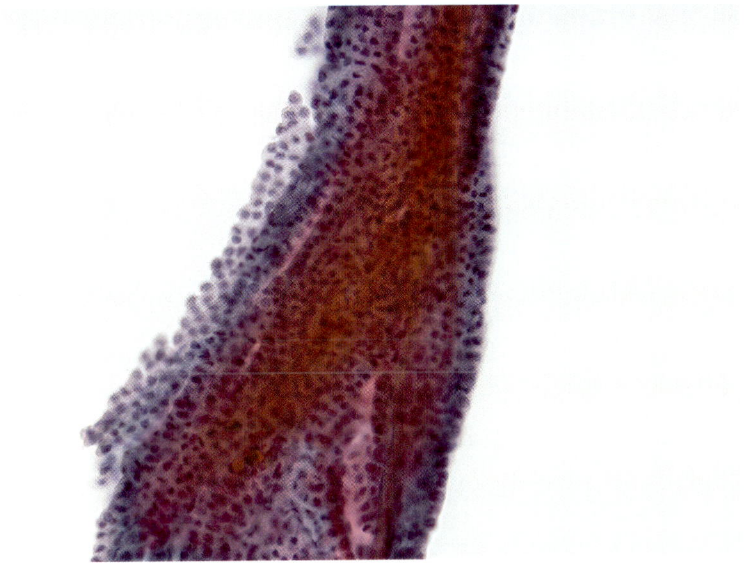

Figure 8.11b — Papillary Thyroid Carcinoma, FNA. The basic architecture of the papillary fragment is illustrated at higher magnification. Note the central zone made up of fibrovascular cores, surrounded by fibrous stroma and enclosed by malignant epithelium with characteristic nuclear features. A peculiar palisading of the nuclei is almost always noticed at the edges of the fragment. (Liquid-based preparation, Papanicolaou stain)

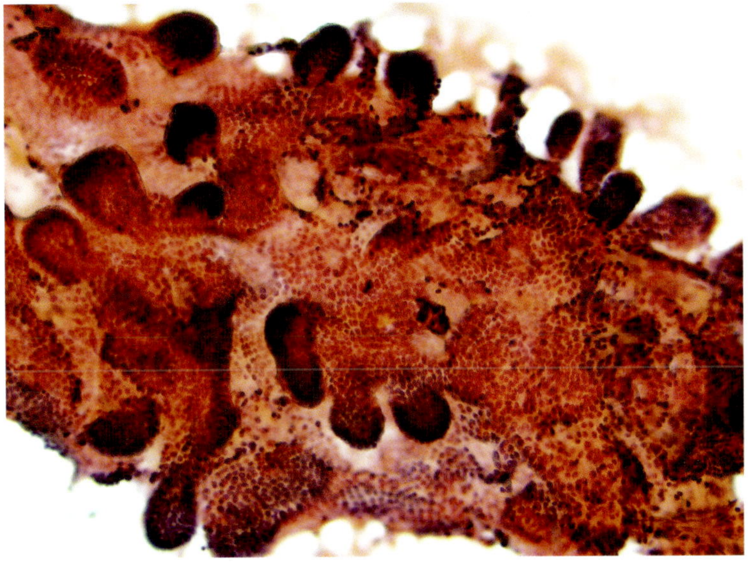

Figure 8.13 — Benign Papillary Hyperplasia, FNA. These papillary projections could be with or without a fibrovascular core; however Graves disease and other hyperplastic thyroid nodules can show benign papillary proliferations. It is critical to look carefully at the cells, especially the nuclear features; a diagnosis of PTC should not be rendered on architecture alone. In this case the patient went to surgery and was found to have papillary hyperplasia in an involuting hyperplastic nodule. (Papanicolaou stain)

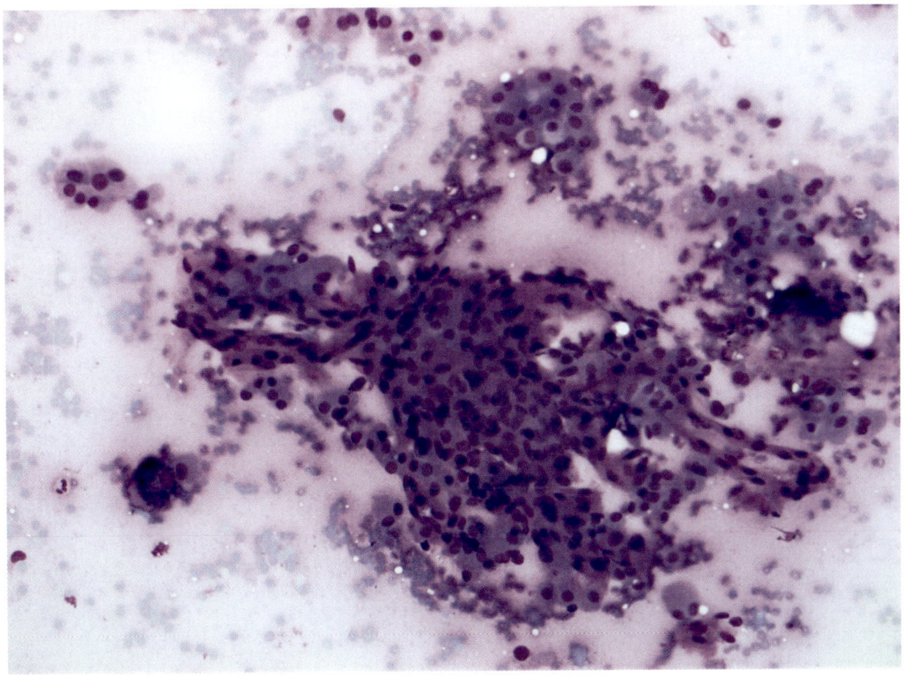

Figure 8.12 — Hürthle Cell Neoplasm, FNA. Vascularity in other neoplasms such as Hürthle cell neoplasm (depicted in this image) should not be mistaken for papillary architecture or PTC. Note the cells around the vessels and in the background—these are Hürthle cells. Bloody aspirates as well as endothelial cells are not unusual in a Hürthle cell neoplasm. Hürthle cells have consistently lower N/C ratios, granular cytoplasm, and round nuclei. FNA is invaluable in the diagnosis of this malignancy. When a cytologic diagnosis of PTC is made by FNA, 96% to 100% are proven to be PTC on histologic follow-up. (Diff Quik stain)

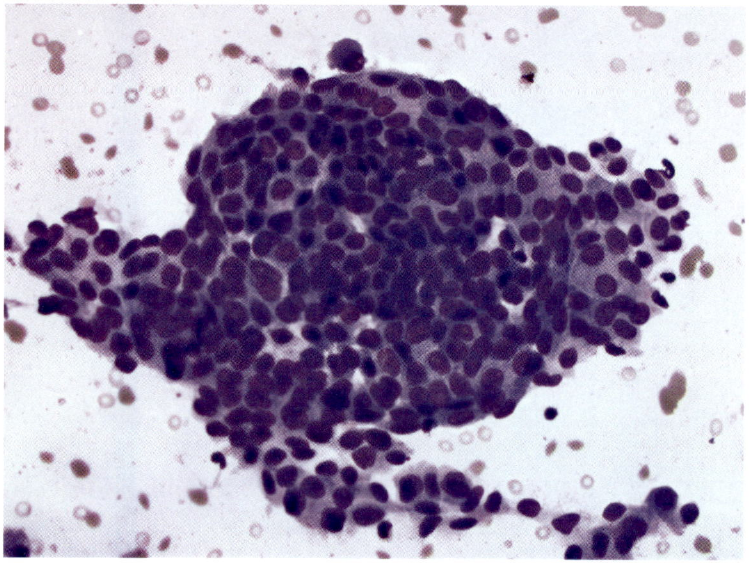

Figure 8.14a — Papillary Thyroid Carcinoma, FNA. A sheet like pattern is one of the most common architectural patterns seen in FNA smears from PTC. The cells are typically arranged in syncytial-like flat pattern ("monolayers") with crowded and overlapping nuclei. In this example, note the syncytial nature of the sheet—there is loss of polarity with enlarged and overlapping nuclei. Some of the nuclei have an elliptical or ovoid shape; change in shape of the nucleus from round (seen in follicular lesions) is an important nuclear diagnostic criterion for PTC. Crowding, overlapping, and molding are important diagnostic features that help distinguish PTC from benign follicular cells. (Diff Quik stain)

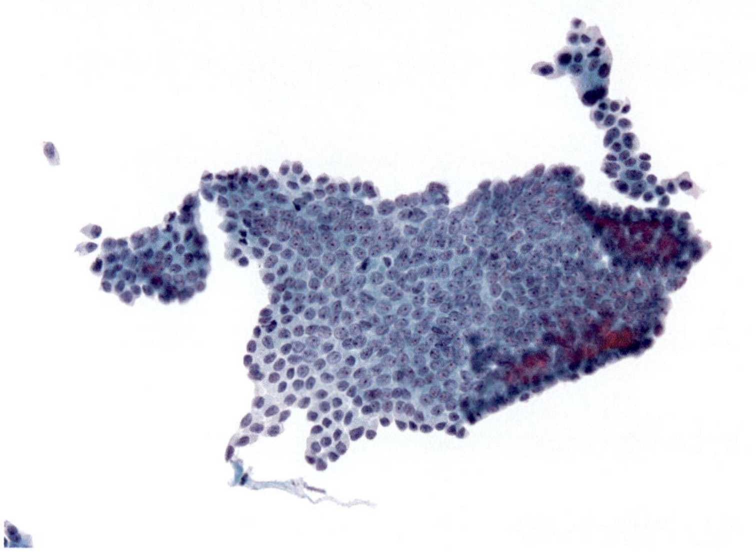

Figure 8.14b — Papillary Thyroid Carcinoma, FNA. A beautiful illustration of the most common architectural pattern of PTC is illustrated here—absolutely flat monolayered fragment. Although focal foldings can be seen at the edges, the central portion of such fragments always displays a flat surface. Note the cellular crowding, oval nuclei, nuclear grooves, and small marginal nucleoli. (Liquid-based preparation, Papanicolaou stain)

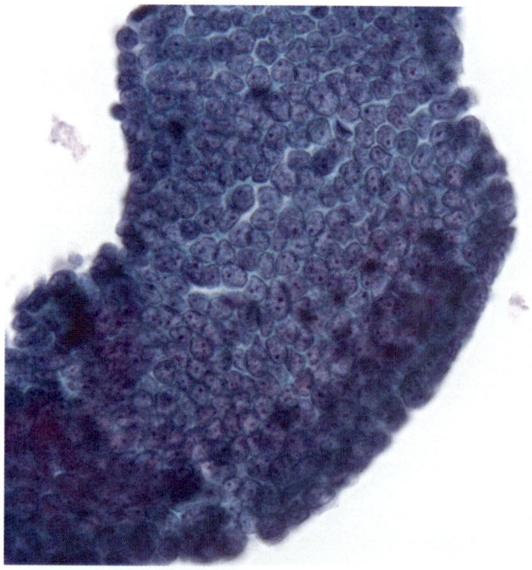

Figure 8.14c — Papillary Thyroid Carcinoma, FNA. Higher magnification shows classic nuclear morphology of PTC: tightly packed ovoid nuclei, powdery chromatin, nuclear membrane irregularity, nuclear grooves, small nucleoli that are mostly submembranous, nuclear molding, and palisading of the nuclei at the edges of the monolayers. All these features are further enhanced on liquid-based preparations, as illustrated in this example. (Liquid-based preparation, Papanicolaou stain)

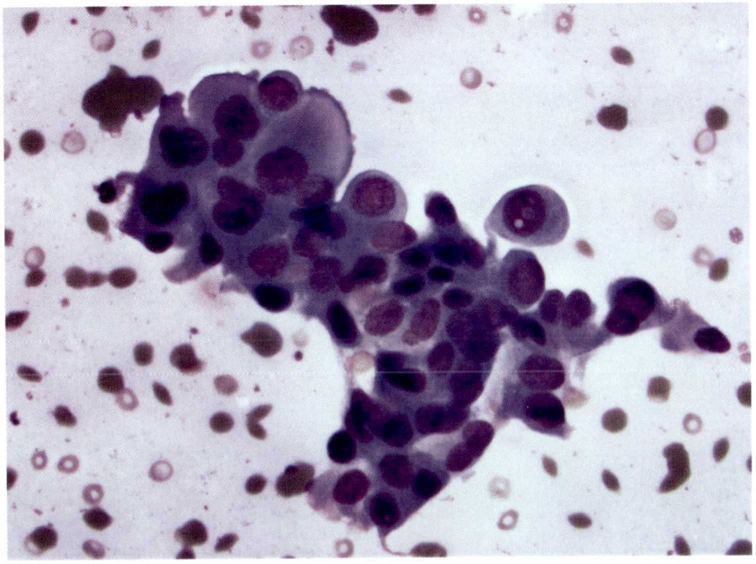

Figure 8.15 — Papillary Thyroid Carcinoma, FNA. It is not unusual for PTC to show pleomorphism of cell size, due to varying quantities of cytoplasm. The cytoplasm can vary from scant to abundant. In cases where there is moderate to abundant cytoplasm, Hürthle cells enter into the differential diagnosis. The cytoplasm in PTC is usually dense, whereas the cytoplasm in Hürthle cells is granular. Note an intranuclear cytoplasmic inclusion on the right. PTC usually presents as a thyroid nodule, often discovered incidentally on routine examination; rarely, patients present with metastatic disease in the cervical lymph nodes. (Diff Quik stain)

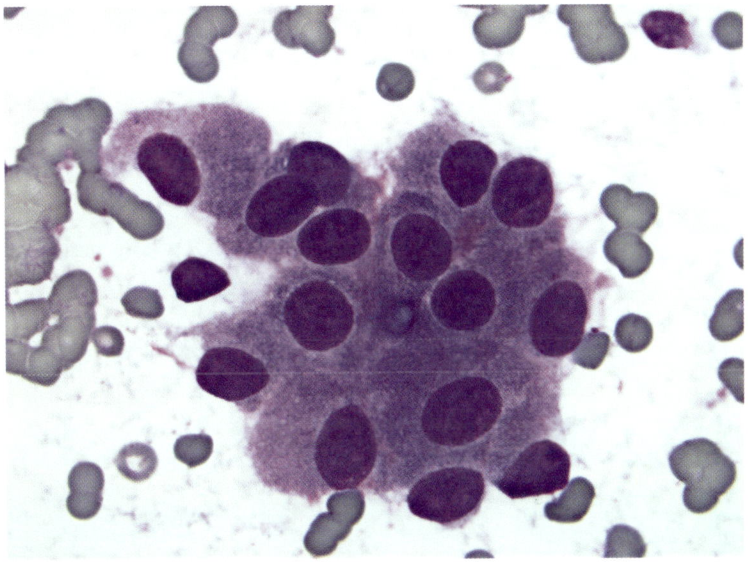

Figure 8.16 — Hürthle Cell Neoplasm, FNA. Hürthle cells showing granular cytoplasm due to abundance of mitochondria, in contrast to the dense cytoplasm of PTC. The nuclear-cytoplasmic ratio tends to be much less variable in Hürthle cells as opposed to PTC. Also note the nuclei in Hürthle cells are round and do not become elongated or oval as in PTC. Nucleoli tend to be more central and larger in Hürthle cells as compared to those in PTC nuclei. (Diff Quik stain)

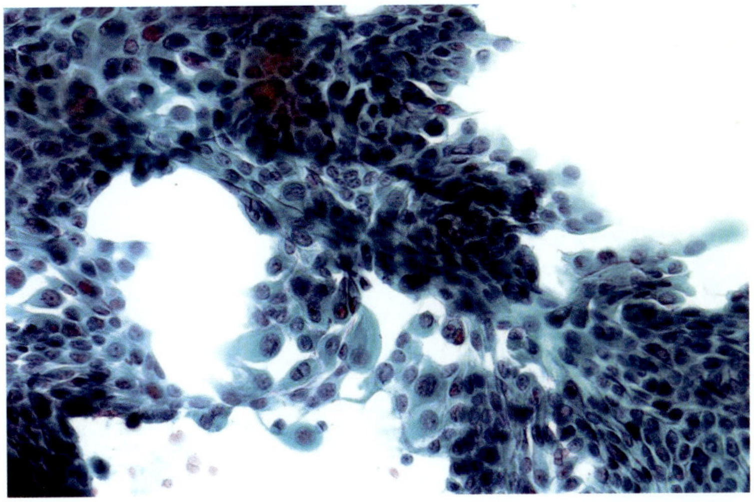

Figure 8.17 — Papillary Thyroid Carcinoma, FNA. In contrast to the previous example, this PTC shows dense, metaplastic-appearing or "squamoid" cytoplasm. The nature of the cytoplasm is a minor diagnostic feature for PTC but is especially useful in separating PTC cells from Hürthle cells. Misdiagnosis of a Hürthle cell neoplasm (HCN) as PTC and vice versa is a well-known pitfall. If the nodule is solitary, the management for these lesions is different—near total thyroidectomy for PTC versus lobectomy for HCN. (Papanicolaou stain)

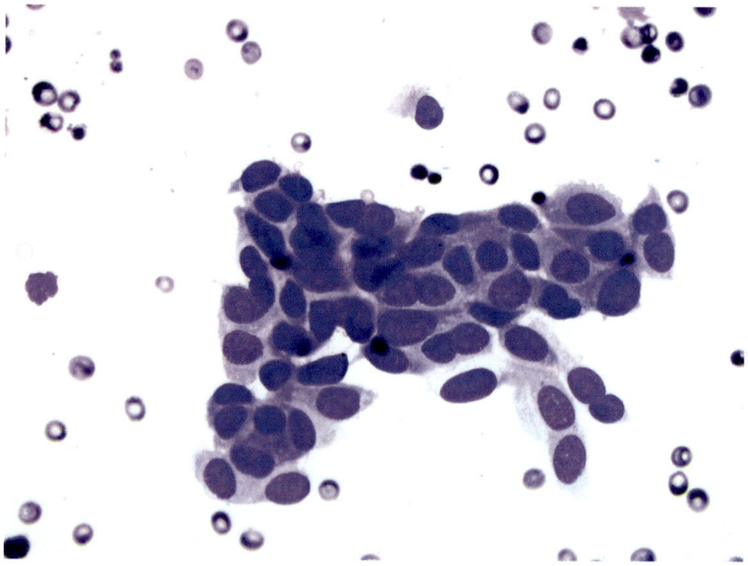

Figure 8.18 — Papillary Thyroid Carcinoma, FNA. One of the most useful features of PTC is variation in shape of the nucleus from round to oval, arrow-head, or elliptical. Note that in the same cluster round as well as oval malignant nuclei are seen. The prognosis of PTC is strongly dependent on many clinical variables: age, tumor size, and histological parameters (extracapsular extension, extrathyroidal extension, lymph node invasion, distant metastasis, and histological variants). (Diff Quik stain)

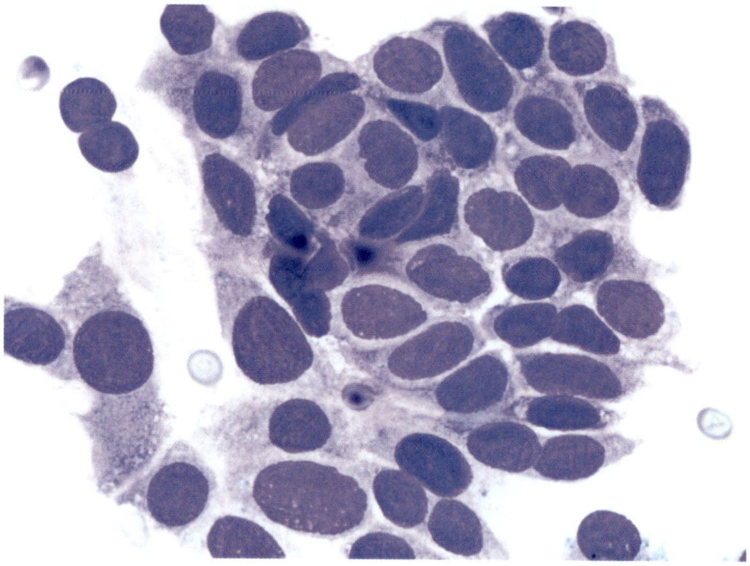

Figure 8.19 — Papillary Thyroid Carcinoma, FNA. Classic PTC nuclear features—nuclear enlargement, oval shape and nuclear grooves are all major diagnostic features for PTC. They can be appreciated well on this air dried smear. The architectural pattern of PTC varies depending on the type of PTC and includes: true papillary fragments with a fibrovascular core, papillary-like fragments lacking a fibrovascular core, microfollicular pattern, cellular swirls (aka "onion-skin" or "cartwheel" pattern), as well as the more common previously illustrated monolayered sheets. (Diff Quik stain)

Figure 8.20 — Papillary Thyroid Carcinoma, FNA. The defining features of PTC are seen in the nuclei and are best appreciated on Papanicolaou staining. The chromatin of a PTC nucleus is usually pale and powdery rather than dark and coarsely textured like a benign follicular cell nucleus. Alcohol fixation enhances the chromatin clearing of the nuclei—a characteristic of PTC nuclei that is also seen on formalin fixed sections and referred to as "orphan Annie" nuclei. Nuclear grooves and small nucleoli, other nuclear features of PTC are also appreciated here. (Papanicolaou stain)

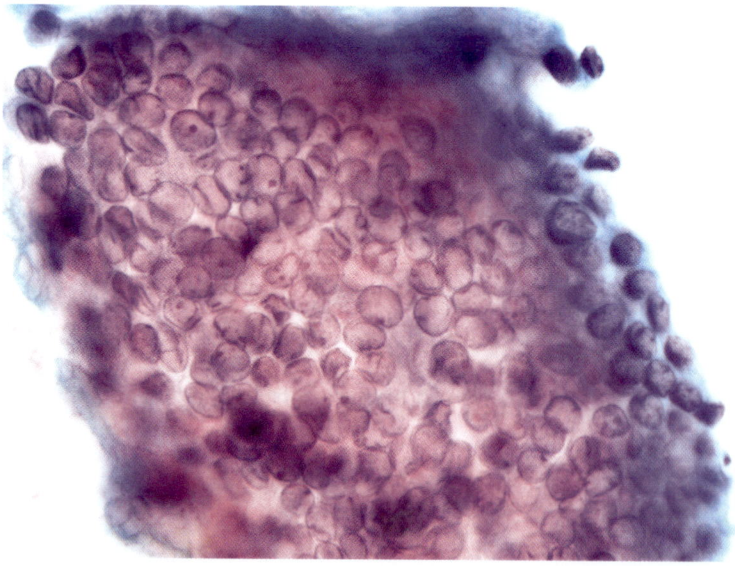

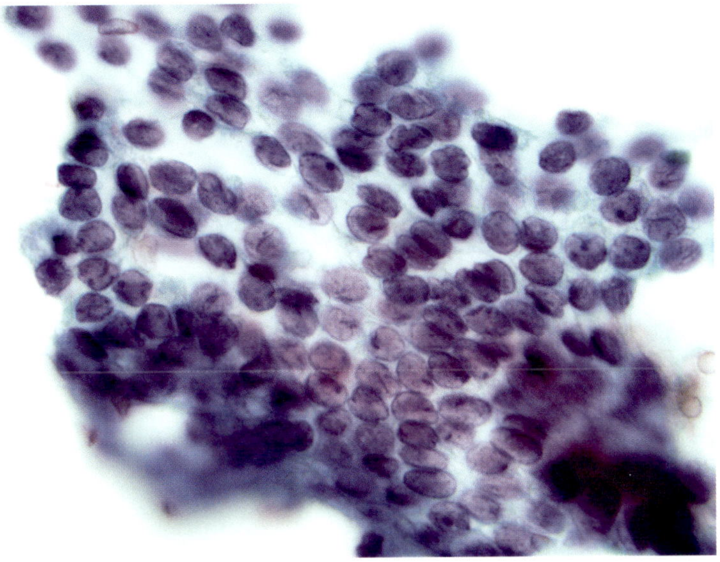

Figure 8.21 — Papillary Thyroid Carcinoma, FNA. Note the change in shape of the nucleus to ovoid, nuclear chromatin clearing, nuclear membrane irregularities, and prominent nuclear grooves in these PTC nuclei. Several molecular alterations have been described for PTC, most common of which is a rearrangement of *RET/PTC* oncogene, particularly in patients who have been exposed to radiation. The activation of the *BRAF* gene accounts for approximately 45% of sporadic mutations resulting from increased *BRAF* kinase activity. (Papanicolaou stain)

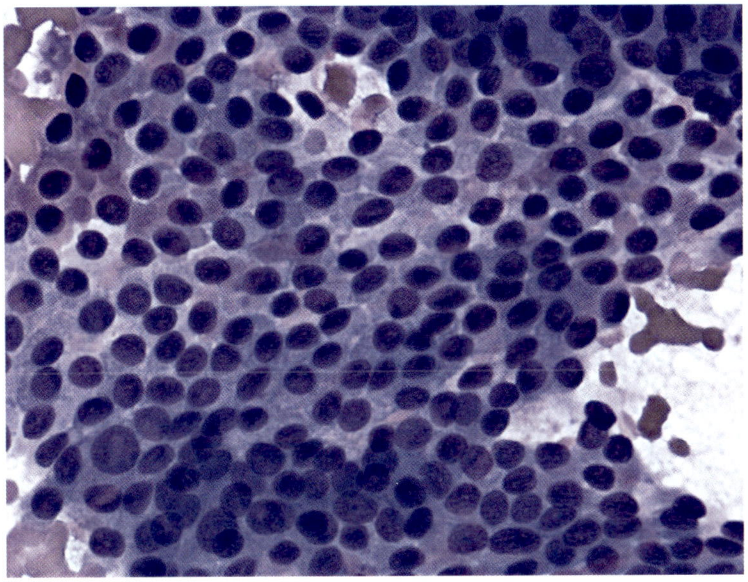

Figure 8.22 — Papillary Thyroid Carcinoma, FNA. PTC is a common malignant neoplasm with excellent clinical behavior, despite the presence of cervical lymph node metastases often seen with this tumor. While nuclear features, especially chromatin clearing, and grooves are better appreciated on alcohol fixed slides; those who routinely use air dried smears for thyroid cytology often appreciate nuclear grooves in these preparations as well. This is well illustrated in this case. (Diff Quik stain)

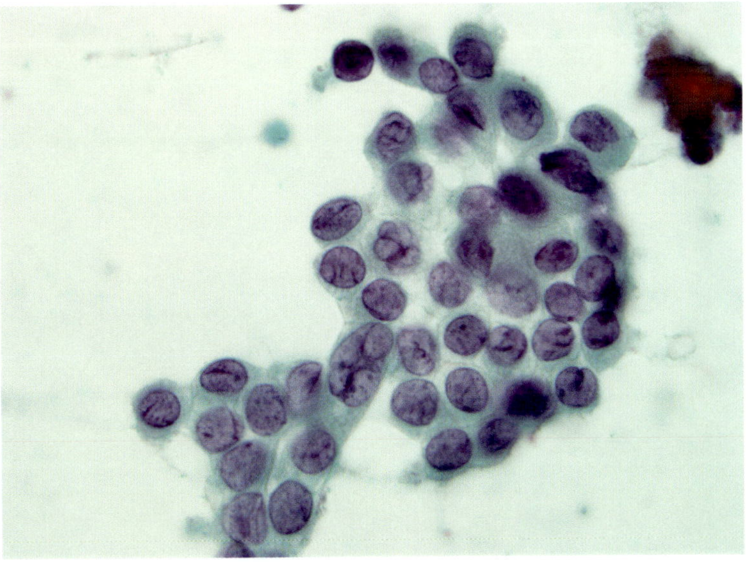

Figure 8.23 — Papillary Thyroid Carcinoma, FNA. This case shows multiple nuclear grooves and nuclear membrane irregularity. The latter is not a major diagnostic feature of PTC but when seen it is helpful in making a definitive diagnosis of PTC. Nuclear grooves are not specific and can be seen in a variety of other thyroid neoplasms and non-neoplastic lesions (such as Hashimoto thyroiditis). A calcification is seen on the right. Nuclear grooves and intranuclear cytoplasmic inclusions (INCI) are manifestations of the increased deformability of the PTC nucleus; resulting from a redundancy in nuclear membrane size causing infoldings. (Papanicolaou stain)

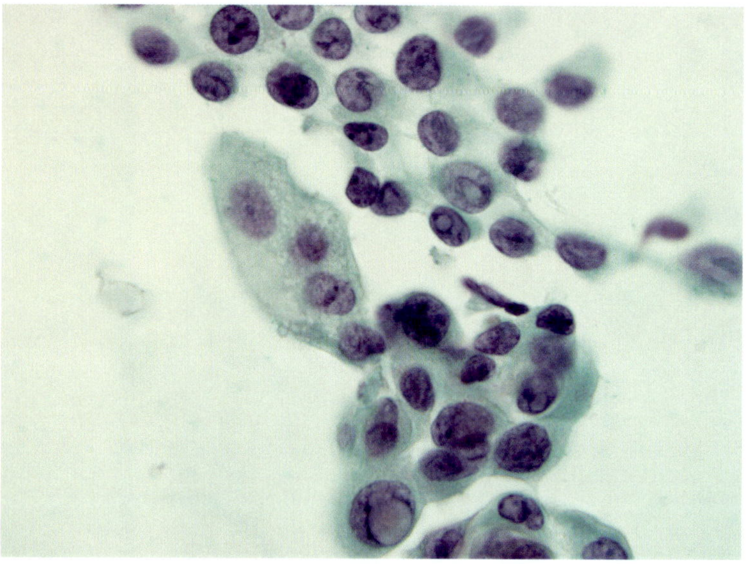

Figure 8.24a — Papillary Thyroid Carcinoma, FNA. INCI are considered to be one of the diagnostic nuclear features of PTC. The characteristic features of a true inclusion are: (a) matches the color and texture of the cytoplasm (b) has a sharply discrete border. While some authors have suggested a size criterion, we do not believe that size is an important feature. The aforementioned features help to distinguish INCIs from their common mimics: degenerative and artifactual vacuoles in the nucleus, fixation artifacts, and superimposed red blood cells (perhaps the most common reason for a "false" INCI). (Papanicolaou stain)

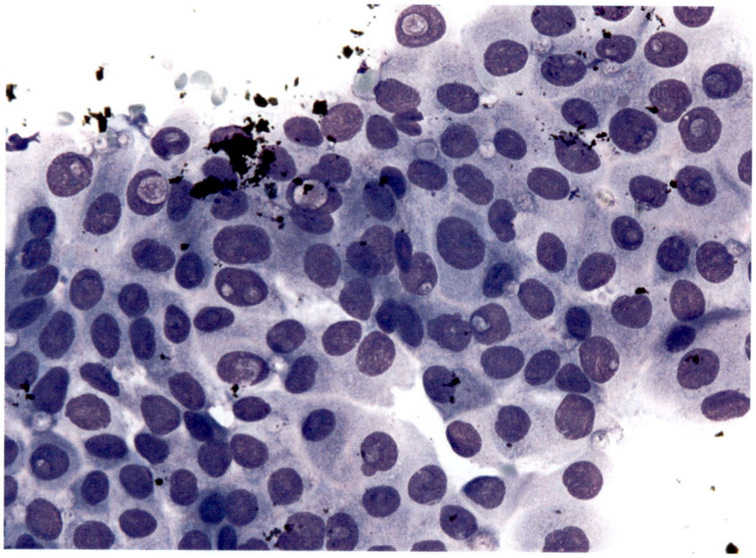

Figure 8.24b — Papillary Thyroid Carcinoma, FNA. Intranuclear inclusions in a PTC are best observed on Papanicolaou stain. However, occasionally PTC may display beautiful intranuclear inclusions on Diff Quik stain (as seen here). Notice the sharply punched out nuclear holes surrounded by margination of the chromatin creating "wire loops." Rare cells have multiple intranuclear inclusions (often considered a feature of tall-cell variant of PTC and referred to as "soap bubble" nucleus). This case, however, turned out to be a classic PTC. (Diff Quik stain)

Figure 8.25 — Papillary Thyroid Carcinoma, FNA. PTC with intranuclear cytoplasmic inclusions is illustrated here. It should be noted that intranuclear inclusions can be seen in medullary carcinoma, anaplastic carcinoma, hyalinizing trabecular adenoma, Hashimoto thyroiditis, and benign mesenchymal or cyst lining cells. Thus, their presence should not be used to diagnose PTC definitively in the absence of other major nuclear and minor diagnostic features. (Diff Quik stain)

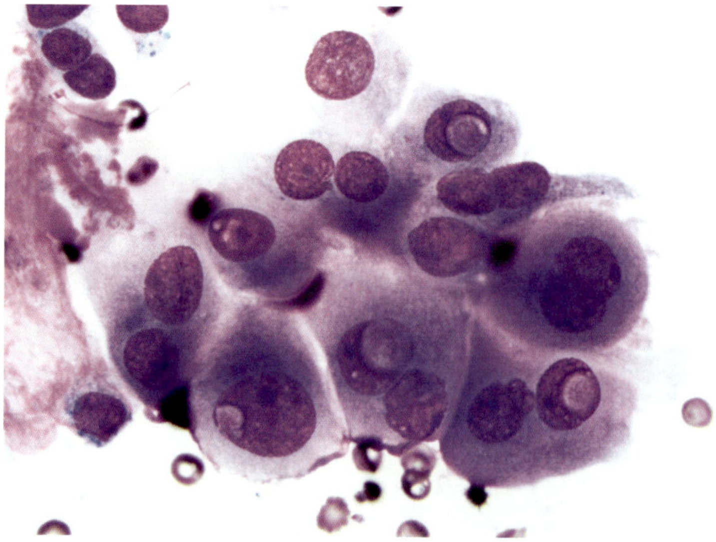

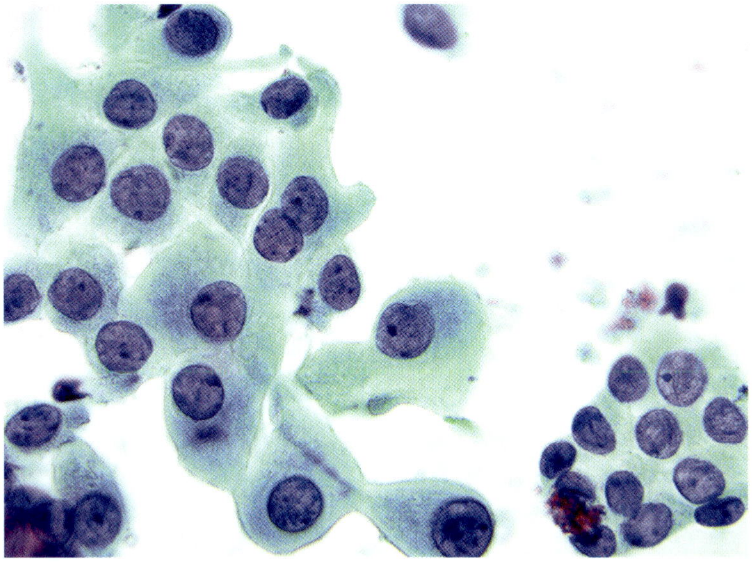

Figure 8.26 — Papillary Thyroid Carcinoma, FNA. PTC with pinpoint small nucleolus is shown here. The small nucleolus is also useful in distinguishing PTC from Hürthle cell neoplasms; Hürthle cells have a round nucleus with larger, centrally located nucleoli. The density of the cytoplasm is squamoid or dense in PTC; and granular in Hürthle cells. There is an oncocytic variant of PTC, however it is not common and for its diagnosis, one should be able to find the characteristic nuclear features of PTC (at least focally). (Papanicolaou stain)

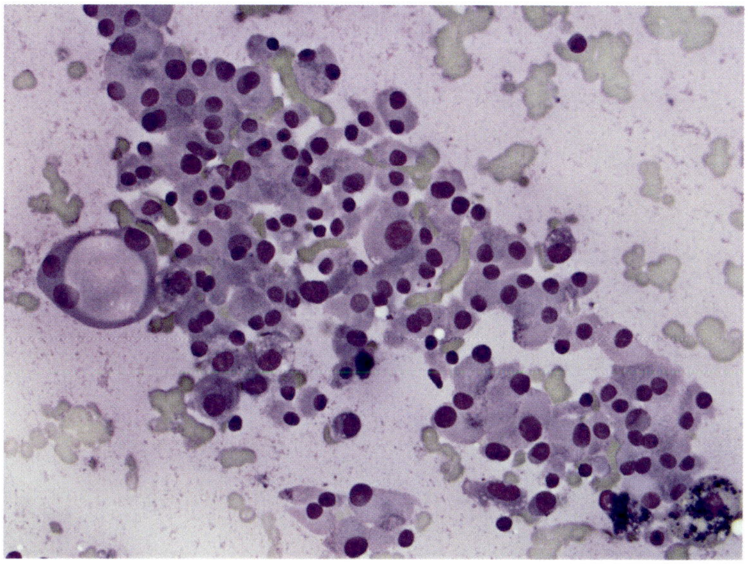

Figure 8.27 — Hürthle Cell Neoplasm, FNA. One of the differential diagnoses of PTC is a Hürthle cell neoplasm. Note the consistently lower N/C ratio of the cells, round nuclei, small to medium sized nucleoli, and cytoplasmic granularity. (Diff Quik stain)

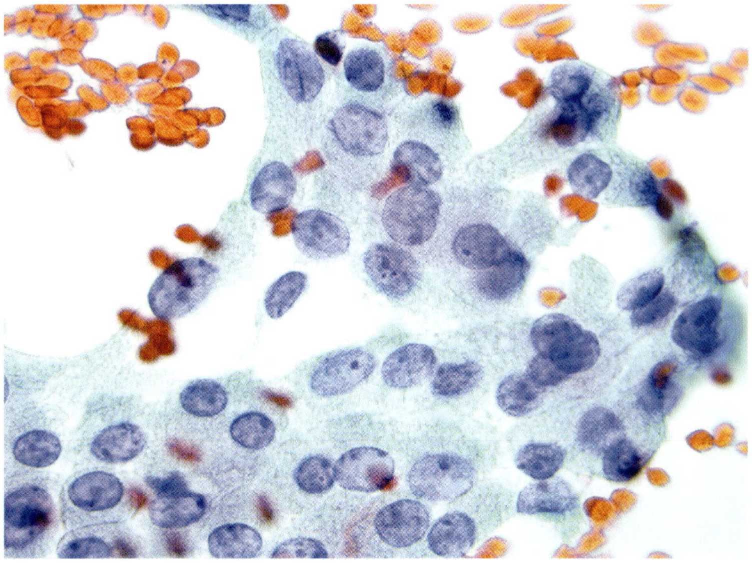

Figure 8.28 — Hashimoto Thyroiditis, FNA. Benign Hürthle cells in a gland with extensive chronic lymphocytic thyroiditis (CLT). The nuclei show features that overlap with PTC. It should be emphasized that Hürthle cells can show nuclear grooves and their presence alone should not elicit concern for PTC. Caution is warranted in diagnosing PTC in the presence of CLT. This case was called atypia of undetermined significance (AUS) and went to surgery. Histology showed florid thyroiditis without any concurrent PTC. Attention to the nuclear shape (mostly round) and cytoplasmic features (granularity) maybe helpful in such cases. (Papanicolaou stain)

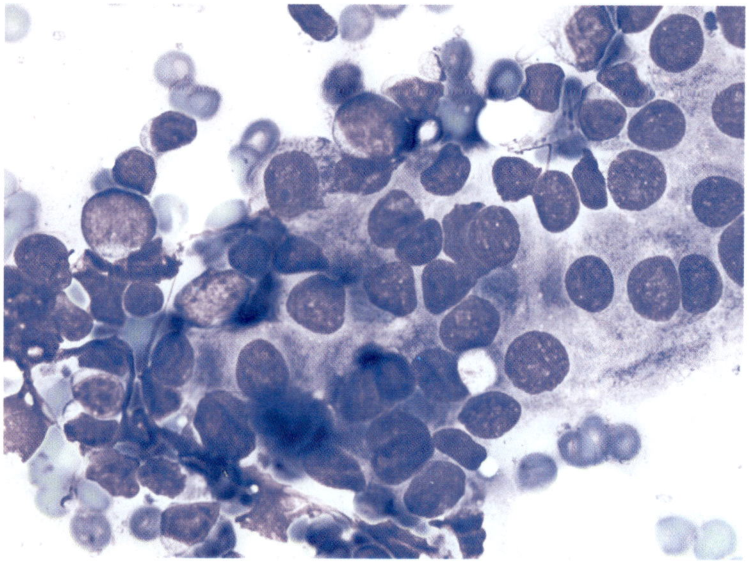

Figure 8.29 — Hashimoto Thyroiditis, FNA. Hürthle cell metaplasia in a case of chronic lymphocytic thyroiditis is illustrated here. Note lymphocytes on left with blue cytoplasmic rim. Hürthle cells can have grooves as seen in this case. Also note round nuclei, moderately large nucleoli, and granular cytoplasm in the Hürthle cells. (Diff Quik stain)

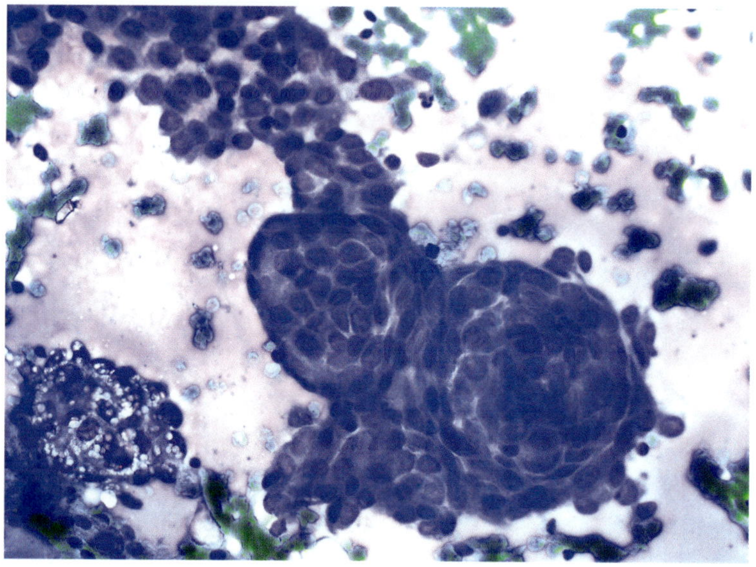

Figure 8.30a — Papillary Thyroid Carcinoma, FNA. Swirling of the tumor cells is a minor architectural diagnostic criterion for PTC. An additional useful diagnostic feature is seen in this and the next figure—flattening of the cells at the edge of the cell clusters. (Diff Quik stain)

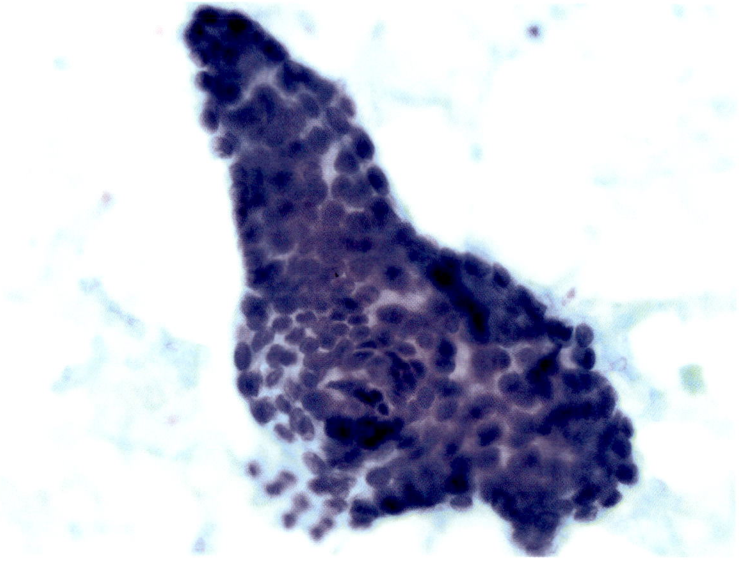

Figure 8.30b — Papillary Thyroid Carcinoma, FNA. This papillary-like fragment displays central swirling of the malignant cells. Another useful diagnostic feature for PTC is seen in this photomicrograph—flattening of the cells at the edge of the fragment. (Papanicolaou stain)

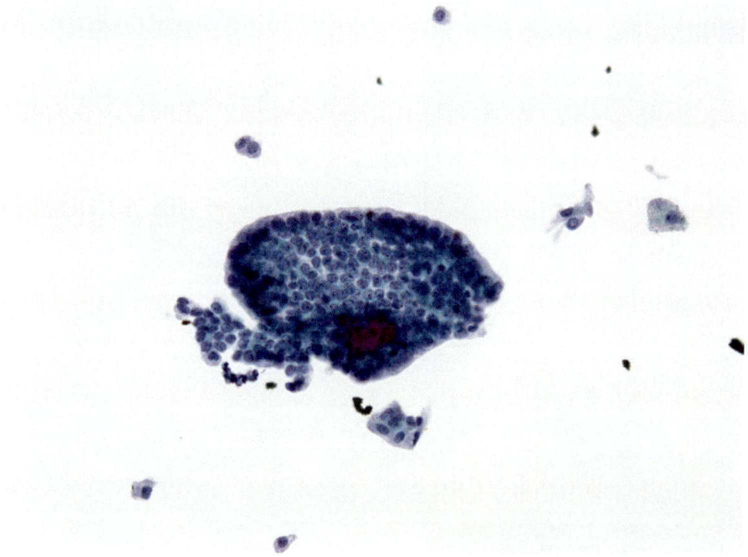

Figure 8.30c — Papillary Thyroid Carcinoma, FNA. A flat monolayered sheet of PTC is seen here. Notice the characteristic peripheral palisading of the nuclei, creating a "picket fence" architecture. (Liquid-based preparation, Papanicolaou stain)

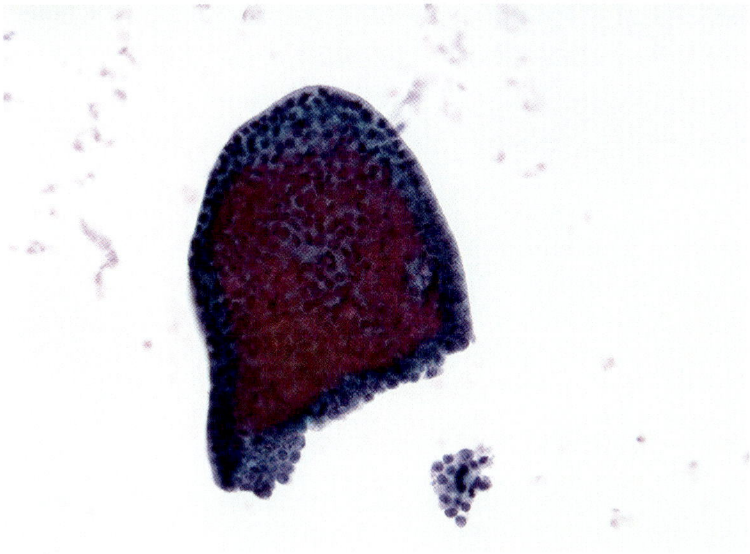

Figure 8.30d — Papillary Thyroid Carcinoma, FNA. This example illustrates the true anatomic edge of a papillary-like fragment of the tumor. Note cellular crowding, oval nuclei, finely granular chromatin, and nuclear palisading at the peripheral edges of the fragment. (Liquid-based preparation, Papanicolaou stain)

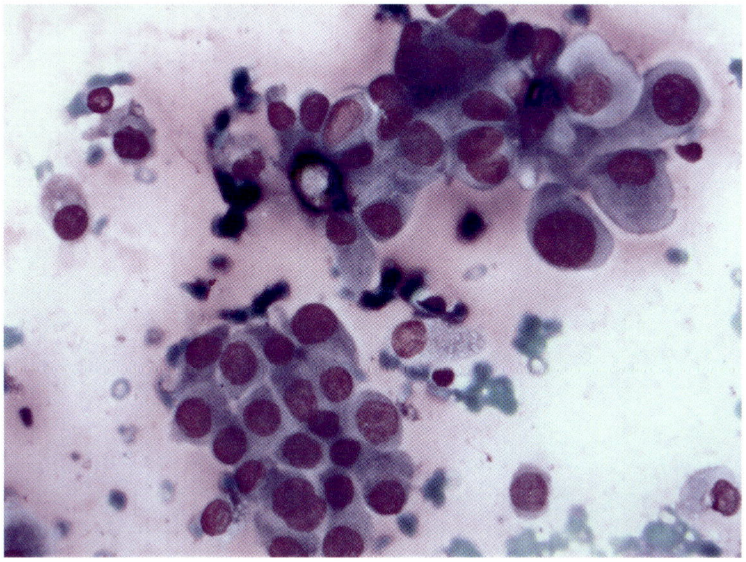

Figure 8.31a — Papillary Thyroid Carcinoma, FNA. Psammoma bodies (PBs) are also a minor diagnostic feature of PTC. They form at the tip of papillae due to avascular necrosis that occurs circumferentially resulting in the concentric lamellations seen in the classic psammoma body. PBs are less frequently observed in FNA samples of PTC (~5%–20% of cases) than in histologic specimens (up to 60%). PBs can be solitary or multiple/confluent, extrafollicular, or inside the follicular lumena. PBs alone are nonspecific and have been described in FNA samples of medullary carcinoma, Hashimoto thyroiditis, Graves disease, and adenomatoid nodules. (Diff Quik stain)

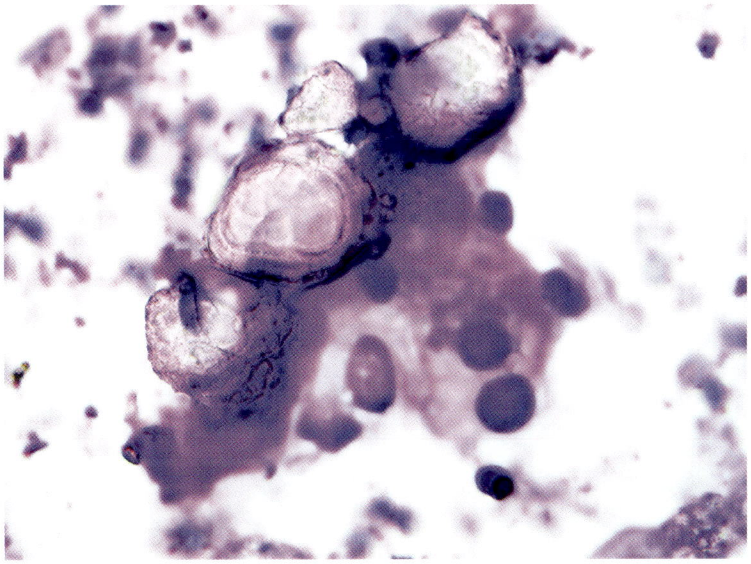

Figure 8.31b — Papillary Thyroid Carcinoma, FNA. While the presence of a psammoma body should elicit a search for cells diagnostic of PTC, by themselves they are not diagnostic of this malignancy. Psammoma bodies (PBs) are nonbirefringent, and composed of calcium phosphate. Studies have estimated the true positive predictive value of PBs for PTC at around 50% (when seen in isolation), whereas when PBs are seen in association with the cytologic features of PTC, the positive predictive value (PPV) goes up to almost 100%. (Diff Quik stain)

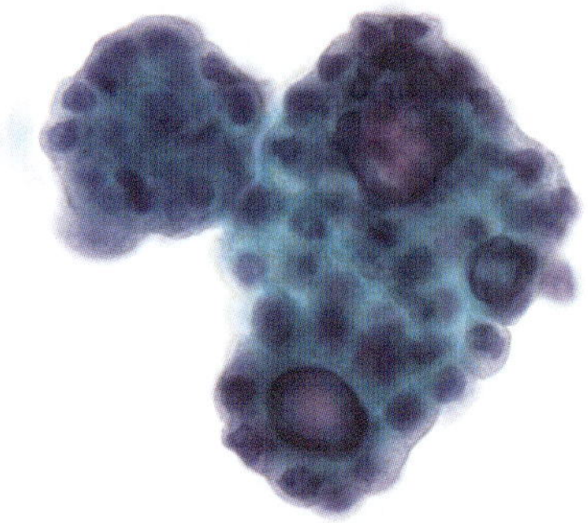

Figure 8.32a — Papillary Thyroid Carcinoma, FNA. Another illustration of multiple psammoma bodies in a PTC is shown here. The psammoma bodies are present within the lumina of the follicular structures. (Liquid-based preparation, Papanicolaou stain)

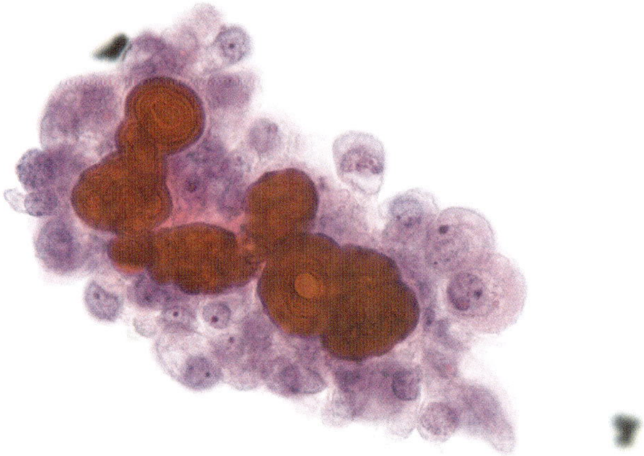

Figure 8.32b — Papillary Thyroid Carcinoma, FNA. The beauty of a liquid-based preparation in thyroid cytology is that it brings out the cellular details from the edges to the central cores of the epithelial fragments, as shown in this fragment of a PTC. Neoplastic cells surround numerous psammoma bodies which display the characteristic concentric lamellations. (Liquid-based preparation, Papanicolaou stain)

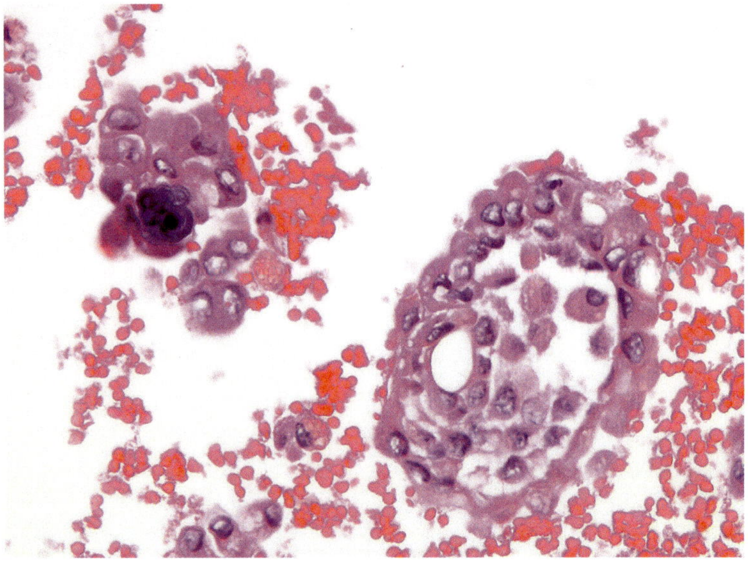

Figure 8.32c — Papillary Thyroid Carcinoma, FNA. Preparation of a cell block, especially in cystic cases is often useful in revealing papillae and/or psammomatous calcifications. Psammoma bodies appear as "microcalcifications" on ultrasound and their presence often triggers an FNA of the nodule. PBs are round microscopic calcific structures and represent a form of necrosis. Necrotic cells form the nidus for surrounding calcific deposition. PBs have a characteristic lammelated, concentric calcified structures and are sometimes large enough to be seen on radiologic scans. (H&E stain)

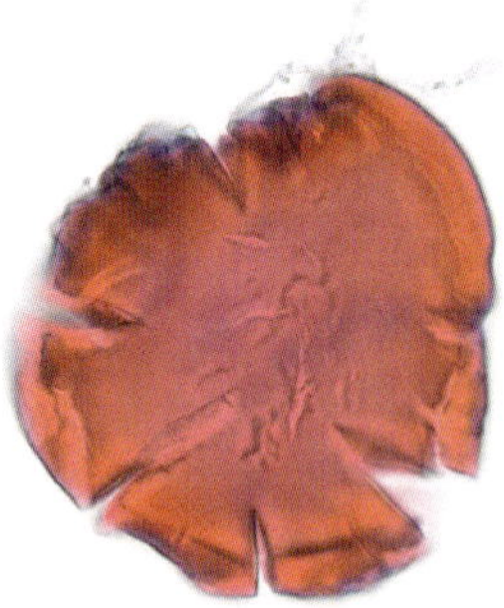

Figure 8.33 — Papillary Thyroid Carcinoma, FNA. Dense colloid in a configuration (radial fractures) may mimic a psammoma body, especially in suboptimally and overstained smears (as shown here). (Papanicolaou stain)

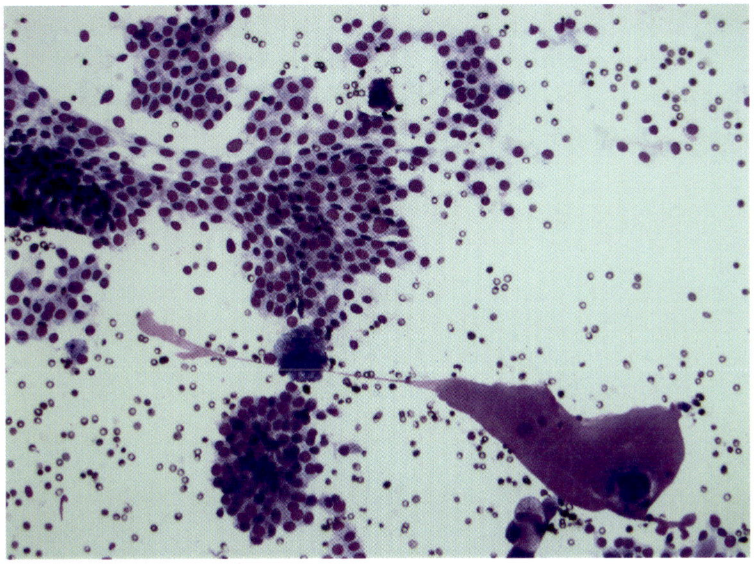

Figure 8.34 — Papillary Thyroid Carcinoma, FNA. Dense colloid, which appears as a magenta pink color on air dried smears and cytospins, can be an extremely useful minor diagnostic feature. It is also called "tooth paste" or "bubble gum" colloid because it "strings out" when smeared. The abnormal tenacious nature prevents an adequate smearing of this colloid on the glass slide, where it simply sits under the cover slip as a sticky glue-like material. This perhaps represents the so-called "bloody" or eosinophilic colloid seen in the histologic sections of PTC. (Diff Quik stain)

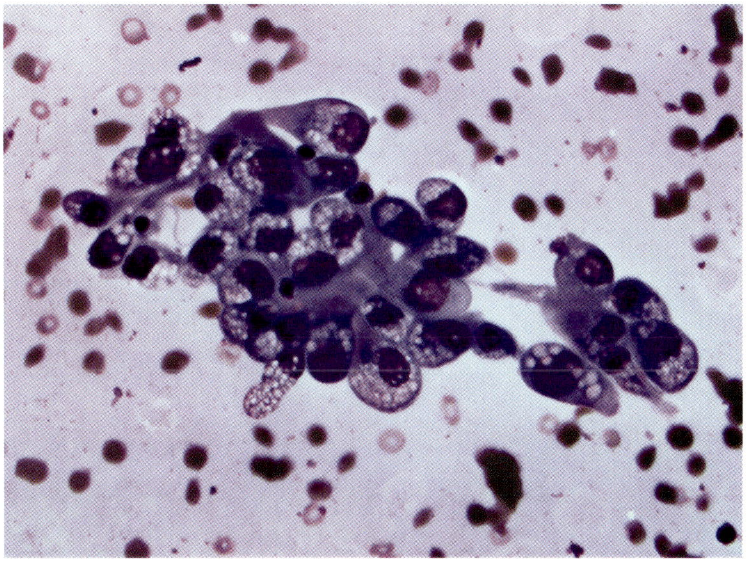

Figure 8.35a — Papillary Thyroid Carcinoma, FNA. "Bubblegum colloid" is specifically useful in cystic cases with a paucity of diagnostic epithelial cells. In this image, the colloid is seen sticking to degenerating tumor cells which contain cytoplasmic vacuoles. The combination should elicit a search for more diagnostic tumor cells. This phenomenon of cytoplasmic clearing is called "hypervacuolization," and is characteristic of PTC, cystic variant. The hypervacuolization is seen on both Diff Quik and Papanicolaou stains on direct smears as well as on liquid-based preparations. (Diff Quik stain)

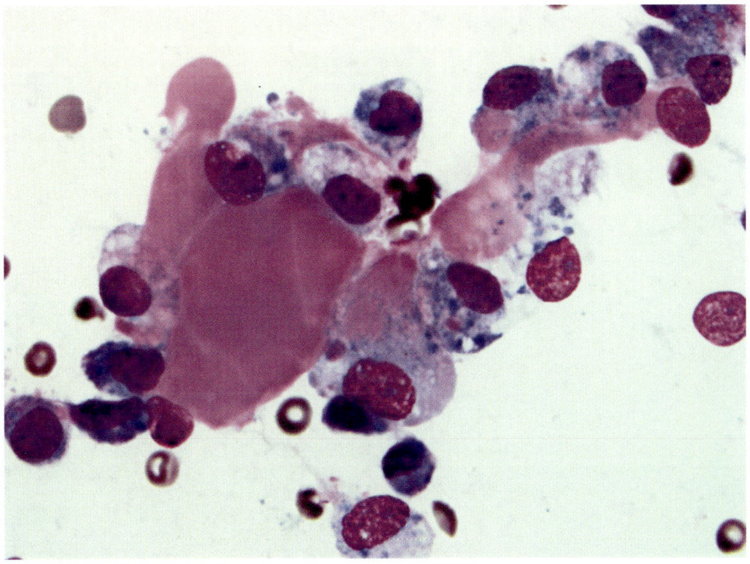

Figure 8.35b — Papillary Thyroid Carcinoma, FNA. On air dried smears the colloid in PTC can show a very specific "pink" color as seen in this image. In this cystic PTC, the "pink bubblegum colloid" is sticking to hemosiderin laden histiocytes. Such a finding is an important clue that the aspirate may represent cystic PTC and such cases should be carefully examined for other diagnostic features of PTC. (Diff Quik stain)

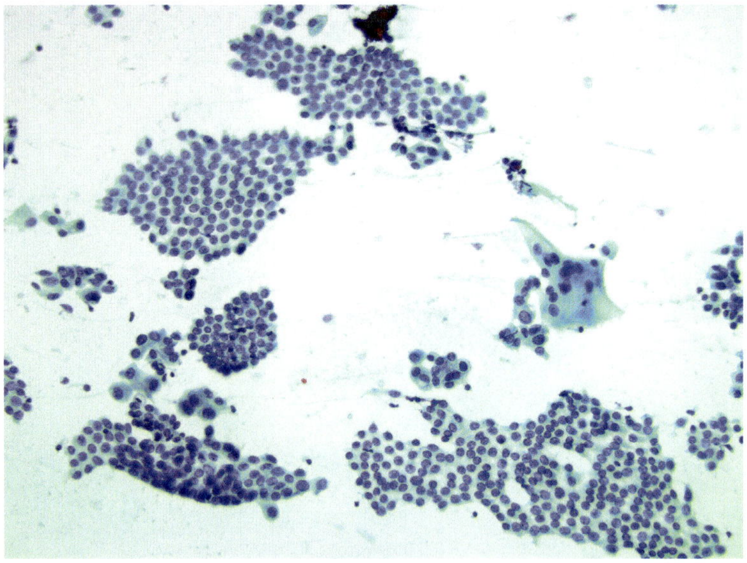

Figure 8.36 — Papillary Thyroid Carcinoma, FNA. Multinucleated giant (MNG) cells are also considered a minor (background) diagnostic feature of PTC. They usually have dense cytoplasm. Immunohistochemical studies have suggested a histiocytic origin; however electron microscopy studies suggest that some of them are tumor giant cells. MNG cells are commonly seen in aspirates of PTC (both in cystic and solid variants). These cells are not specific for PTC and have been observed routinely in other benign and malignant lesions of the thyroid. MNG cells can be very large, containing few to many nuclei and represent response of the host immune system to the lesional cells. (Papanicolaou stain)

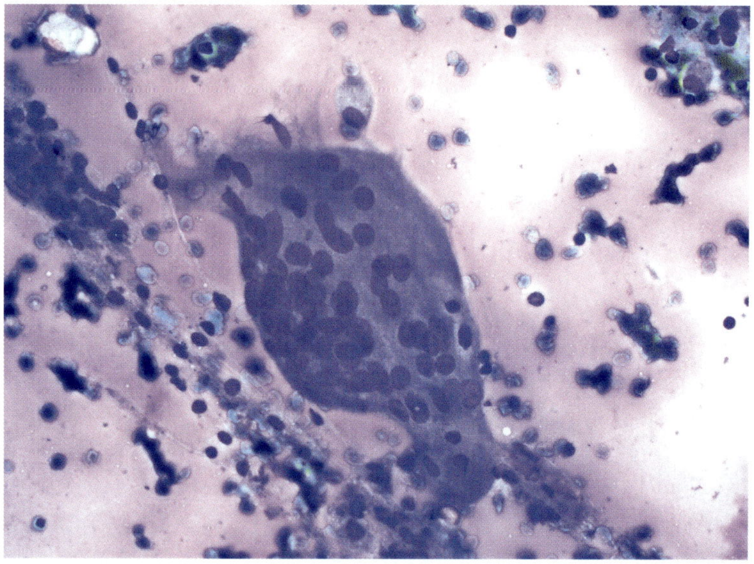

Figure 8.37 — Papillary Thyroid Carcinoma, FNA. Multinucleated giant cells are not specific for any thyroid entity. They can be seen in several benign and malignant thyroid lesions including chronic lymphocytic thyroiditis, DeQuervain's (subacute thyroiditis), cystic change in benign or neoplastic nodules, and anaplastic carcinoma. This particular giant cell is from a PTC. (Diff Quik stain)

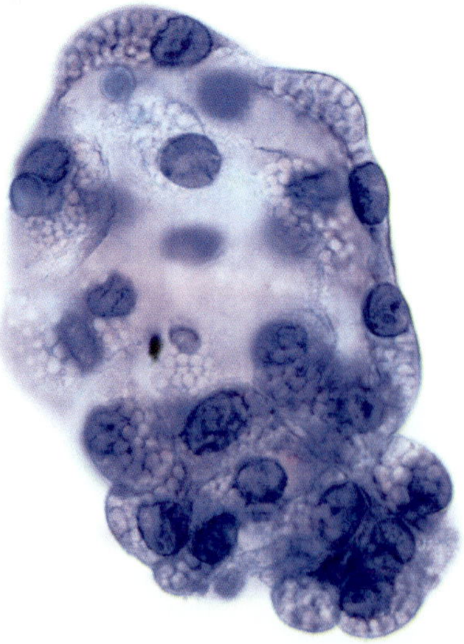

Figure 8.38a — Papillary Thyroid Carcinoma, FNA. Cystic PTC cells often show degenerative vacuoles or cellular "hypervacuolization." Some authors have described these cells to be "histiocytoid" in nature. A useful feature in recognizing these cells correctly and distinguishing them from histiocytic cells is that the vacuoles often have sharply defined edges as opposed to the "fluffy" vacuoles in histiocytes. Nuclei may display some or all of the features of PTC including well-formed INCIs. Notice the clean and transparent smear background reflecting the presence of thin degenerated cystic fluid which is often hard to retain or fix on the glass slide surface. (Papanicolaou stain)

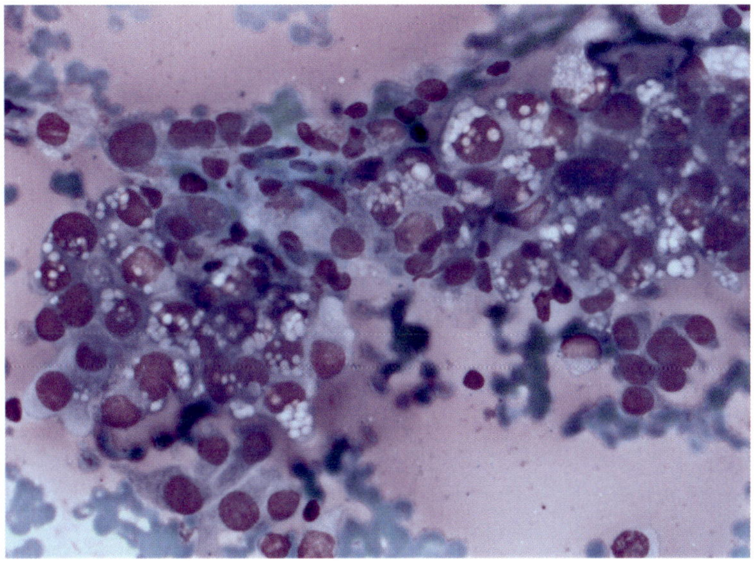

Figure 8.38b — Papillary Thyroid Carcinoma, FNA. PTC, cystic variant is seen here. Notice the hypervacuolization of cell cytoplasm due to the presence of innumerable small vacuoles. Neoplastic cells disclose some nuclear features of PTC (oval nuclei, fine chromatin, and occasional grooves). A second component of macrophages is often present with cytoplasmic vacuolization; however, the histiocytic nuclei appear markedly different from the nuclei of PTC cells. (Diff Quik stain)

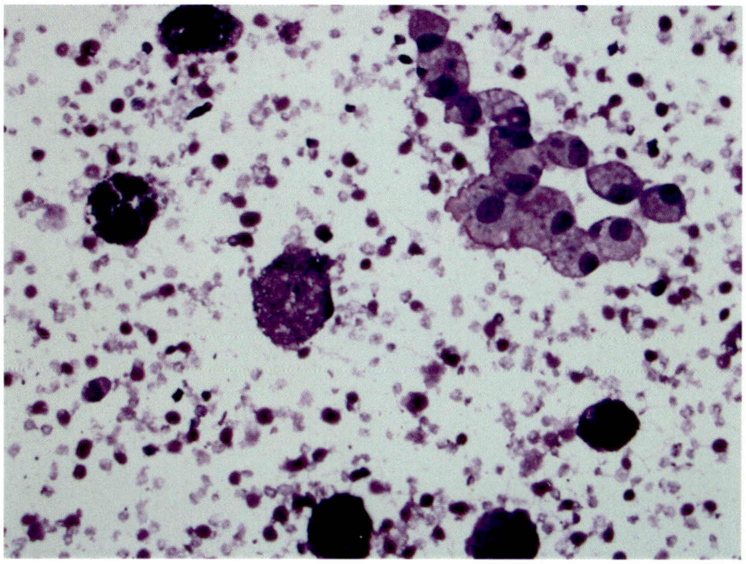

Figure 8.39a — Papillary Thyroid Carcinoma, FNA. The cystic variant of PTC is shown here. "Histiocytoid" cells are degenerated PTC cells that resemble histiocytes. A useful feature is that the nuclei are too plump to be histiocytes and some similar cells have denser cytoplasm than would be expected in histiocytes. A combination of several minor diagnostic features—sharply delineated cytoplasmic vacuoles, "bubble gum" colloid and psammomatous calcifications, and histiocytoid cells are useful clues in diagnosing a cystic papillary carcinoma. (Diff Quik stain)

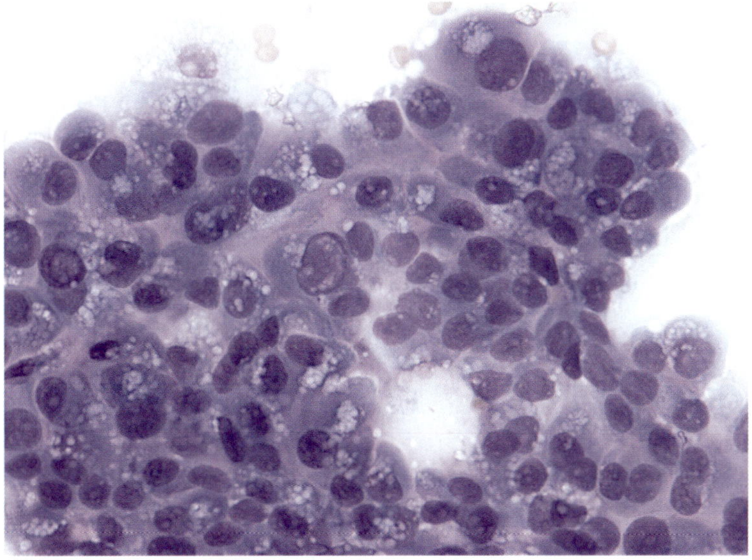

Figure 8.39b — Papillary Thyroid Carcinoma, FNA. In this particular example, the nuclei of the hypervacuolated "histiocytoid" cells have convincing resemblance to the nuclei of PTC. Multiple intranuclear inclusions are nicely visualized. Few hemosiderin-laden macrophages and thin cystic fluid are observed in the smear background. (Diff Quik stain)

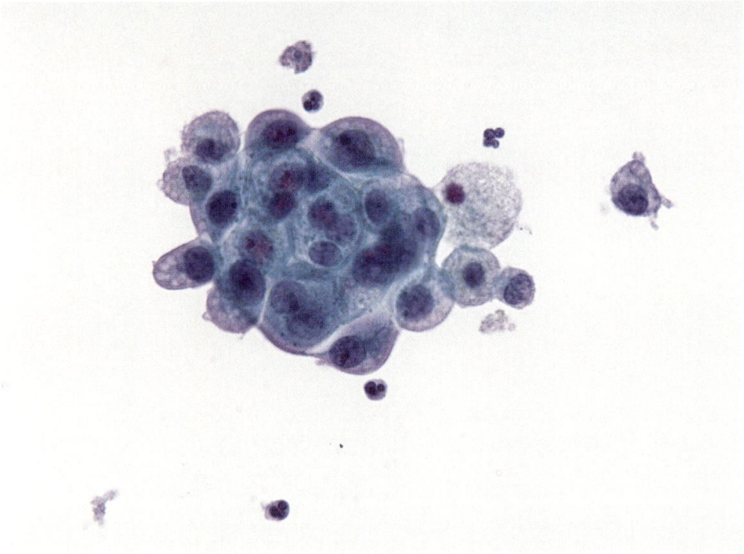

Figure 8.39c — Papillary Thyroid Carcinoma, FNA. The histiocytoid nature of the cystic variant of PTC is further enhanced in liquid-based preparations, as seen here. Notice the soap bubble cytoplasm resembling a macrophage. However, nuclear features clearly support an epithelial cell origin. Occasionally, cells at the edges of the fragments display focal nuclear protrusions creating a "hob nail" appearance. (Liquid-based preparation, Papanicolaou stain)

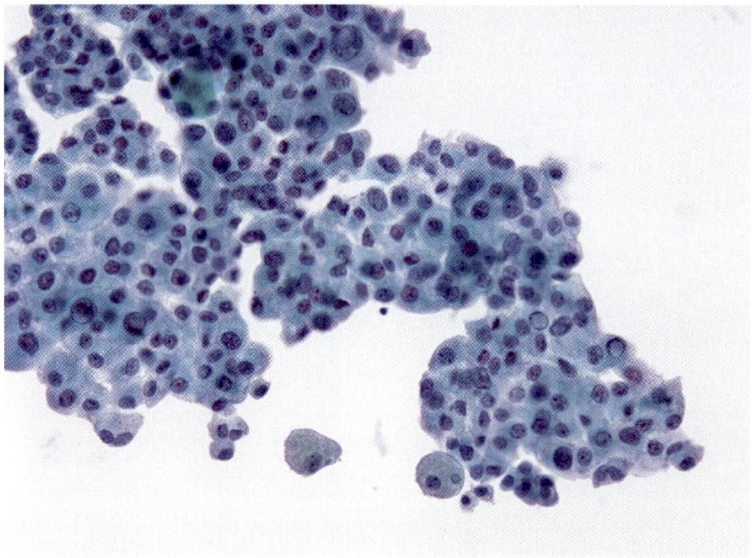

Figure 8.39d — Papillary Thyroid Carcinoma, FNA. Classic appearance of a cystic variant of PTC is illustrated here. Cells have an amazing resemblance to macrophages due to voluminous, finely vacuolated cytoplasm. However, numerous eye catching intranuclear inclusions dominate this image. (Liquid-based preparation, Papanicolaou stain)

Figure 8.39e — Papillary Thyroid Carcinoma, FNA. Similar to the previous case, this cystic PTC shows a cystic smear background with clear watery fluid and contains rare loose aggregates of histiocytoid cells depicting the phenomenon of "hypervacuolization." Diagnostic feature however, are the numerous intranuclear inclusions. (Papanicolaou stain)

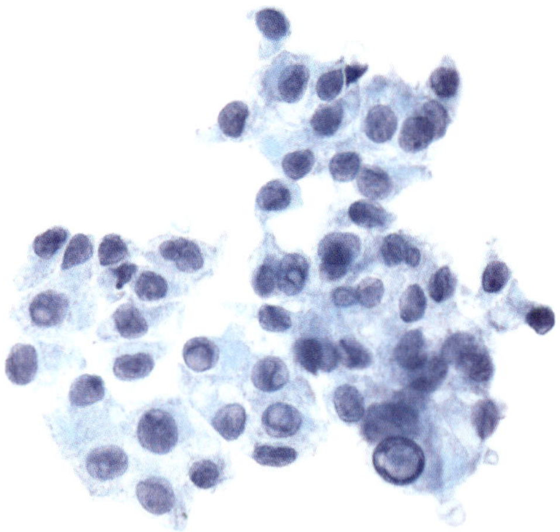

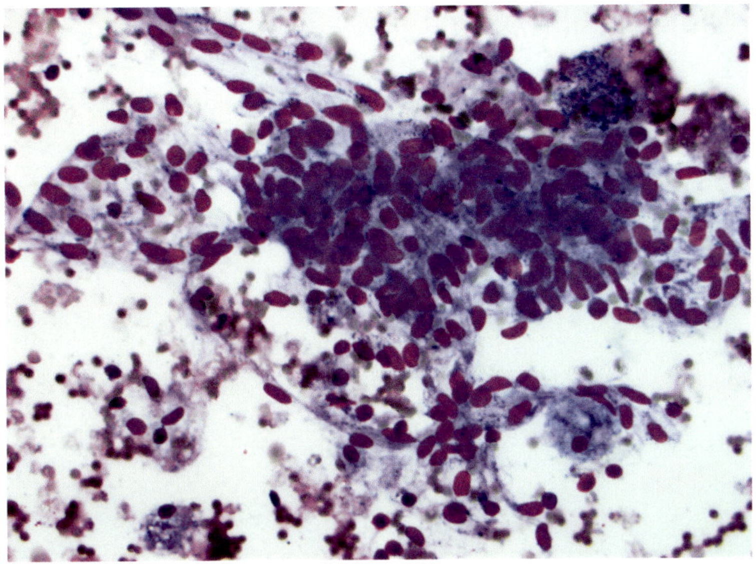

Figure 8.40 — Reactive Fibroblasts (in repair), FNA. Benign mesenchymal cells containing hemosiderin pigment in a cystic aspirate are shown here. This is a manifestation of repair and can be seen in any benign or malignant case with cystic change. The elongated cells are characteristic of mesenchymal cells and should not be confused with ovoid PTC cells. Some of them display blue granules in their cytoplasm. Mesenchymal cells can have nuclear grooves and rarely, intranuclear inclusions. (Diff Quik stain)

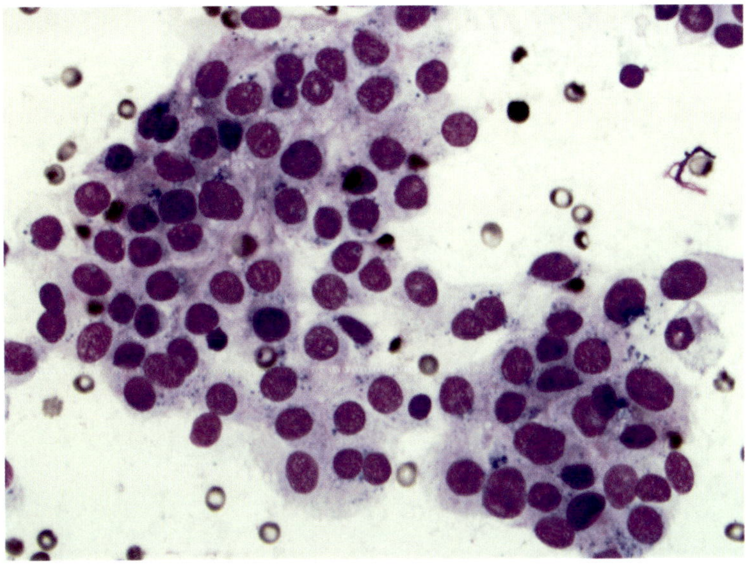

Figure 8.41 — Papillary Thyroid Carcinoma, FNA. PTC tumor cells can contain the intracytoplasmic "blue granules," as illustrated in this case. The presence of the "blue granules" should not detract from making a diagnosis of PTC. Note the PTC nuclear features and a flat monolayered architecture. (Diff Quik stain)

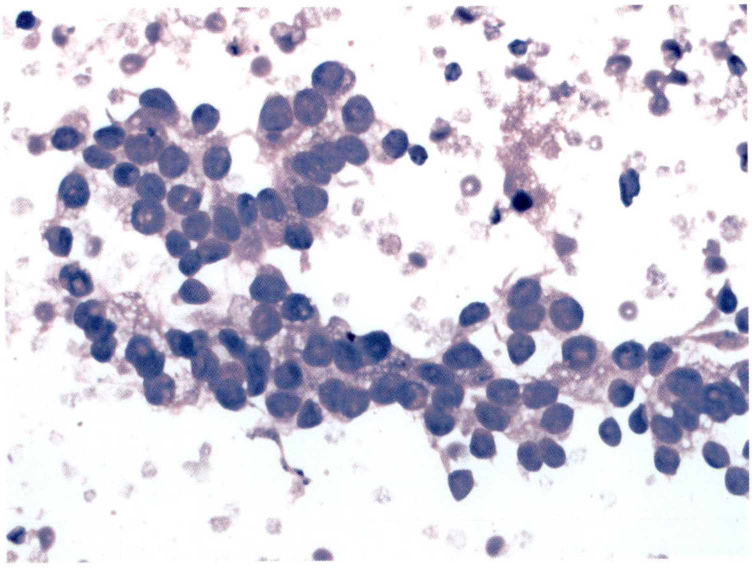

Figure 8.42 — Papillary Thyroid Carcinoma, FNA. Degenerative nuclear pseudoinclusions in a cystic PTC are seen here. The border is not well defined and the color does not match that of the cell cytoplasm. Smear background suggest cystic degeneration. (Diff Quik stain)

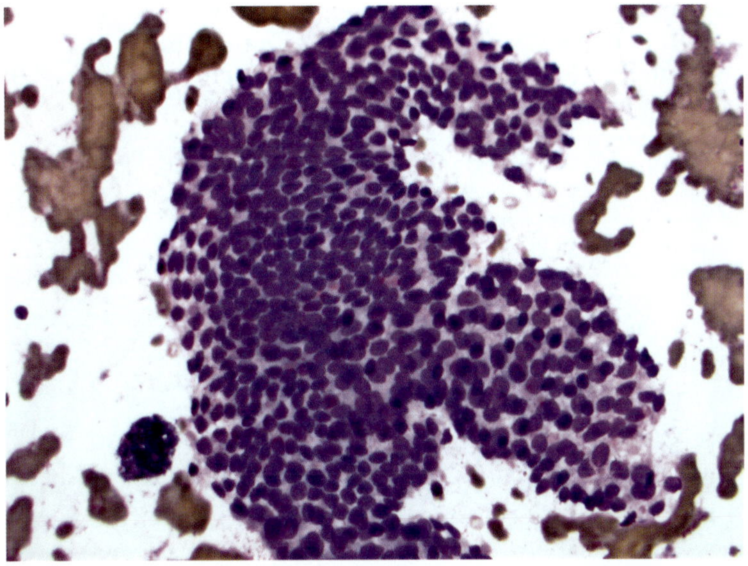

Figure 8.43 — Papillary Thyroid Carcinoma, FNA. PTC showing a syncytial sheet in the center with focal cellular swirls, as well as microfollicle formations at the edges. Admixture of various architectural patterns is not unusual in PTC. (Diff Quik stain)

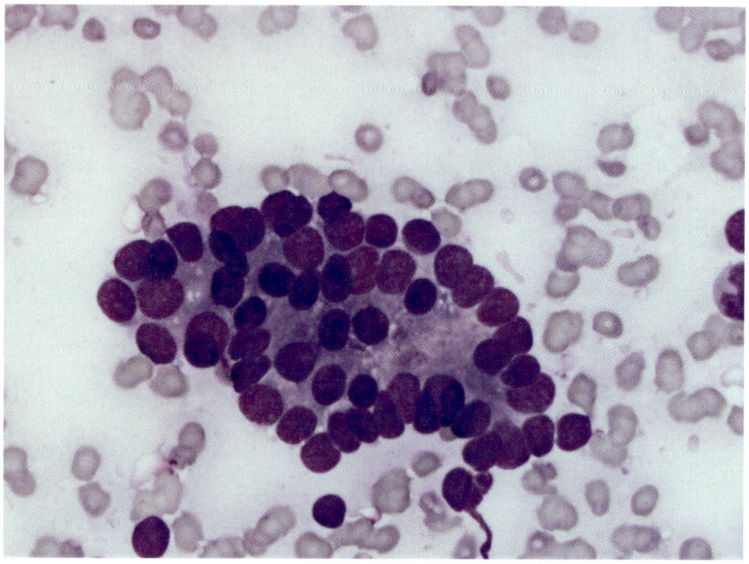

Figure 8.44 — Papillary Thyroid Carcinoma, FNA. TBSRTC defines the follicular variant of PTC (FVPTC) as "a variant of PTC in which the tumor is completely or almost completely composed of small to medium-sized follicles lined by cells with the nuclear features of a PTC." Patients with follicular variant of PTC often present with a larger tumor size and at a younger age than patients with conventional PTC. This image from a FVPTC case displays a microfollicle with enlarged, overlapping nuclei, many of which are elongated. Based only on architecture, assuming this were the predominant pattern, such a case may be called follicular neoplasm. However, attention to the nuclear features—shape, chromatin, grooves, inclusions—will allow a more specific diagnosis of follicular variant of PTC, cytologic and histologic diagnosis was FVPTC. FVPTC is the third most common type of PTC, following conventional papillary thyroid carcinoma and papillary microcarcinoma. (Diff Quik stain)

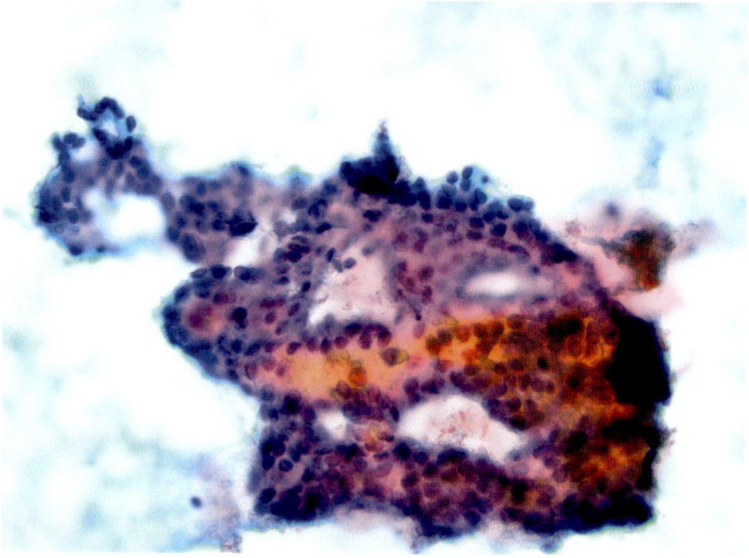

Figure 8.45 — Papillary Thyroid Carcinoma, FNA. Trabecular pattern of follicular variant of PTC is shown here. At low magnification this is often called follicular neoplasm. Assessment of nuclear features of PTC is essential. These may be focal in FVPTC; and certain features, particularly nuclear inclusions and psammoma bodies and multinucleated giant cells are less frequently seen than in the follicular variant of PTC. FVPTC tends to display more favorable clinicopathological features than conventional PTC. However, the long-term clinical outcome of FVPTC patients is somewhat similar to that of conventional PTC patients. (Papanicolaou stain)

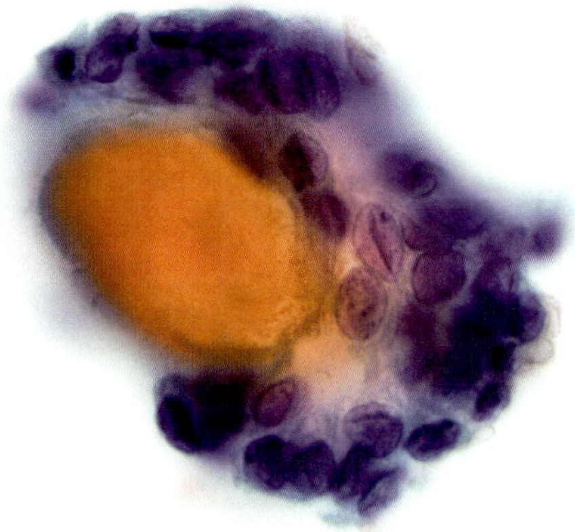

Figure 8.46a — Papillary Thyroid Carcinoma, FNA. Additional high power examination is warranted to make a diagnosis of PTC in cases of the follicular variant. At higher magnifications, the oval shape of the nucleus, nuclear grooves, and chromatin clearing are diagnostic of PTC. This is an important step for the pathologist to take because in the case of a solitary nodule, lobectomy is done for follicular neoplasm and a near total thyroidectomy for a follicular variant of PTC in most centers in the United States. (Papanicolaou stain)

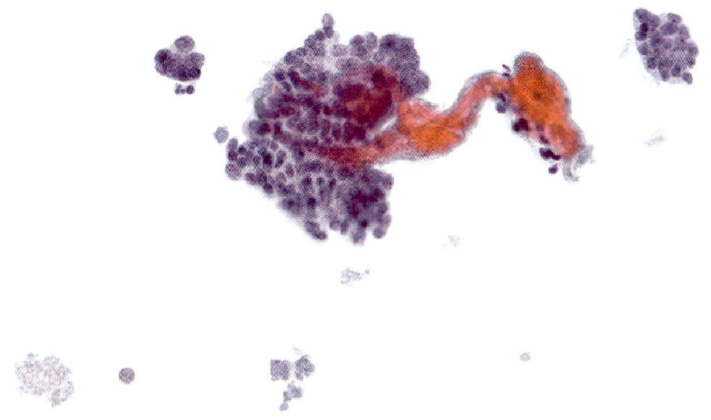

Figure 8.46b — Papillary Thyroid Carcinoma, FNA. FVPTC displays the thick tenacious and stringy colloid resembling a fibrous core, associated with fragments of malignant cells. Notice the vague microfollicular pattern. Nuclear features are well-developed. (Liquid-based preparation, Papanicolaou stain)

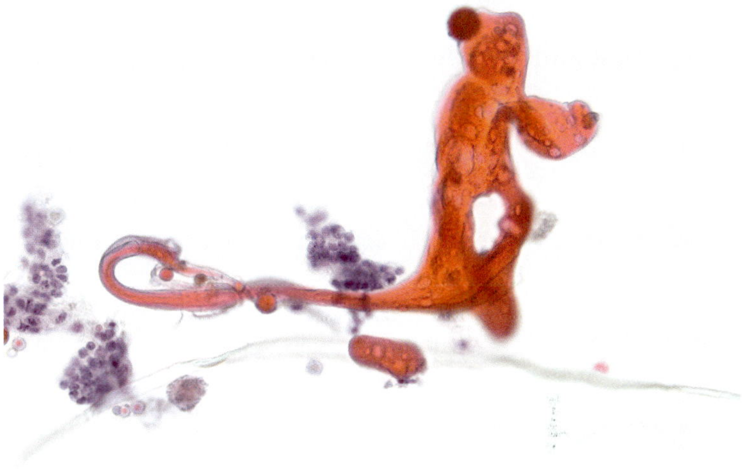

Figure 8.46c — Papillary Thyroid Carcinoma, FNA. Another field from the previous case demonstrates the appearance of the abnormally thick and sticky colloid often observed in FVPTC. Few fragments of malignant cells are present in the background. (Liquid-based preparation, Papanicolaou stain)

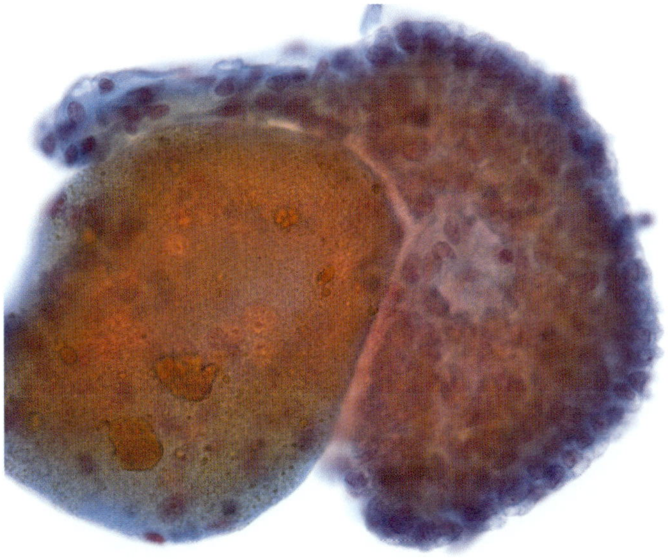

Figure 8.46d — Papillary Thyroid Carcinoma, FNA. FVPTC illustrating a thick and sticky glob of colloid juxtaposed to a follicle-forming fragment of malignant epithelium showing classic PTC nuclear features. (Liquid-based preparation, Papanicolaou stain)

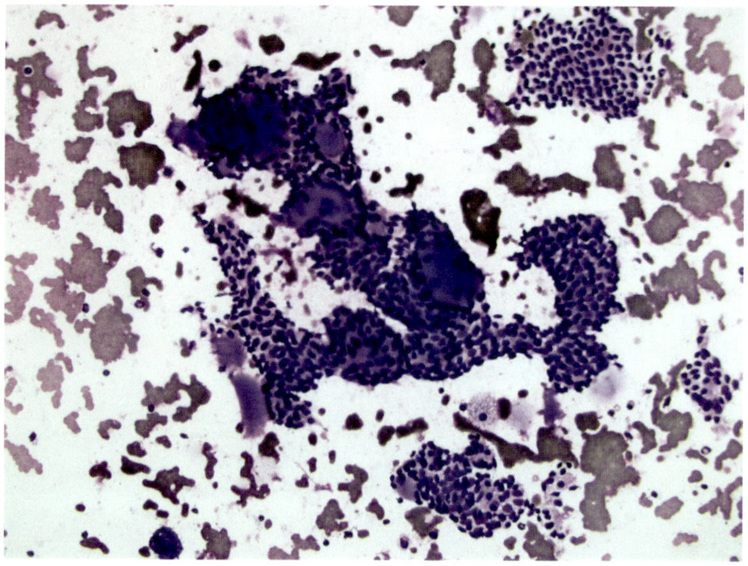

Figure 8.47a — Papillary Thyroid Carcinoma, FNA. A low power image of a follicular variant of PTC is shown here. There is scant colloid and a microfollicular pattern. Nuclei are clearly oval in shape and display features of PTC (pale chromatin, longitudinal grooves). Some studies have shown that managing these patients with total thyroidectomy is not necessary in all cases, thereby decreasing the number of total thyroidectomies. However, there is other evidence to support total thyroidectomy in FVPTC patients. The latter studies clearly demonstrate that recurrence rates are lower after total thyroidectomy because PTC may be characterized by a multinodular and bilobar disease. (Diff Quik stain)

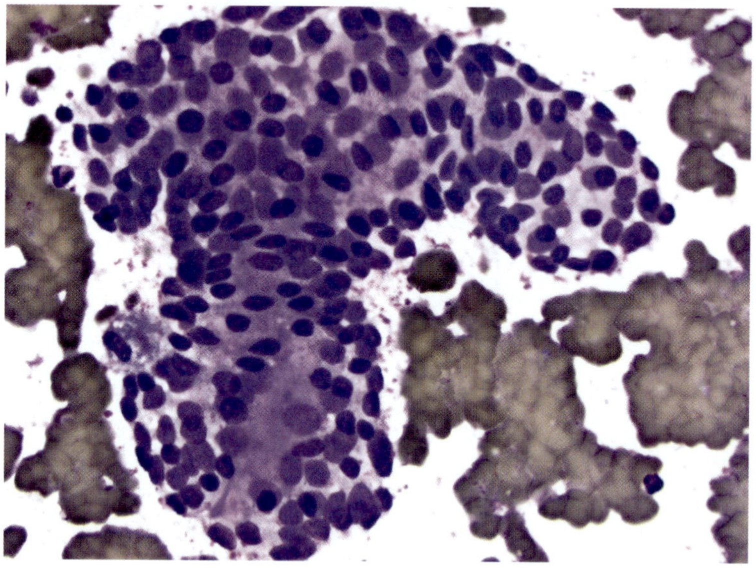

Figure 8.47b — Papillary Thyroid Carcinoma, FNA. A higher magnification of the previous case of a follicular variant of PTC displays nuclei that are oval and have other features of PTC (pale chromatin, longitudinal grooves). FVPTC is not an easy interpretation at the microscope even in surgical pathology. Studies have demonstrated the concordance rate for the diagnosis of FVPTC amongst endocrine pathologists to be less than 40%. Therefore, it's not surprising that almost 15% to 22% of cases that are diagnosed as "suspicious for a follicular neoplasm" on FNA eventuate in a FVPTC diagnosis. The vast majority of FVPTC are composed of microfollicles; however, some FVPTCs are composed of normal-sized follicles. (Diff Quik stain)

Figure 8.47c — Papillary Thyroid Carcinoma, FNA. A classic appearance of FVPTC is shown here. Malignant cells clearly form a follicular pattern and contain central globs of inspissated colloid. However, nuclei are oval and focally display PTC characteristics. A substantial number of FVPTC cases are initially misdiagnosed as "suspicious for a follicular neoplasm" before a lobectomy is done. (Diff Quik stain)

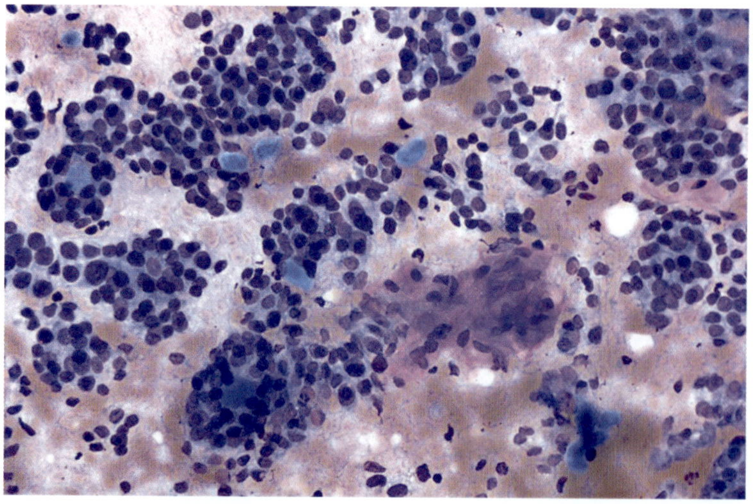

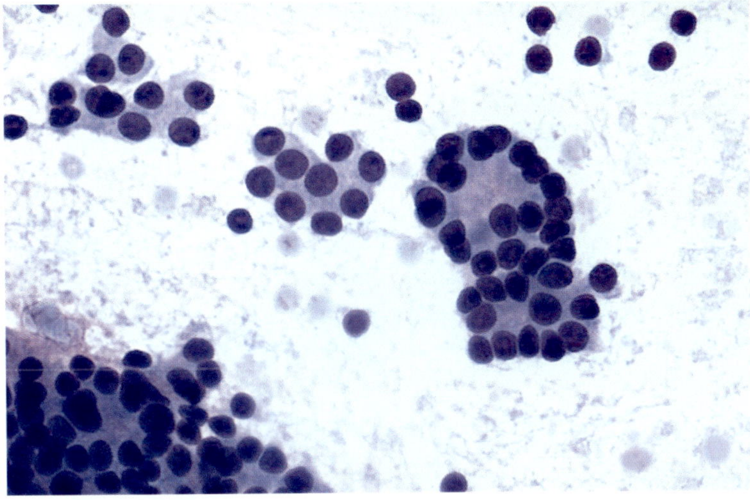

Figure 8.47d — Papillary Thyroid Carcinoma, FNA. Another example of FVPTC is shown here at higher magnification. This case was initially misdiagnosed as a follicular neoplasm on FNA due to a predominant microfollicular architecture. Occasional nuclei are ovoid in shape. Nuclear features of PTC were only focally noticed on retrospective review in this difficult case. (Diff Quik stain)

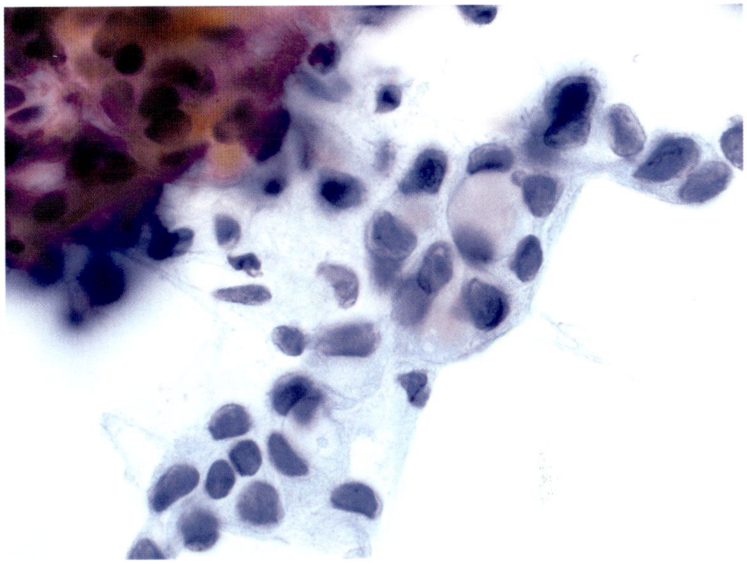

Figure 8.48a — Papillary Thyroid Carcinoma, FNA. This case of follicular variant of PTC shows clear cytoplasm that appears almost "mucinous." However the intracellular appearing substance is colloid in the lumen of microfollicles. Nuclei display characteristic features of a PTC. (Papanicolaou stain)

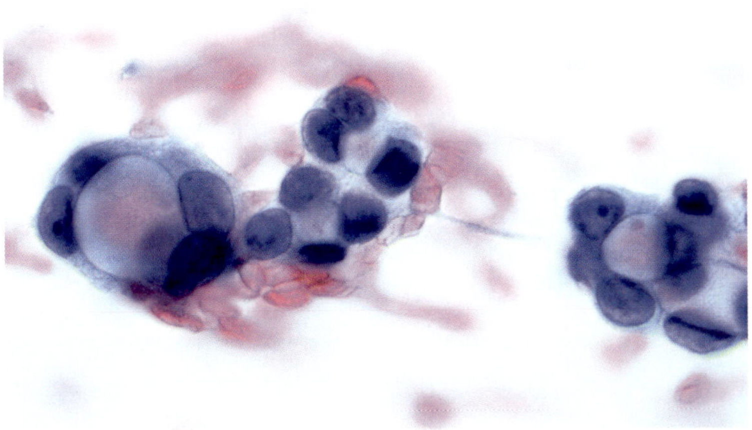

Figure 8.48b — Papillary Thyroid Carcinoma, FNA. FVPTCs are composed primarily, if not exclusively, of follicles rather than papillae. At higher magnification, these microfollicles show nuclear features diagnostic of PTC. FVPTC is an important member of a group of thyroid lesions known as "follicular patterned lesions" (adenomatoid nodule, follicular neoplasm, and FVPTC). There is a huge variation in the amount of nuclear features seen in a FVPTC cases. Some FVPTCs have qualitatively and quantitatively abundant classic nuclear features of PTC whereas, in others the features are only partially and focally observed. (Papanicolaou stain)

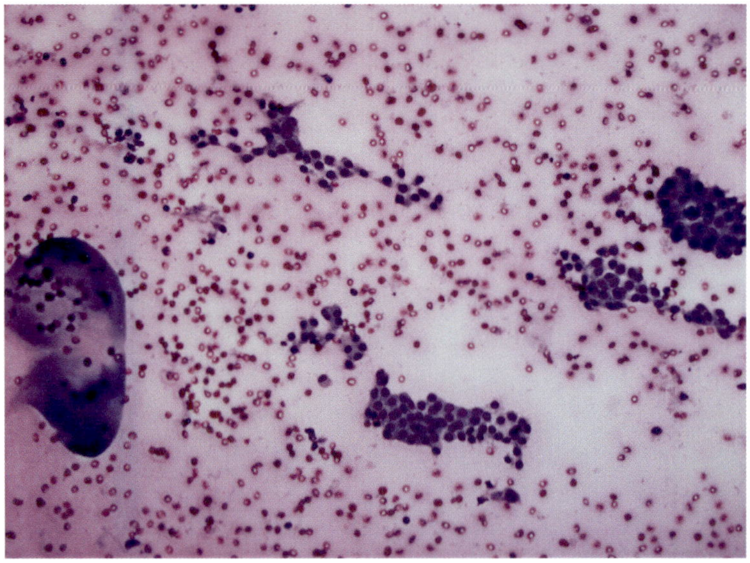

Figure 8.49 — Papillary Thyroid Carcinoma, FNA. Abundant colloid and sheets of follicular cells seen at low magnification can be misinterpreted as a benign hyperplastic/adenomatoid nodule. However when looking at it critically, the sheets show nuclear enlargement and overlap, warranting further high power examination to exclude a macrofollicular neoplasm. (Diff Quik stain)

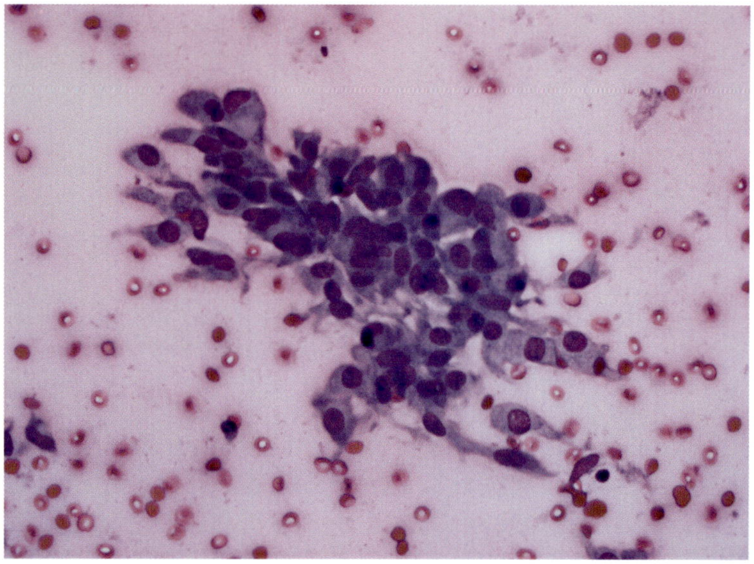

Figure 8.50 — Papillary Thyroid Carcinoma, FNA. Higher magnification shows elongated, enlarged nuclei with nuclear grooves. This was diagnosed as suspicious for macrofollicular variant of PTC, which also turned out to be the final surgical diagnosis. Macrofollicular variant of PTC is rare; however it represents an important cause of false negative diagnosis in PTC. The interobserver reproducibility is also poor on histology since diagnostic features tend to be very focal and the low power macrofollicular architecture suggests a benign nodule. (Diff Quik stain)

Figure 8.51a — Papillary Thyroid Carcinoma, FNA. Occasionally PTC may present in a predominantly dissociated cell pattern as seen here. Distinction from medullary carcinoma is important in such cases, since intranuclear inclusions and giant cells can be seen in both tumors. Attention to the chromatin is the key in distinguishing PTC from medullary carcinoma. (Papanicolaou stain)

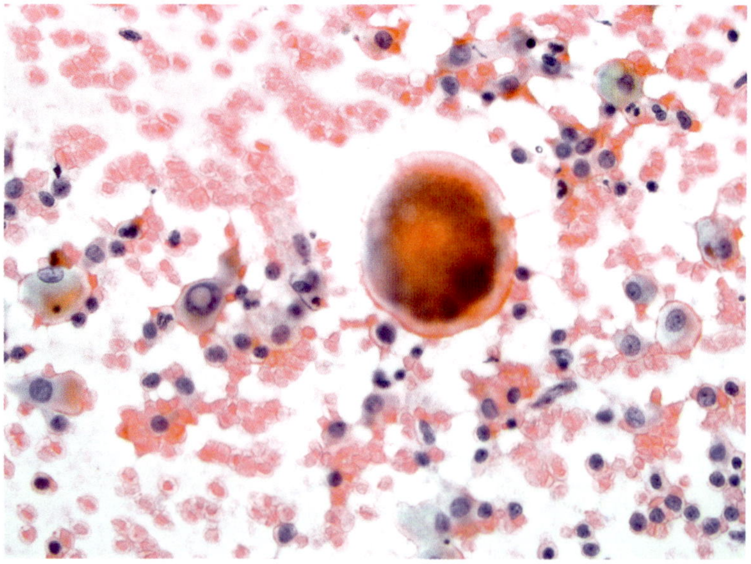

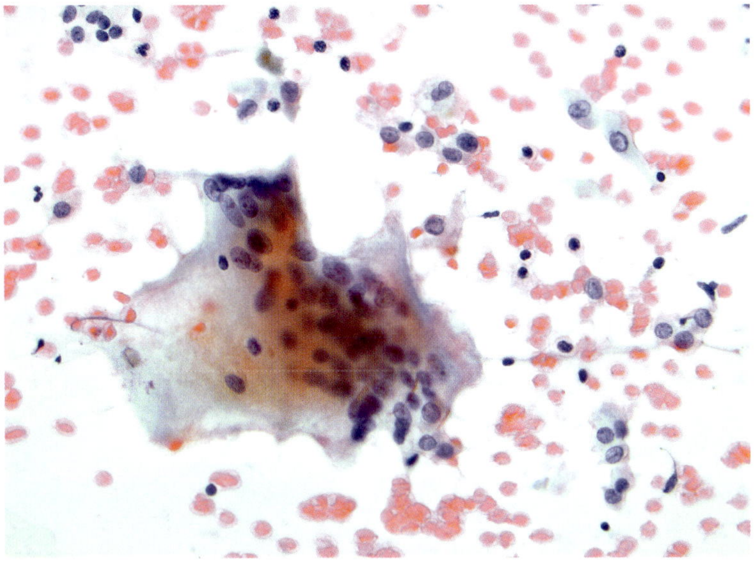

Figure 8.51b — Papillary Thyroid Carcinoma, FNA. Multinucleated giant (MNG) cells are not uncommon in PTC, as shown here. The diagnostic malignant cells are present in the smear background displaying classic nuclear features. Besides being commonly seen in adenomatoid nodule and Hashimoto thyroiditis, MNG cells are also seen in medullary carcinoma and anaplastic carcinoma. (Papanicolaou stain)

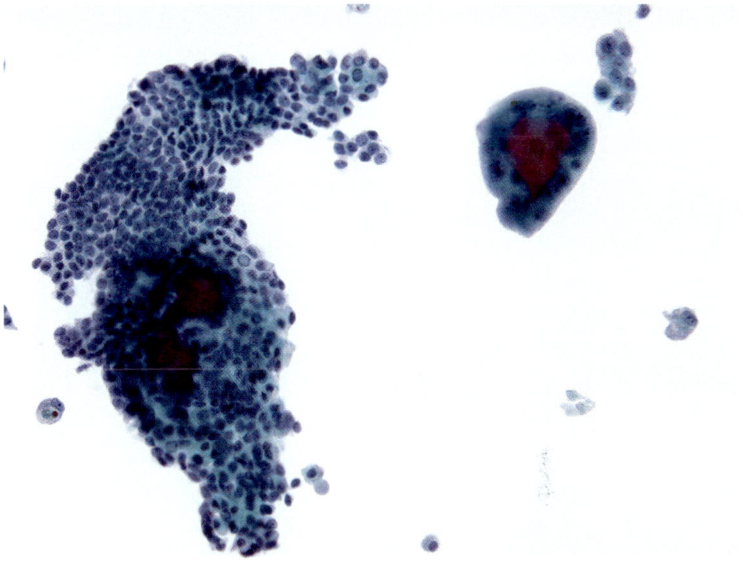

Figure 8.51c — Papillary Thyroid Carcinoma, FNA. A monolayered fragment of PTC is shown here associated with an epithelial fragment with Hürthleoid features (left of the field). Occasionally fused cytoplasmic borders in such fragments give an impression of a giant multinucleated histiocyte. Cells display characteristic nuclear morphology with few intranuclear inclusions. (Liquid-based preparation, Papanicolaou stain)

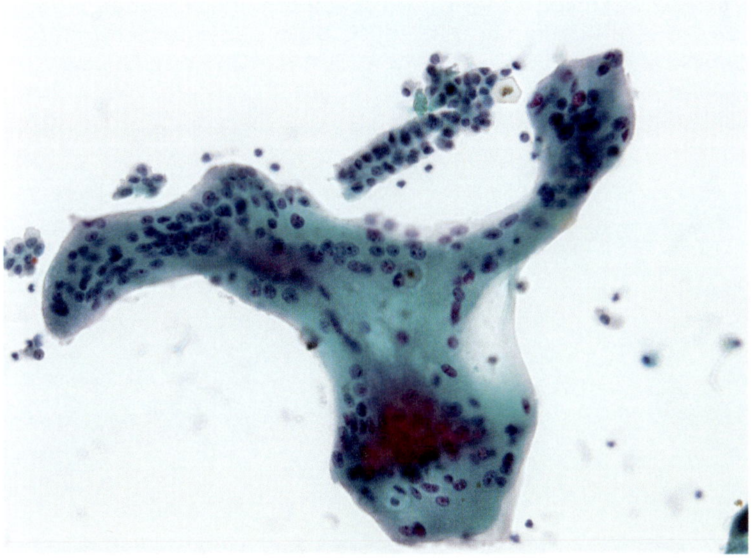

Figure 8.51d — Papillary Thyroid Carcinoma, FNA. A bizarre giant multinucleated (MNG) cell is seen here with innumerable small uniform nuclei haphazardly distributed throughout the cell. A small fragment of PTC cells is seen above the MNG cell. (Liquid-based preparation, Papanicolaou stain)

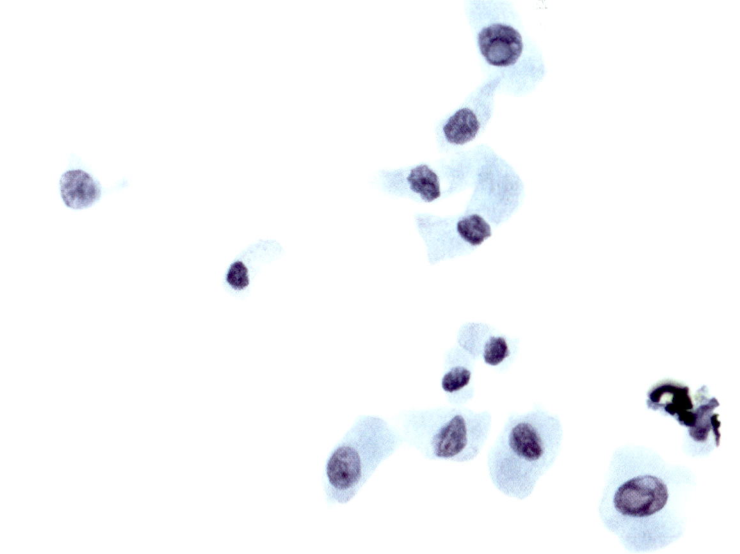

Figure 8.52a — Papillary Thyroid Carcinoma, FNA. Tall-cell variant of PTC (TCV-PTC) is shown in this example. Most of the cells seen here are singly placed and have a distinct columnar appearance. Intranuclear inclusions are prominently present. (Liquid-based preparation, Papanicolaou stain)

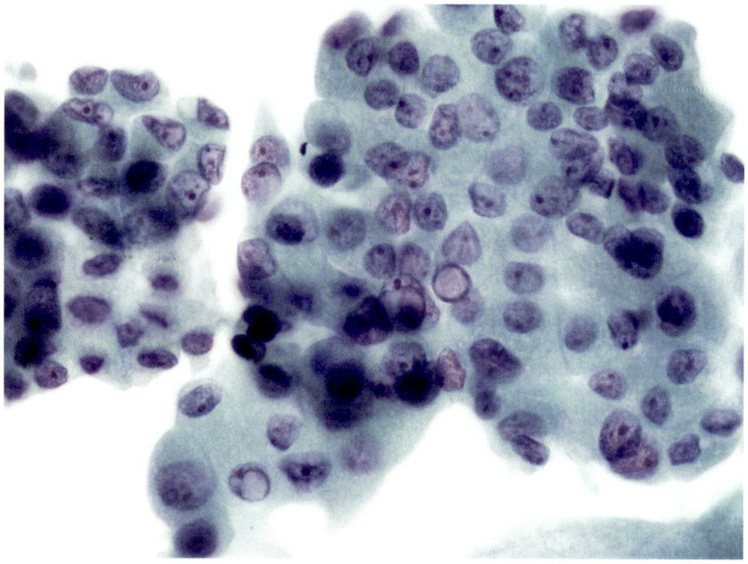

Figure 8.52b — Papillary Thyroid Carcinoma, FNA. As opposed to the previous example, this TCV-PTC displays malignant cells in a sheet-like architecture. Note the oncocytic cytoplasm and well-formed intranuclear inclusions. Columnar cell shapes are difficult to appreciate in flat sheets. (Liquid-based preparation, Papanicolaou stain)

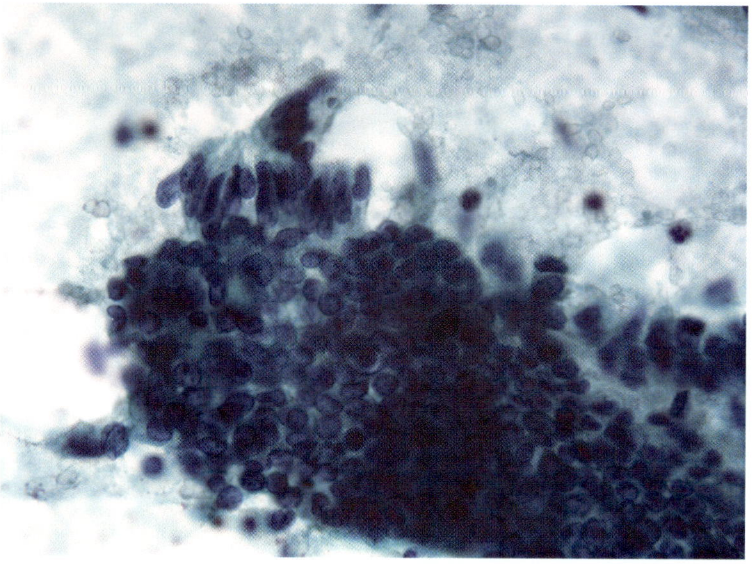

Figure 8.52c — Papillary Thyroid Carcinoma, FNA. At the top of the field is a beautiful illustration of the tall columnar-shaped nuclei, tightly stratified with well-formed grooves. The rest of the fragments display the classic nuclear morphology of PTC. Columnar cell/nuclear shapes are not always present in a TCV-PTC. Even when they are observed, they usually are a focal finding in a tumor with an otherwise typical PTC morphology. An FNA diagnosis of TCV is not absolutely required. If such a diagnosis is made it may guide the surgeon in determining the extent of surgery since TCV-PTC behaves in a much more aggressive manner than the conventional papillary carcinomas. (Papanicolaou stain)

Figure 8.52d — Papillary Thyroid Carcinoma, FNA. In this TCV-PTC, the cells lining the edges of the fragments display tall columnar shapes without the nuclei being elongated (as seen in the previous example). Note the dense cytoplasmic opacity. (Diff Quik stain)

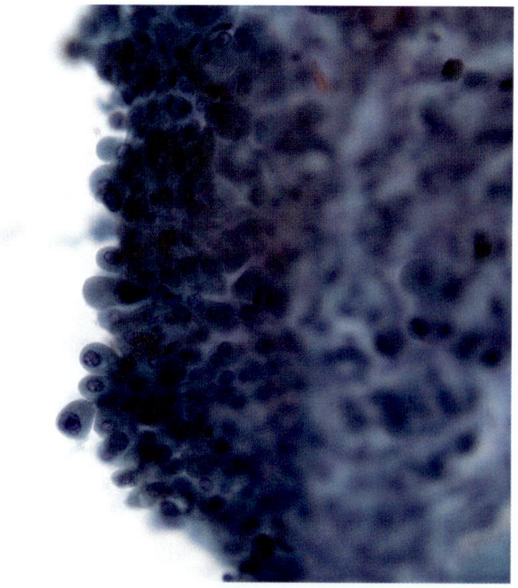

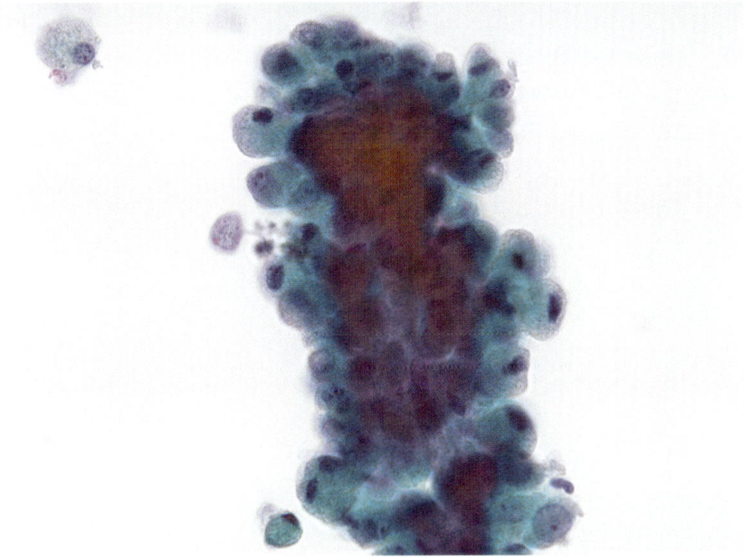

Figure 8.53a — Papillary Thyroid Carcinoma, FNA. Oncocytic variant of PTC (OCV-PTC) is exceedingly difficult to diagnose on FNA, particularly in liquid-based preparations, as shown here. In a significant number of cases, the FNA diagnosis is that of a Hürthle cell neoplasm. Nuclear features of PTC are not well-developed and are only present focally. In this example, the cells display cytoplasmic features of Hürthle cells, however, the nuclei are elongated and display grooves. Macronucleoli characteristic of Hürthle cell neoplasms are absent. Rarely intranuclear inclusions may be observed and are highly supportive of a PTC diagnosis as Hürthle cell neoplasms do not harbor INCIs. The other differential diagnosis would be an oncocytic variant of medullary carcinoma. (Liquid-based preparation, Papanicolaou stain)

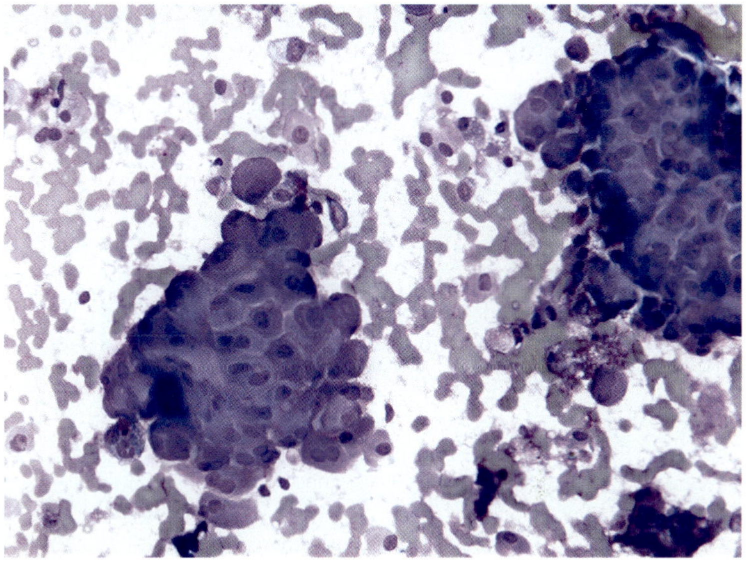

Figure 8.53b — Papillary Thyroid Carcinoma, FNA. Most studies have not indicated differences between OCV-PTC and conventional PTC, whereas other published data suggests that OCV-PTC is more aggressive than conventional PTC. OCV-PTC display predominantly tissue fragments, rather than single cells which are often a feature of Hürthle cell neoplasms. Notice the combination of Hürthleoid cytoplasm and oval-shaped nuclei with grooves. Only rare single cells are present in the background. OCV-PTC typically display clear nuclei, prominently irregular nuclear membranes with a distinct peripheral margination of chromatin and inconspicuous or absent nucleoli. Hürthle cell neoplasm (the major differential here) would have cells with prominent nuclear hyperchromasia, round vesicular nuclei, prominent centrally placed nucleoli, and binucleation, features most often absent in OCV-PTC. (Diff Quik stain)

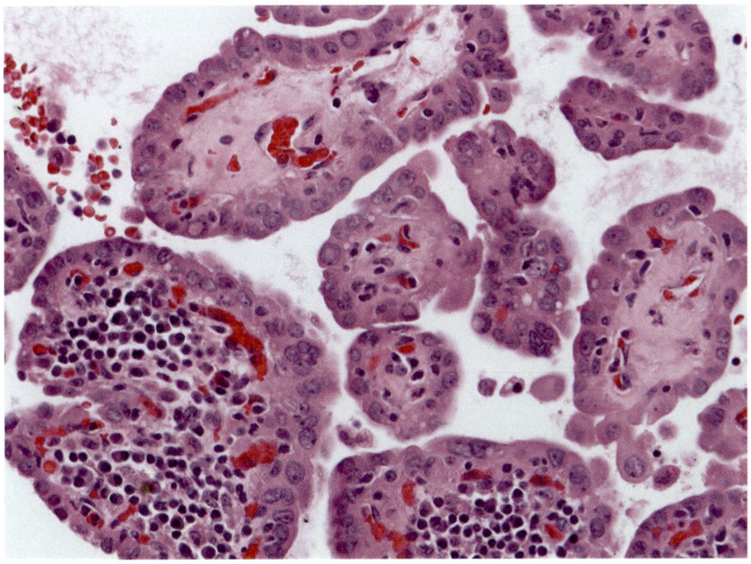

Figure 8.53c — Oncocytic Variant of Papillary Thyroid Carcinoma, Histologic Section. While the cytoplasm of the cells lining the papillary fronds have a distinct oncocytic flavor, the nuclear characteristics (eg, prominent intranuclear inclusions) are more in keeping with papillary carcinoma. (H&E stain)

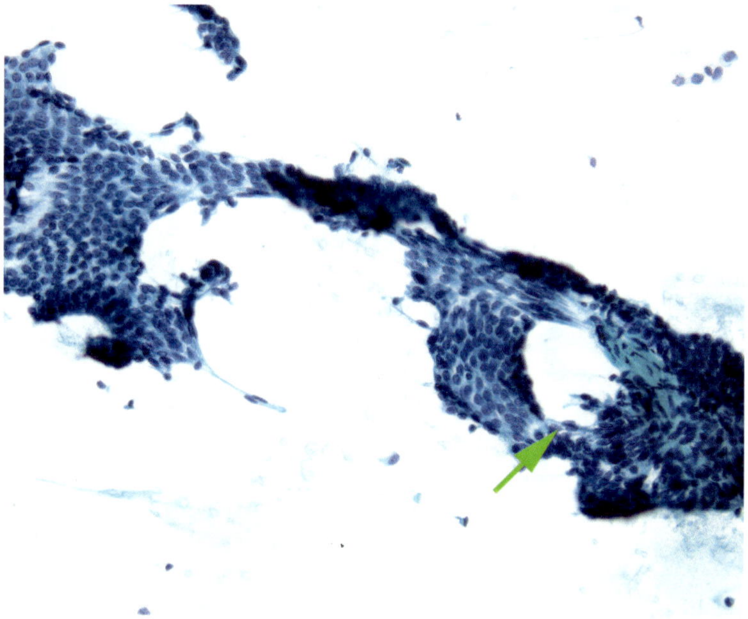

Figure 8.54a — Papillary Thyroid Carcinoma, FNA. While most cases of PTC are sporadic, the cribriform-morular variant of PTC (CMV-PTC) is a rare form that usually arises in individuals with familial adenomatous polyposis (FAP). There is significant overlap between the architectural and nuclear features of CMV-PTC and conventional PTC. Studies have shown that papillary configurations, nuclear elongation, grooves, and overlap and intranuclear inclusions are all easily identified in CMV-PTC. In this example, along with the classic architectural and nuclear features of PTC, well-formed cribriform spaces (arrow) were noticed. (Papanicolaou stain)

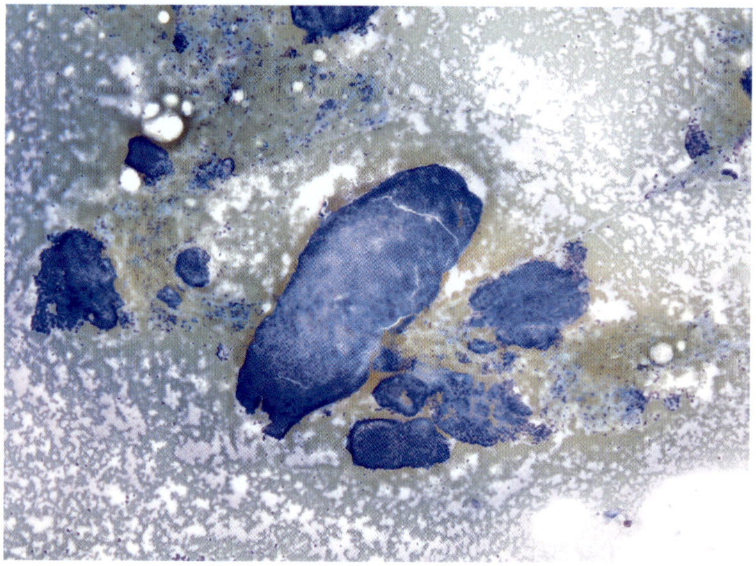

Figure 8.54b — Papillary Thyroid Carcinoma, FNA. Another case of cribriform-morular variant of PTC is shown here. CMV-PTC is a rare morphologic entity, which is more common in young females usually less than 30 years of age. Although the clinical prognostic and survival data on CMV-PTC are limited, the distinction between conventional and CMV-PTC probably has little impact on disease-specific long-term prognosis or surgical management. This image illustrates the tightly packed "morule" formation by the malignant epithelium (especially at 6 o'clock). Well-developed squamoid morules are rarely seen on FNA material. The morular cells are positive with Bcl-2 and negative or weakly positive for beta-catenin. (Diff Quik stain)

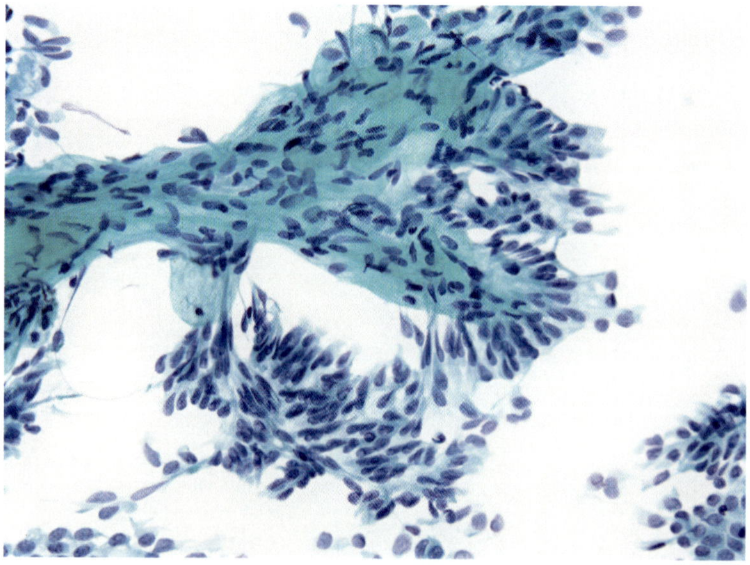

Figure 8.54c — Papillary Thyroid Carcinoma, FNA. Occasionally, nuclear elongation in cribriform-morular variant of PTC suggests the more aggressive tall-cell variant. In our experience, the cytologic interpretation of malignancy in FNA material from patients with CMV-PTC is straightforward because the smears are cellular, and the classical architectural and nuclear changes of PTC are easily identified. However, the greater challenge in these cases is to recognize the additional features that would suggest CMV-PTC and should warrant beta-catenin immunostaining either on the cytological or histological material. The nuclear beta-catenin indicates a mutation of the adenomatous polyposis coli (APC) gene that defines FAP. (Papanicolaou stain)

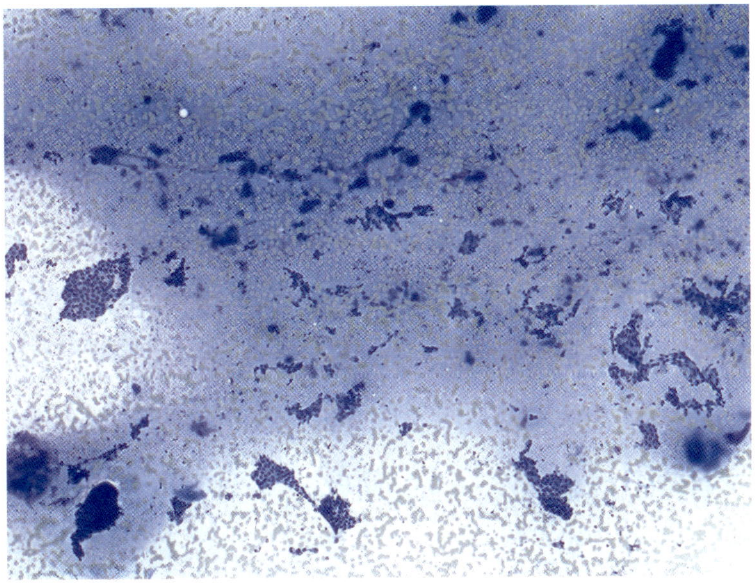

Figure 8.55a — Papillary Thyroid Carcinoma, FNA. A macrofollicular variant of PTC is illustrated here. This often becomes a difficult diagnosis on FNA since the low power appearance suggests a benign nodule due to an overabundance of colloid. However, even at this magnification, the flat monolayered architecture is hard to ignore. (Diff Quik stain)

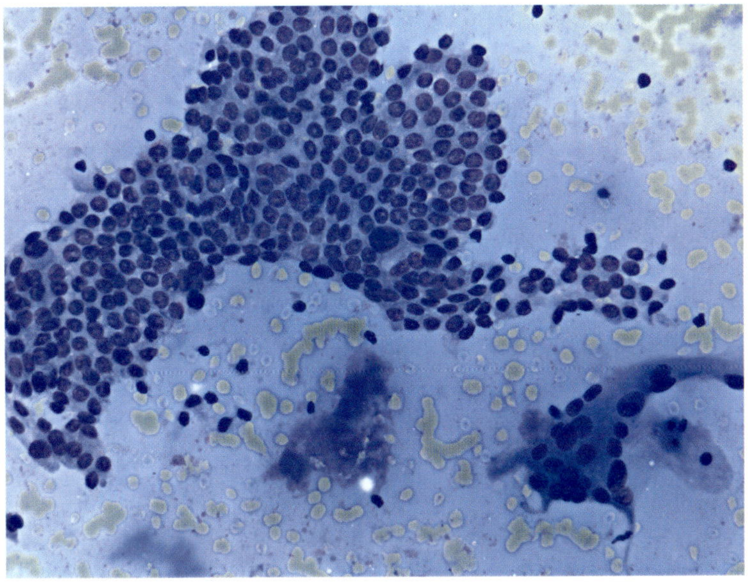

Figure 8.55b — Papillary Thyroid Carcinoma, FNA. At higher magnification of this macrofollicular variant of PTC, the monolayered sheet displays classic nuclear features of PTC. Notice the abundant background colloid, which often leads to underdiagnosis of such cases. A careful evaluation at higher magnification is needed especially if clinical/family history or radiologic findings suggest malignancy. (Diff Quik stain)

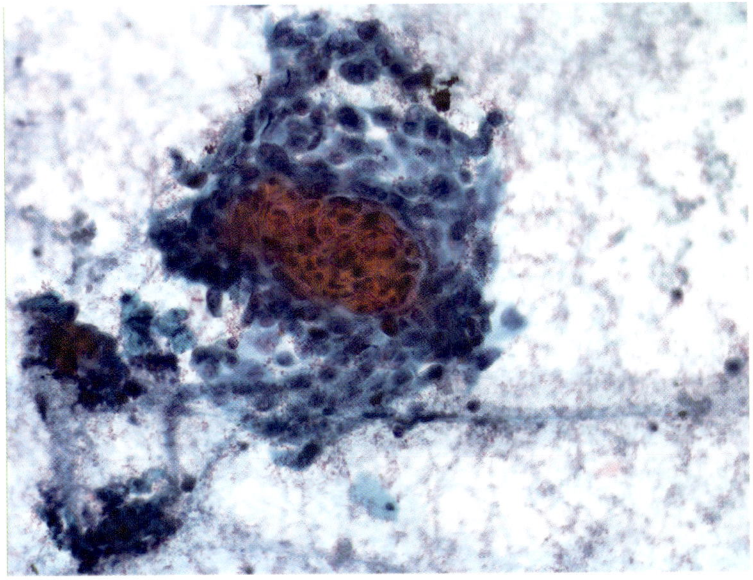

Figure 8.56 — Papillary Thyroid Carcinoma, FNA. Squamous change in a PTC is an under reported phenomenon and can occur in up to 25% of the cases. In this PTC, a group of keratinized squamous cells are surrounded by malignant cells displaying classic nuclear morphology. (Papanicolaou stain)

9

Medullary Thyroid Carcinoma

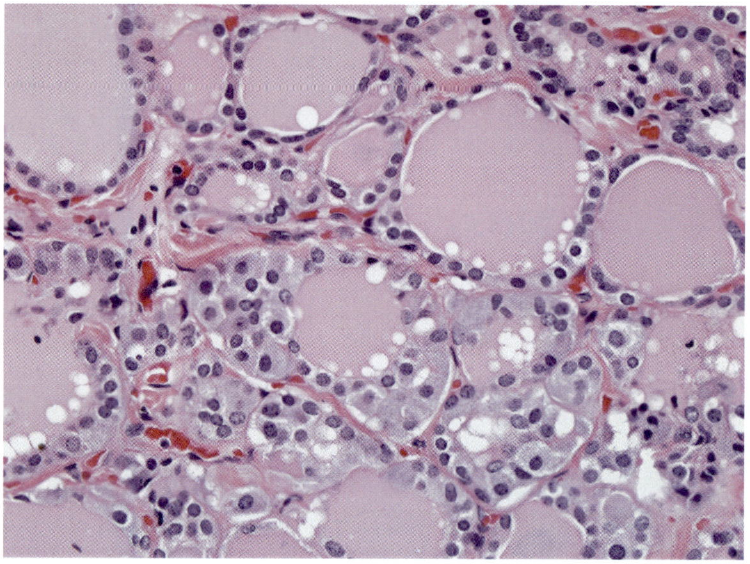

Figure 9.1a — C Cell Hyperplasia, Histologic Section. C-cells reside in an intrafollicular location between the follicular epithelium and the limiting follicular basement membrane. Compared to the follicular epithelial cell, C-cells tend to have larger nuclei and more abundant pale cytoplasm. They are not easily identified in the normal thyroid gland, but they become more conspicuous in the proliferative condition known as C-cell hyperplasia. In C-cell hyperplasia, the proliferating C-cells envelope the central follicular cells and then progressively encroach on the follicular spaces. Continued proliferation results in filling and expansion of the follicles by solid nodules of C-cells. (H&E stain)

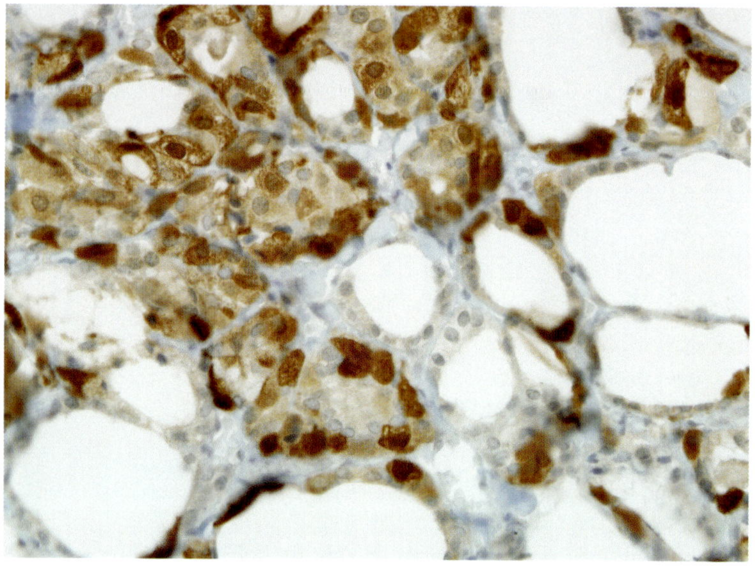

Figure 9.1b — C Cell Hyperplasia (Calcitonin Staining), Histologic Section. Immunohistochemical staining for calcitonin is useful in distinguishing C-cells from follicular epithelial cells. (Immunostain)

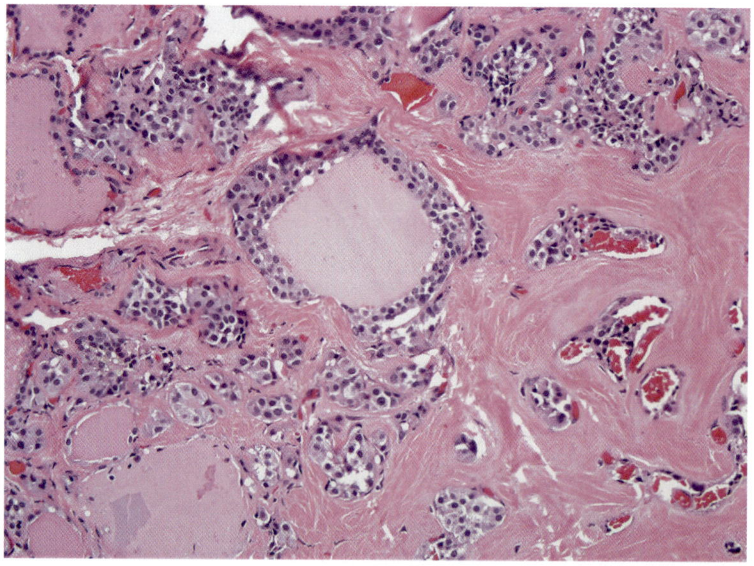

Figure 9.2 — Microinvasive Medullary Thyroid Carcinoma, Histologic Section. In C-cell hyperplasia, the proliferative process is confined by the basement membrane surrounding the thyroid follicles. In microinvasive medullary carcinoma, cords of neoplastic C-cells penetrate the follicular basement membrane and extend into the interstitium between the follicles. Infiltration of the interstitium tends to elicit some degree of stromal fibrosis. (H&E stain)

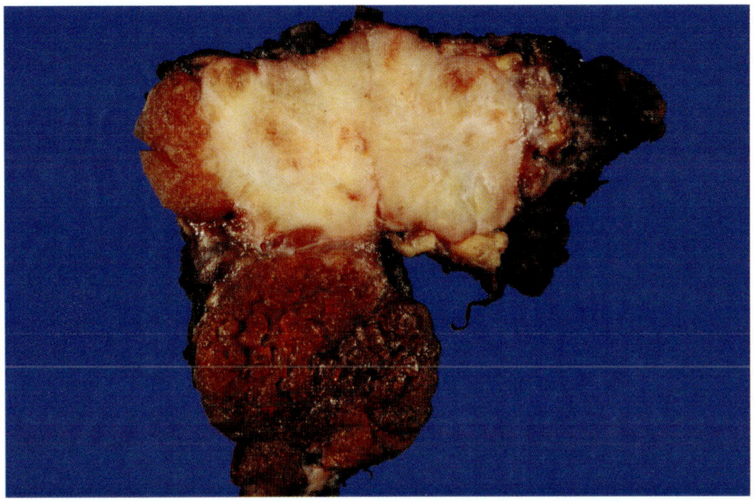

Figure 9.3a — Medullary Thyroid Carcinoma, Gross Appearance. This medullary carcinoma is highly infiltrative and replaces most of the right thyroid lobe. On cut section, its surface is solid, firm, and white to tan. Careful inspection should be made of both lobes for additional tumors as familial forms of medullary carcinomas are often multifocal.

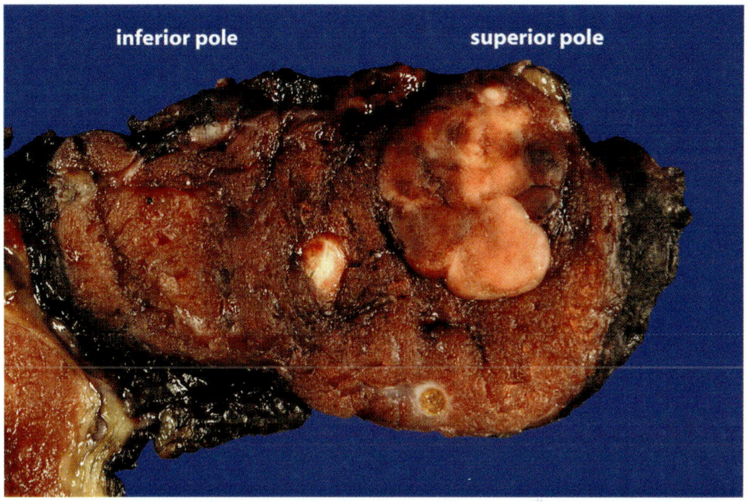

Figure 9.3b — Medullary Thyroid Carcinoma, Gross Appearance. Medullary carcinomas are nonencapsulated, but their border can sometimes be circumscribed. The location of this medullary carcinoma is typical in that they usually arise from the junction of the middle and upper thirds of the thyroid lobes—the region of the thyroid where the C-cells are most densely dispersed.

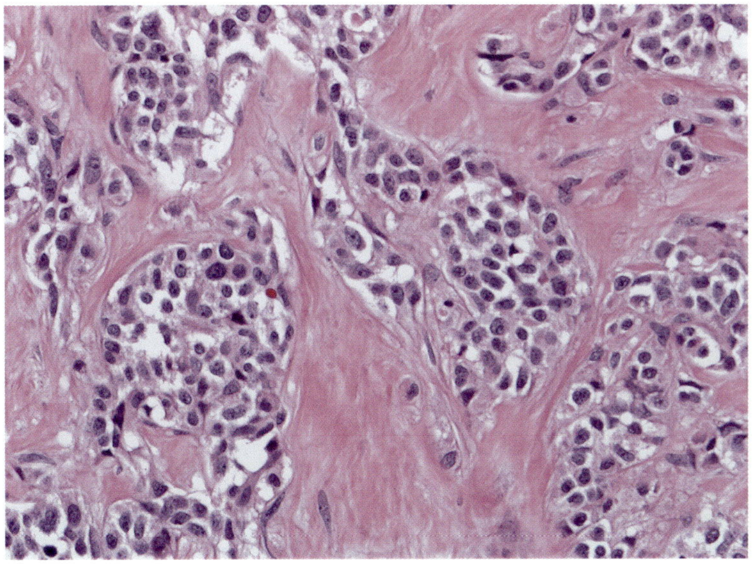

Figure 9.4a — Medullary Thyroid Carcinoma, Histologic Section. Although medullary carcinomas can demonstrate a wide range of growth patterns, the prototypic medullary carcinoma grows in a nested pattern. The shapes of the tumor cells range from round to polygonal to slightly spindled. Their cytoplasm tends to be pale and slightly eosinophilic or amphophilic. The nuclei are round to oval with a uniformly stippled chromatin pattern and inconspicuous nucleoli. Most medullary carcinomas have the appearance of well differentiated neuroendocrine neoplasms, but they can sometimes exhibit more advanced histologic grades characterized by high mitotic activity and tumor necrosis. Immunohistochemical studies may be helpful in distinguishing these higher grade medullary thyroid carcinomas from poorly differentiated carcinomas of follicular epithelial origin such as insular carcinoma. In contrast to insular carcinoma, medullary carcinomas are consistently immunoreactive for carcinoembryonic antigen (CEA) and/or calcitonin, and they are not immunoreactive for thyroglobulin. (H&E stain)

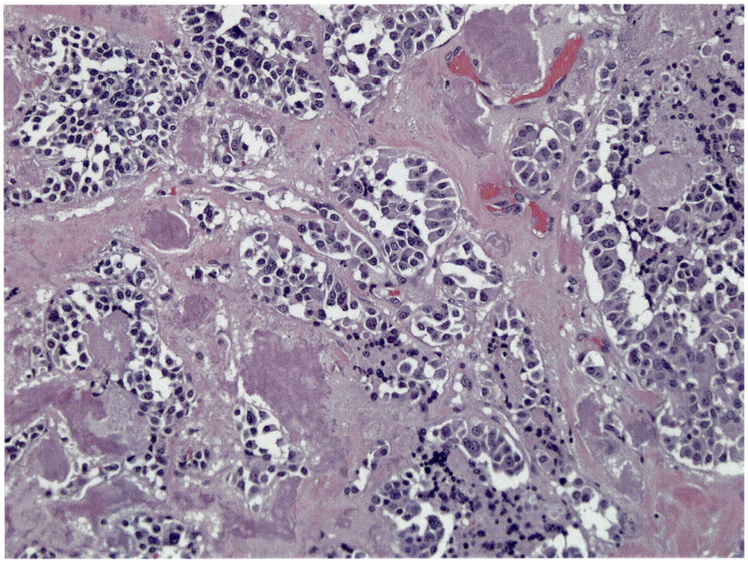

Figure 9.4b — Medullary Thyroid Carcinoma, Histologic Section. Tumor stroma surrounding the nests of medullary thyroid carcinoma is often densely hyalinized. The hyalinized stroma often contains nodular deposits of amorphous eosinophilic material representing amyloid. (H&E stain)

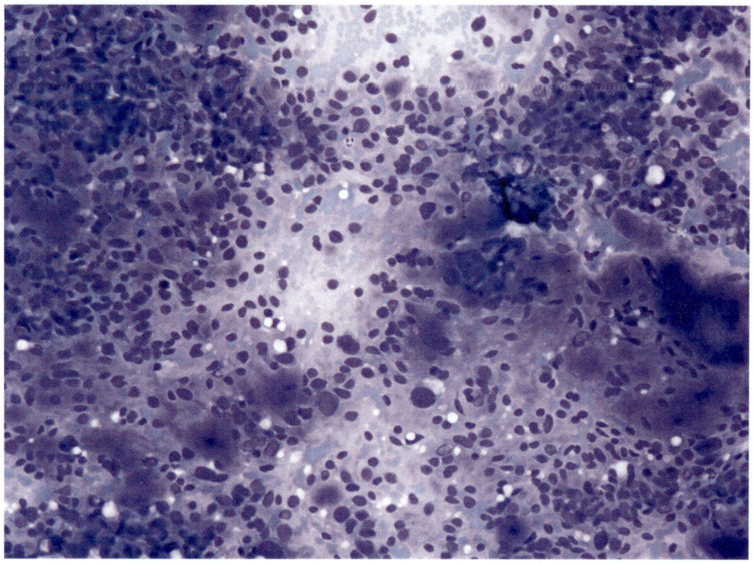

Figure 9.5 — Medullary Thyroid Carcinoma, Fine Needle Aspiration (FNA). Medullary thyroid carcinoma (MTC) is defined as "a malignant neoplasm derived from and/or morphologically recapitulating the parafollicular cells of the thyroid gland." MTC smears are typically hypercellular and display a variety of architectural patterns. Numerous single cells are commonly present. Also observed are numerous loose tissue fragments often displaying syncytial architecture. Amorphous material representing amyloid is commonly identified and aids in the cytologic diagnosis. Amyloid should not be confused with colloid. Follicle formations are not seen and papillary formations are exceedingly rare. (Diff Quik stain)

Figure 9.6 — Medullary Thyroid Carcinoma, FNA. MTC typically is comprised of a uniform and monotonous cell population. Focal mild to moderate pleomorphism can be observed, as in this case, which also displays a large amount of amyloid. Some cells here suggest a nested pattern; however, true follicle formations are not seen. The giant nucleus in the middle of the field also shows an intranuclear inclusion, which is not an uncommon finding in MTC. After papillary thyroid carcinoma, intranuclear inclusions are most commonly observed in MTC. (Diff Quik stain)

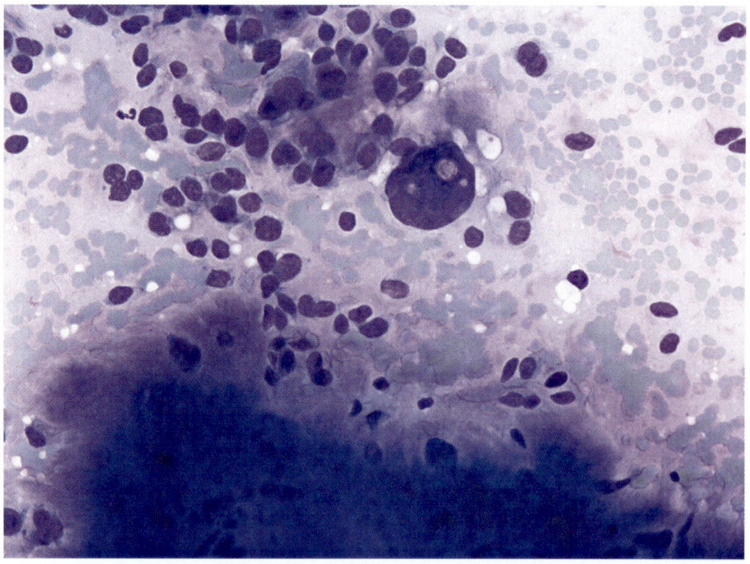

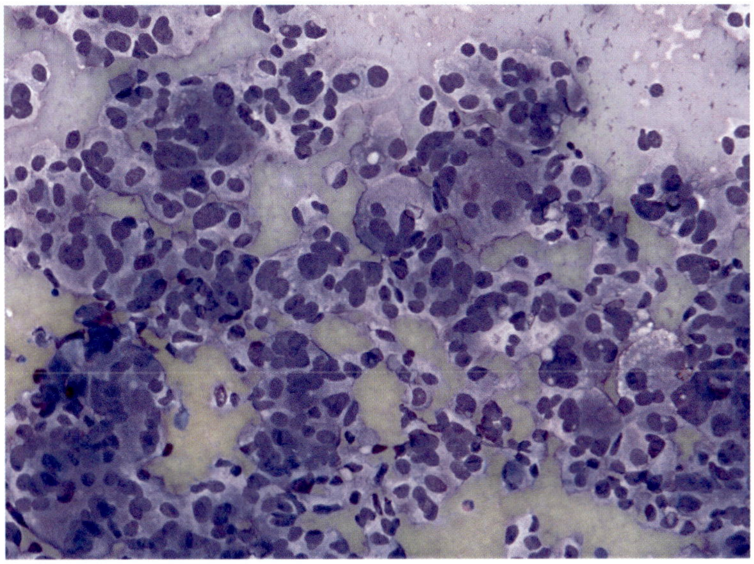

Figure 9.7 — Medullary Thyroid Carcinoma, FNA. Medullary thyroid carcinoma accounts for 5% to 8% of all thyroid cancers and develops in either sporadic (75%) or hereditary form (25%). This case displays a nested and trabecular pattern with mostly epithelioid type cells. Cytoplasm shows basophilic granularity and contains eccentrically placed nuclei. The nested pattern can be confused with microfollicular proliferation, occasionally leading to a misdiagnosis of a "follicular neoplasm." (Diff Quik stain)

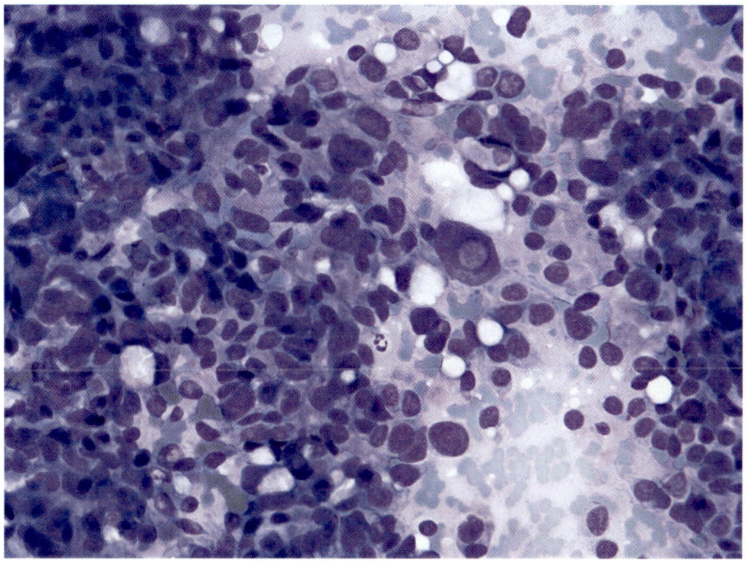

Figure 9.8 — Medullary Thyroid Carcinoma, FNA. Higher magnification of a uniform population of mostly epithelioid malignant cells, few oval to spindled nuclei, focal anisonucleosis, and distinct basophilic granularity of the cytoplasm reflecting a high content of dense core neurosecretory granules in the tumor cells. A well-formed intranuclear inclusion is present in the middle of the field. None of the cells display prominent nucleoli. (Diff Quik stain)

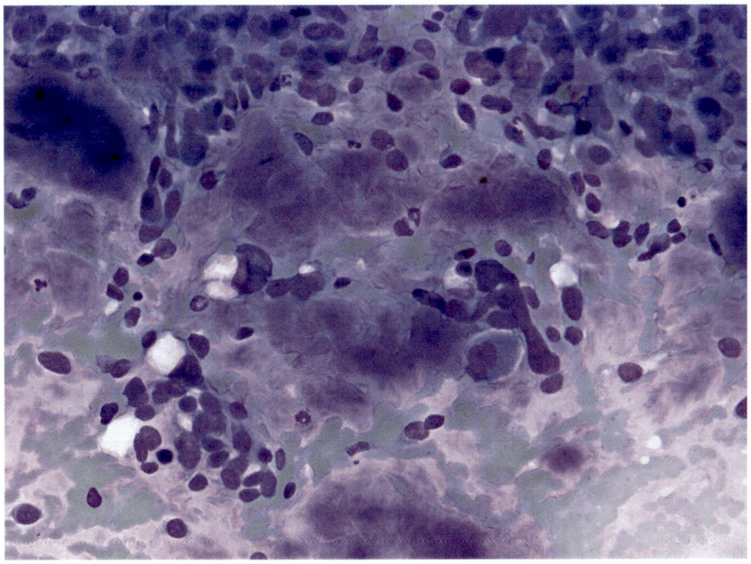

Figure 9.9 — Medullary Thyroid Carcinoma, FNA. Amyloid is often present in smears of MTC cases. It tends to have an amorphous to fine fibrillary appearance on Diff Quik stain and needs to be accurately distinguished from colloid. Presence of amyloid is highly supportive of an MTC diagnosis. Rarely, well-formed multinucleated giant cells are associated with amyloid deposits in MTC as seen in the center of this image. Also observed is focal anisonucleosis with round to spindled nuclei. (Diff Quik stain)

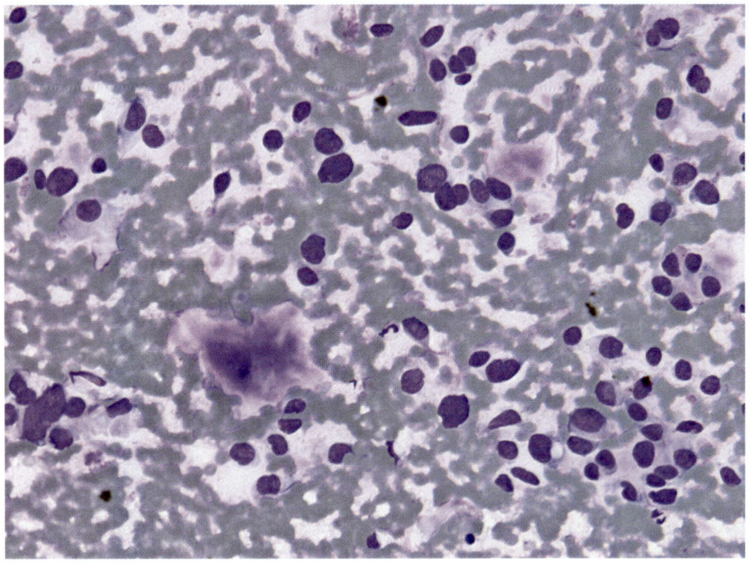

Figure 9.10 — Medullary Thyroid Carcinoma, FNA. A predominant single cell architectural pattern was observed in this case. Cells are monotonous with round to oval nuclei, finely wispy cytoplasm displaying faint and focal basophilic granularity. Also seen are amyloid deposits. MTC is a biologically aggressive malignancy that spreads by hematogenous and lymphatic routes. Common sites of metastasis include cervical lymph nodes, lung, liver, bone, and adrenal glands. (Diff Quik stain)

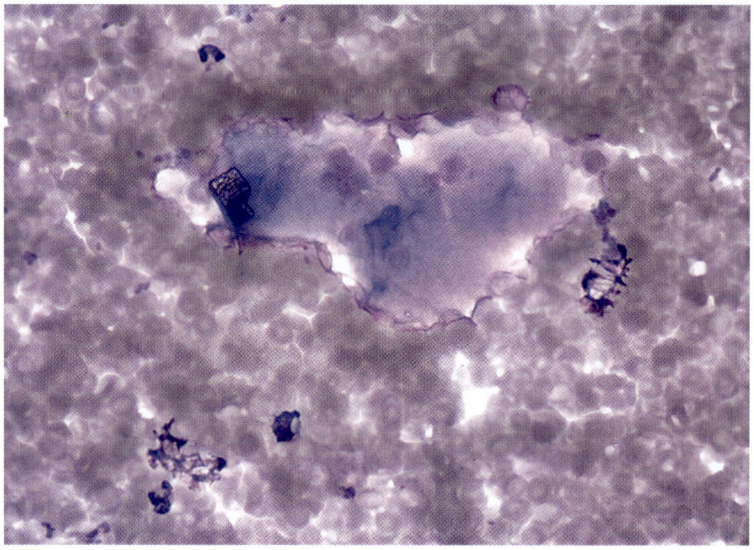

Figure 9.11 — Medullary Thyroid Carcinoma, FNA. An amyloid deposit is seen at higher magnification and appears as metachromatic amorphous material. This case was hypocellular with only few malignant cells but was diagnosed as MTC due to the presence of abundant amyloid material. Studies have estimated the frequency of amyloid in MTC varies from 50% to 80% of cases. (Diff Quik stain)

Figure 9.12 — Medullary Thyroid Carcinoma, FNA. A monotonous single cell pattern characterizes this case of MTC. Neoplastic cells predominantly appear as bare nuclei with finely granular or "neuroendocrine-type" chromatin, lacking nucleoli. Well-defined globular fragments of refractile amyloid are readily identified in this case. (Papanicolaou stain)

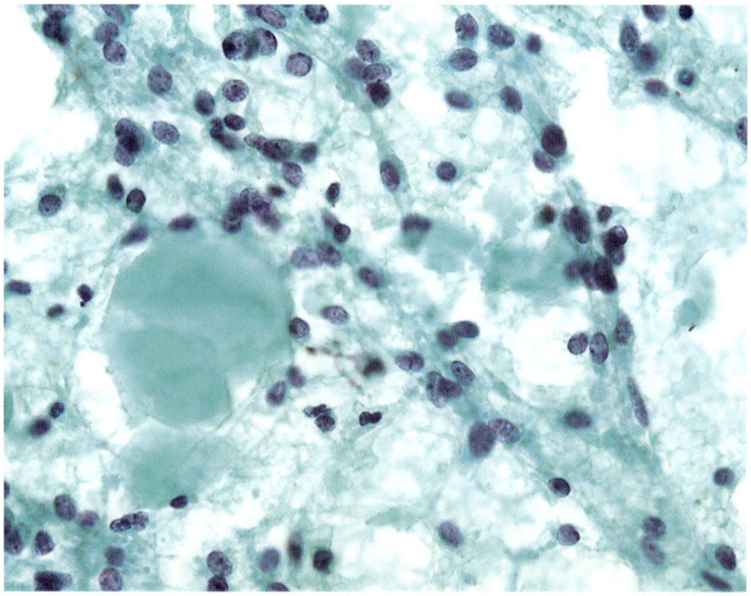

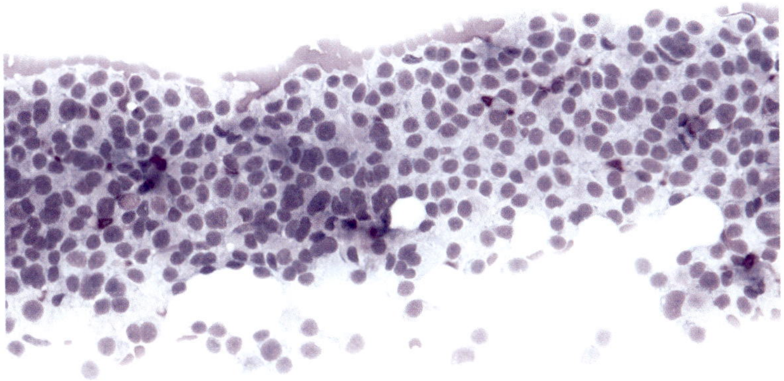

Figure 9.13 — Medullary Thyroid Carcinoma, FNA. Numerous loosely cohesive malignant cells are depicted in this case with uniform round nuclei and small punctate nucleoli. The cytoplasm is vacuolated to finely granular. Faint cytoplasmic basophilia is apparent in some cells. There was a total lack of colloid. It's important to remember that clinically, up to 50% of patients with MTC present with cervical nodal metastases, and in these patients the primary tumor can be occult. Hence, the possibility of metastatic MTC should be kept in mind in a patient with a positive cervical lymph node of unknown primary. (Diff Quik stain)

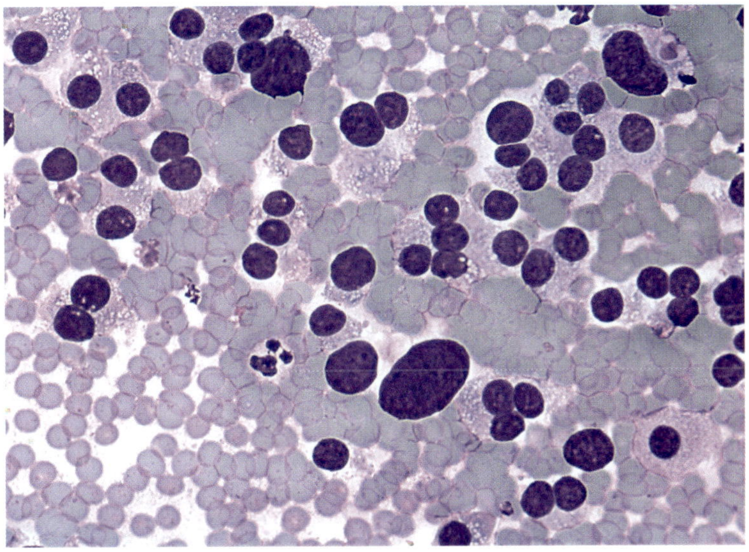

Figure 9.14 — Medullary Thyroid Carcinoma, FNA. On higher magnification, this example of MTC displays mostly uniform and round nuclei. Aggregation of cells may give suggestion of microfollicular pattern (1 o'clock), which may lead to an erroneous interpretation. Cytoplasm is mostly finely vacuolated or "histiocyte-like." (Diff Quik stain)

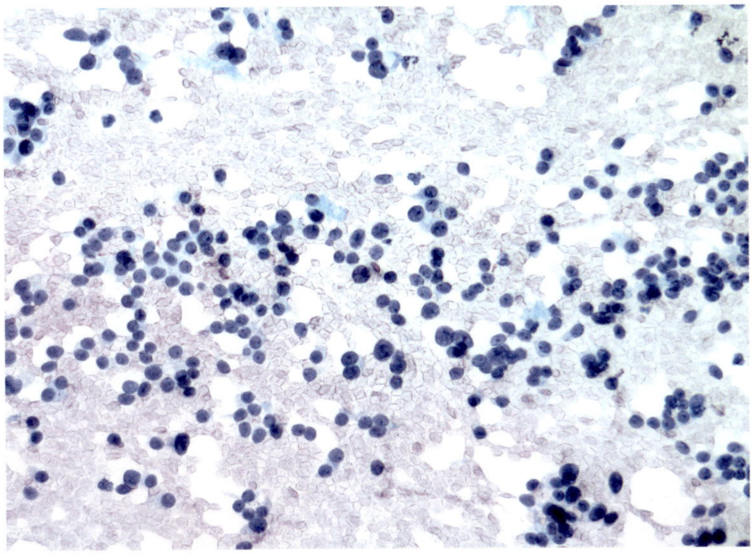

Figure 9.15 — Medullary Thyroid Carcinoma, FNA. The smears in this case were diffusely hypercellular and almost exclusively showed a single cell pattern. Most cells have lost their cytoplasm and appear as bare nuclei. If such cytomorphologic pattern predominates, a parathyroid lesion should also be considered in the differential diagnosis. Serum calcitonin, CEA, and parathyroid hormone level determination is extremely crucial. A total lack of colloid will make a follicular neoplasm an unlikely diagnosis in this case. Also notice the finely granular chromatin and small inconspicuous nucleoli. (Papanicolaou stain)

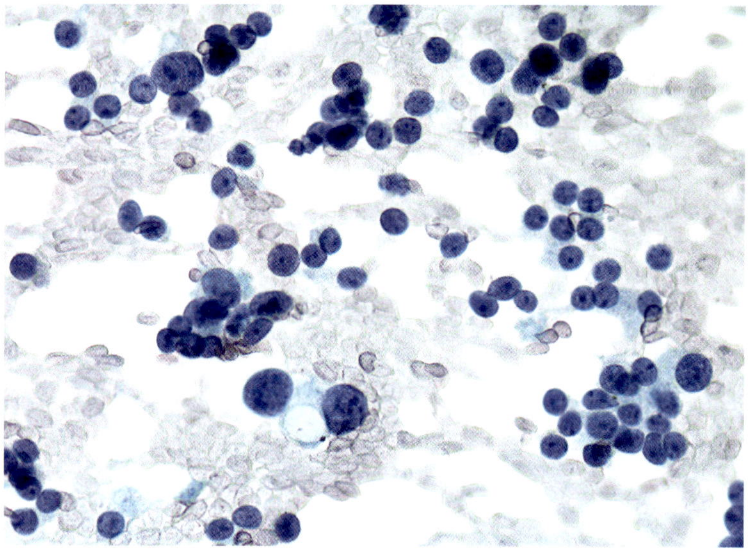

Figure 9.16 — Medullary Thyroid Carcinoma, FNA. The neuroendocrine chromatin pattern is nicely observed at higher magnification. Most cells appear as bare nuclei. Note the micronucleoli. Presence of macronucleolus in malignant cells usually argues against the diagnosis of MTC in a thyroid aspirate. (Papanicolaou stain)

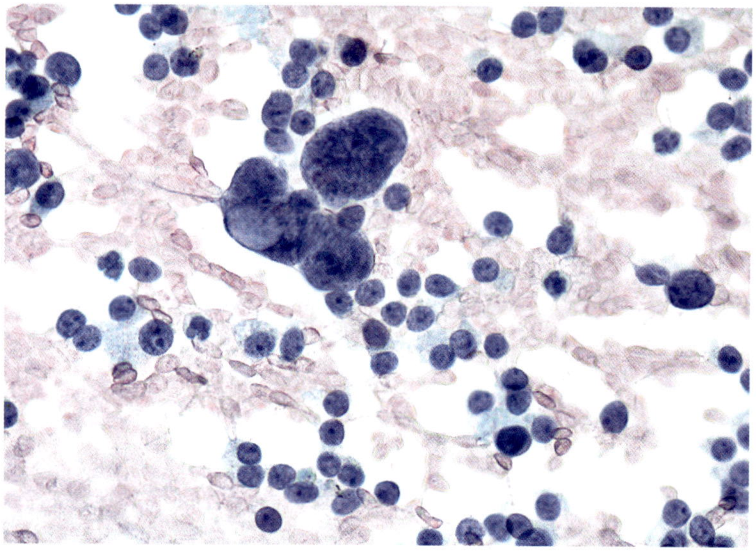

Figure 9.17 — Medullary Thyroid Carcinoma, FNA. Along with mostly bare nuclei, this case displays focal extreme anisonucleosis, which is not entirely uncommon in aspirates of MTC. One giant nucleus displays an intranuclear inclusion. Surgical treatment of MTC is usually total extracapsular thyroidectomy with lymph node dissection. (Papanicolaou stain)

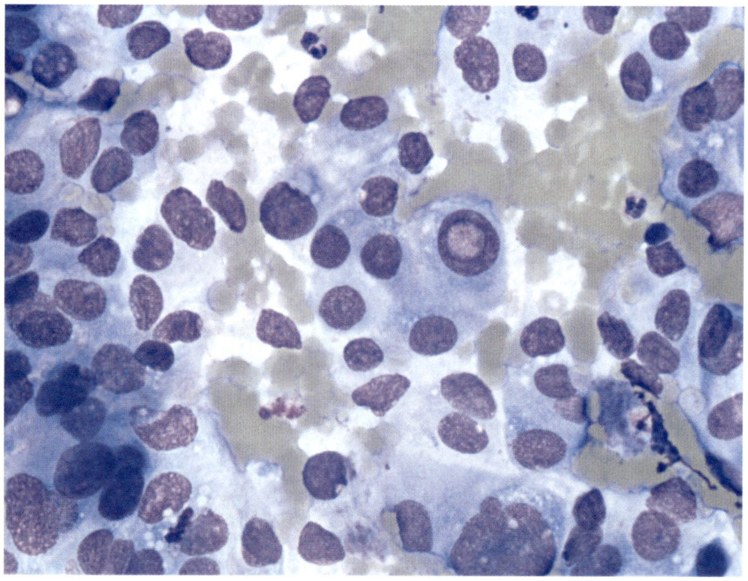

Figure 9.18 — Medullary Thyroid Carcinoma, FNA. A beautiful illustration of plasmacytoid cells, a well-formed intranuclear inclusion, dense basophilic cytoplasmic granularity and uniform round to oval nuclear shapes. Intranuclear inclusions (indistinguishable from those seen in papillary carcinoma) are encountered in one-half of the cases of MTC. (Diff Quik stain)

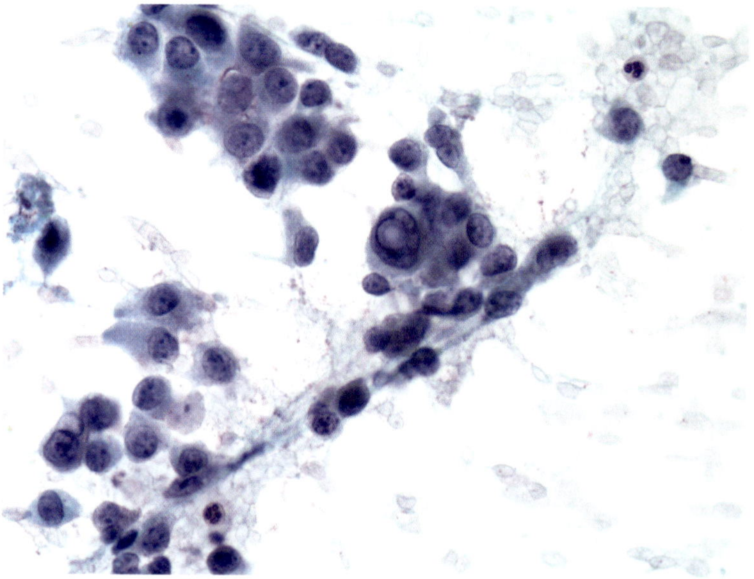

Figure 9.19 — Medullary Thyroid Carcinoma, FNA. Malignant cells show markedly enlarged, round to oval nuclei with fine dusty chromatin. Although papillary thyroid carcinoma often displays a similar chromatin texture, it is characterized by well-formed nuclear grooves and small marginal nucleoli. Additionally, eccentric nuclear placement strongly supports MTC in this case. (Papanicolaou stain)

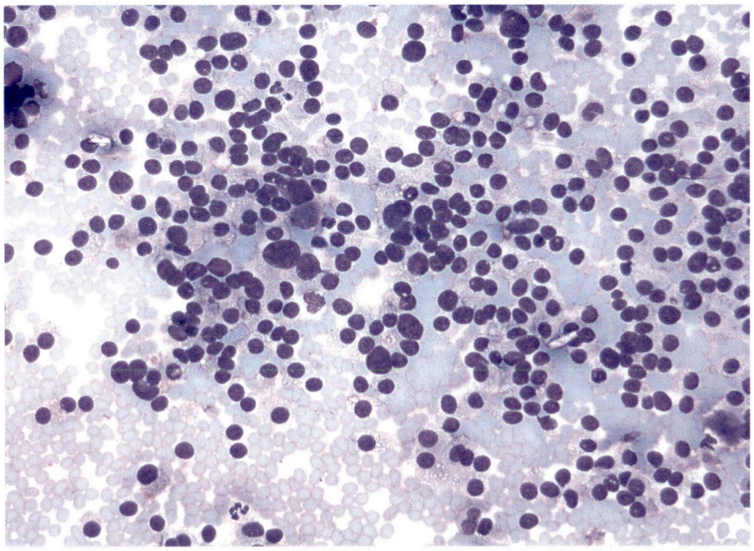

Figure 9.20 — Medullary Thyroid Carcinoma, FNA. A single cell dispersed pattern is quite commonly observed in MTC. Note the cellular monotony with only focal anisonucleosis, bare nuclei, finely vacuolated fragile cytoplasm, basophilic cytoplasmic granularity, and amyloid deposits. In most cases of MTC, the majority of the neoplastic cells are uniform in appearance, with only mild to moderate pleomorphism. (Diff Quik stain)

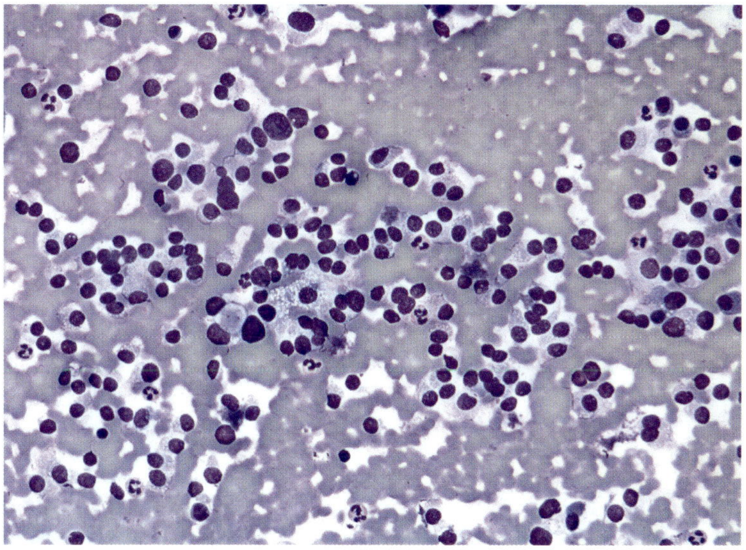

Figure 9.21 — Medullary Thyroid Carcinoma, FNA. A prominent plasmacytoid appearance is highlighted in this case. Occasional cells have a nested pattern which should not be confused with microfollicular pattern of a follicular neoplasm. Note a total lack of any colloid. In doubtful cases, the cytomorphologic findings should be correlated with serum calcitonin levels and/or immunoperoxidase staining for neuroendocrine markers. (Diff Quik stain)

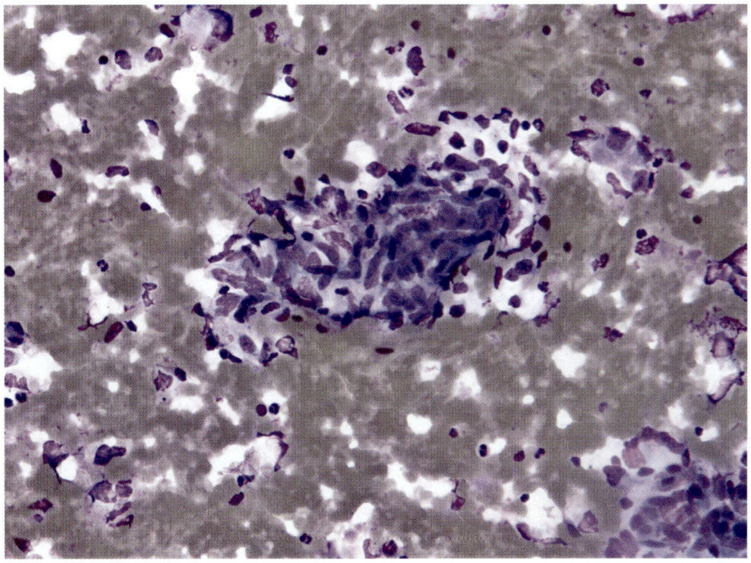

Figure 9.22 — Medullary Thyroid Carcinoma, FNA. A slightly less prevalent pattern of MTC is a pure "spindle cell" phenotype, as seen in this case. Malignant cells have nicely developed fusiform nuclei, which may occasionally show palisading, raising the possibility of a mesenchymal lesion. MTC more often will show a predominantly epithelioid or a mixed epithelioid and spindle cell pattern rather than a predominantly spindled architecture, as in this case. Other entities in differential diagnosis would be hyalinizing trabecular neoplasm and paraganglioma. (Diff Quik stain)

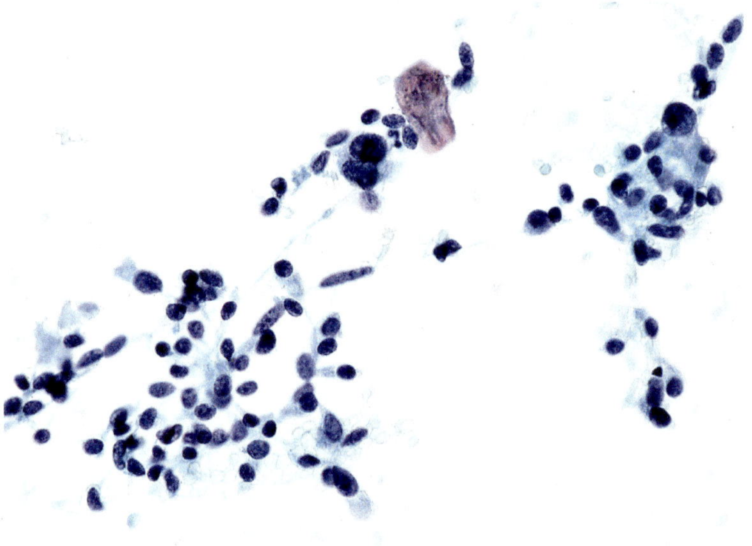

Figure 9.23 — Medullary Thyroid Carcinoma, FNA. In contrast to the previous example, this MTC smear shows a biphasic or mixed pattern of round (or epithelioid) cells and spindle cells. Notice the characteristic "neuroendocrine" chromatin pattern. While MTCs are characterized by a high rate of locoregional metastases, they tend to progress indolently and are associated with 10-year survival rates of approximately 80%. (Papanicolaou stain)

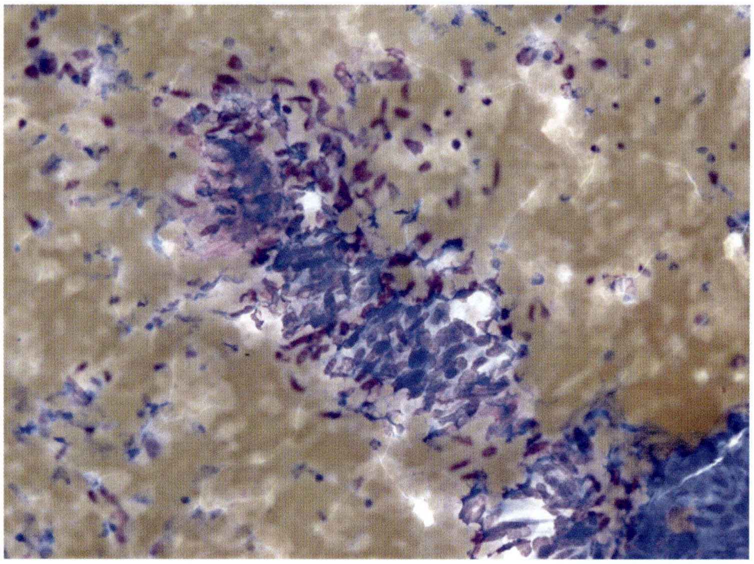

Figure 9.24 — Medullary Thyroid Carcinoma, FNA. The spindle cell pattern was so pronounced in this case that the initial cytomorphologic impression was a "nerve sheath tumor." The well-developed spindle cells are tightly palisaded against each other. The other differential diagnoses of spindle cell variant of MTC include anaplastic carcinoma, solitary fibrous tumor, spindle cell metastatic melanoma and nodular fasciitis-like variant of papillary carcinoma. (Diff Quik stain)

Figure 9.25 — Medullary Thyroid Carcinoma, FNA. This MTC displays an exclusive epithelioid phenotype. Notice the diffuse hypercellularity, mostly nested/syncytial pattern with few single cells and a prominent plasmacytoid appearance. Few structures suggest rosette-like formations. There is total lack of colloid. Nearly all the hereditary MTCs are associated with the MEN 2 syndromes. Recent advances in genetic screening have enabled early detection of hereditary MTCs and prophylactic thyroidectomy for affected kindred. (Papanicolaou stain)

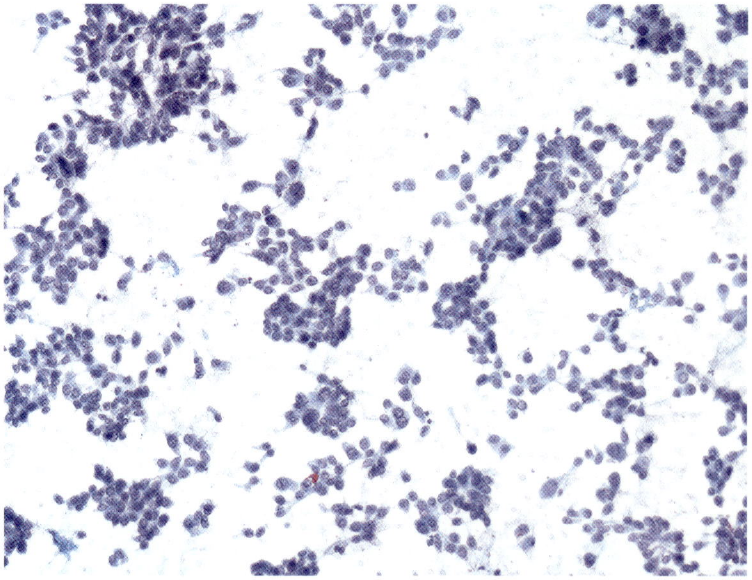

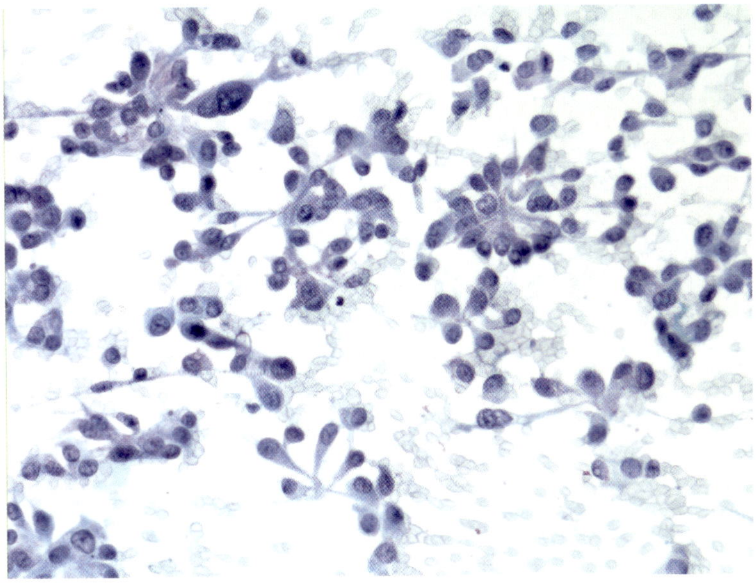

Figure 9.26 — Medullary Thyroid Carcinoma, FNA. Although the cells have round nuclei, they display long tapering cytoplasmic processes. There is suggestion of rosetting. Finely granular nuclear chromatin is quite apparent as well as plasmacytoid appearance and mild focal anisonucleosis. Cytoplasm shows abundant granularity, however, these cells should not be confused with a Hürthle cell neoplasm, which is often a close differential diagnosis of MTC. In contrast to MTC, Hürthle cell neoplasm often displays centrally placed nuclei and macronucleoli, with most cells frequently displaying bi-nucleation. (Papanicolaou stain)

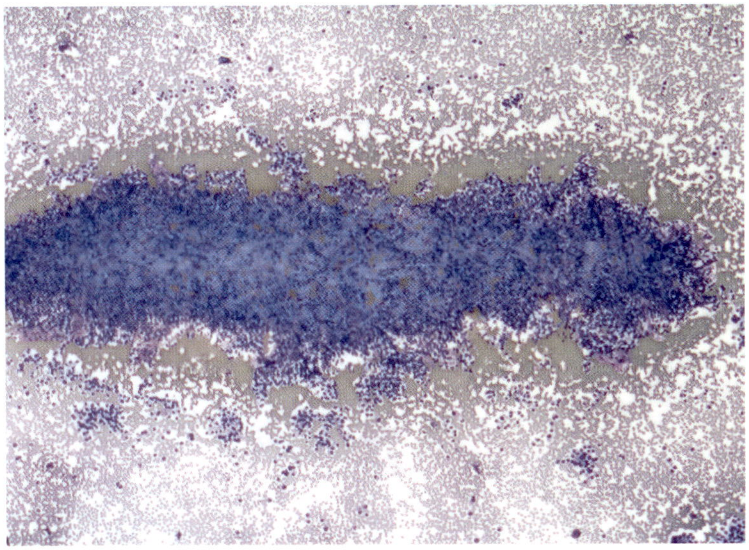

Figure 9.27 — Medullary Thyroid Carcinoma, FNA. The more common sporadic MTCs typically present with a solitary thyroid nodule. They show a median age of approximately 50 years, with a male:female ratio of 1:1.4. This diffusely hypercellular aspirate from MTC was initially interpreted as a follicular neoplasm due to a cohesive trabecular architecture, vascularity, and occasional dispersed microfollicular-type structures. (Diff Quik stain)

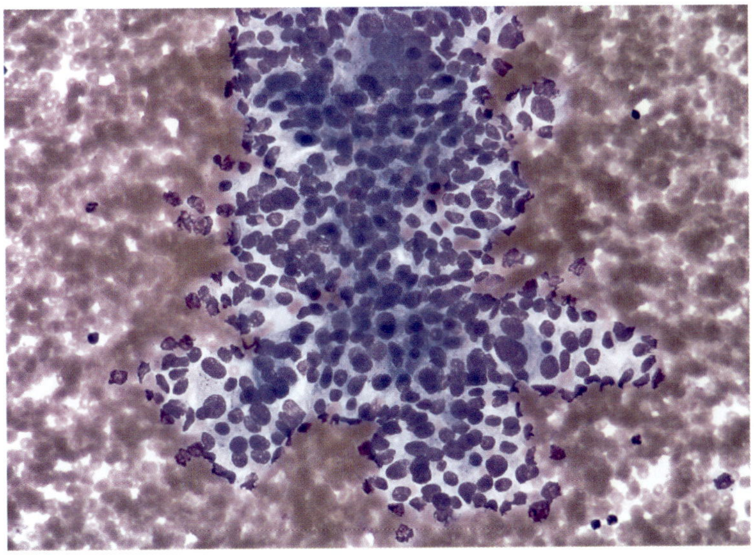

Figure 9.28 — Medullary Thyroid Carcinoma, FNA. The diagnosis of MTC is often challenging when a predominantly cohesive architecture is present, as in this case. Malignant cells have round to oval nuclei, which appear to be tightly palisaded. Oval nuclear shapes, especially when associated with intranuclear inclusions may also suggest a papillary thyroid carcinoma. However, when intranuclear inclusions are seen in MTC, they tend to be far fewer than in papillary carcinoma. (Diff Quik stain)

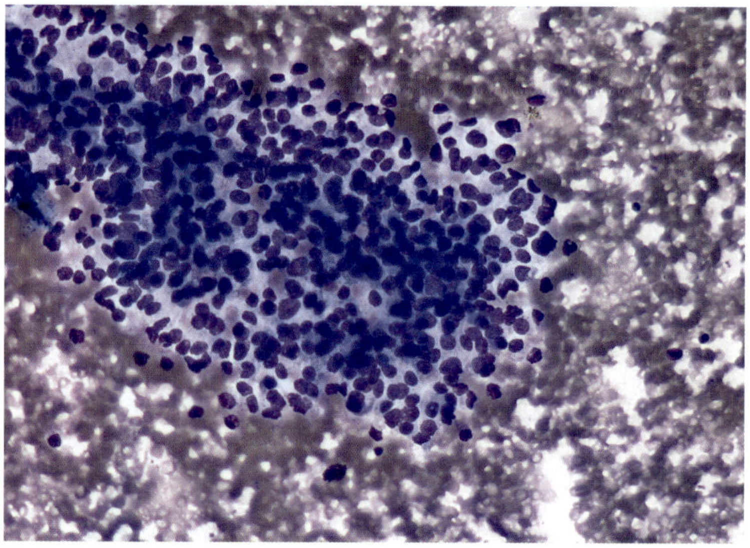

Figure 9.29 — Medullary Thyroid Carcinoma, FNA. Another example of MTC displaying a cohesive syncytial-like pattern of malignant cells is shown here. Initial impression in this case was a "follicular neoplasm." The typical differential diagnosis of MTC includes a Hürthle cell neoplasm, papillary carcinoma, anaplastic carcinoma, hyalinizing trabecular tumor (HTT), plasma cell myeloma, and metastatic melanoma. (Diff Quik stain)

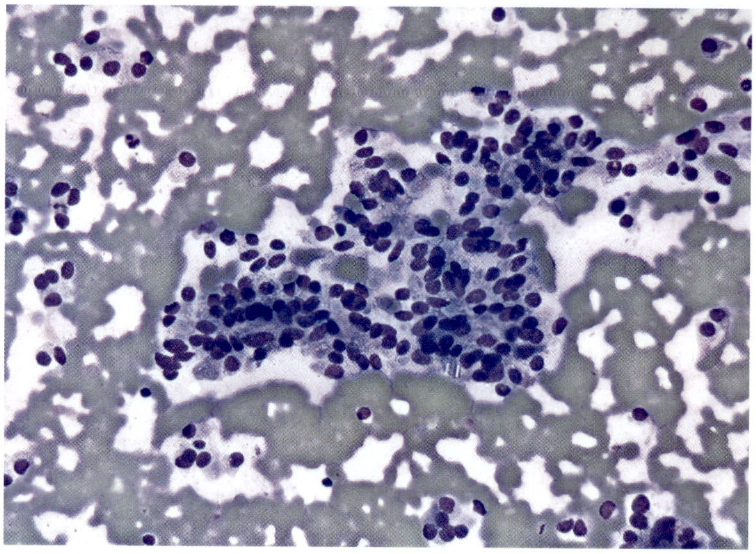

Figure 9.30 — Medullary Thyroid Carcinoma, FNA. Basophilic granularity is markedly pronounced in this case with mostly epithelioid cells in a loose syncytium. Cytoplasm also displays fine vacuolization. Most tumors occur in the upper and central areas of the thyroid where C-cells are present in higher concentrations. (Diff Quik stain)

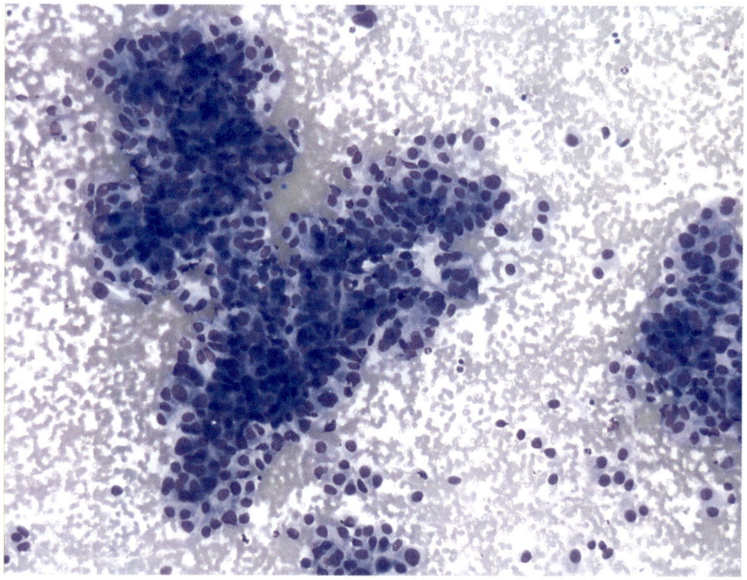

Figure 9.31 — Medullary Thyroid Carcinoma, FNA. Well-formed syncytia of tumor cells with epithelioid morphology are shown. Single cells in the background depict plasmacytoid features. MTCs are multicentric in most hereditary cases and in up to 30% of sporadic cases. (Diff Quik stain)

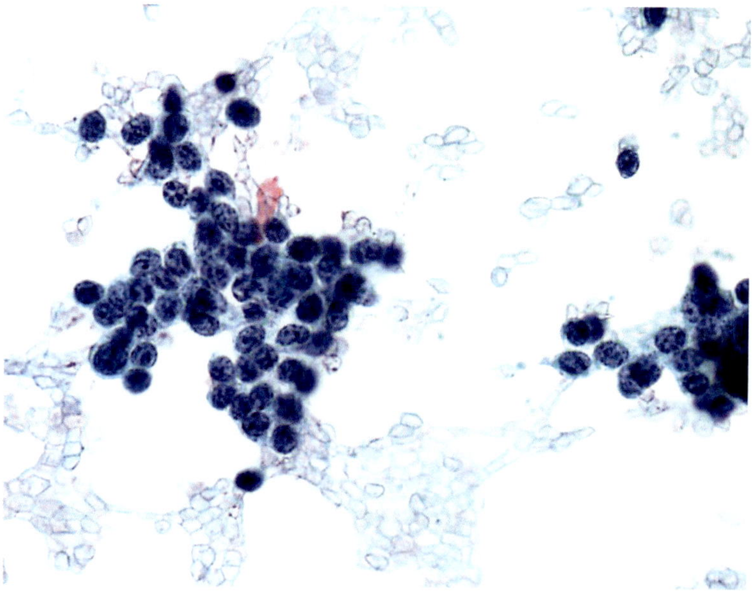

Figure 9.32 — Medullary Thyroid Carcinoma, FNA. Depicted here are malignant cells appearing almost as naked nuclei forming loose clusters. Chromatin shows the typical speckled appearance. These naked nuclei should not be confused with lymphocytes. Other differential diagnosis would include parathyroid lesion and less likely a poorly differentiated carcinoma (insular type). (Papanicolaou stain)

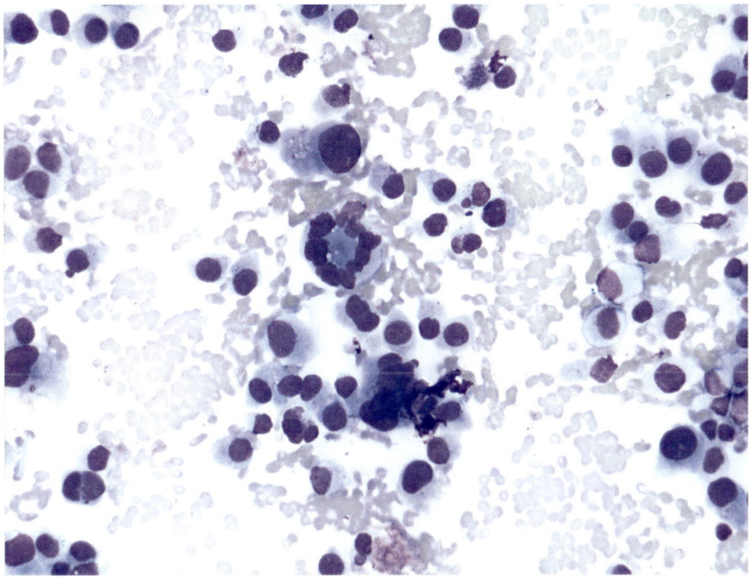

Figure 9.33 — Medullary Thyroid Carcinoma, FNA. A bizarre multinucleated cell is seen in the middle of the field. Such cells are often associated with the presence of amyloid in MTC. The most eye catching feature in this case is eccentric nuclear placement. Some metachromatic material (6 o'clock) suggests amyloid. (Diff Quik stain)

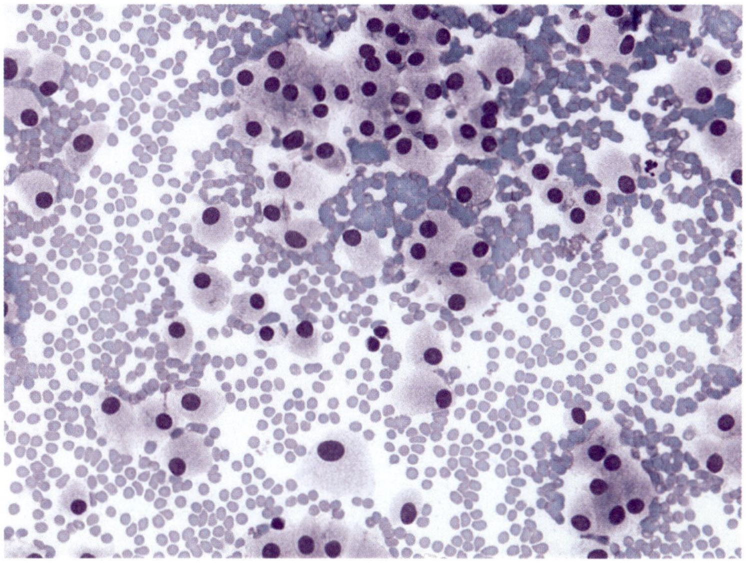

Figure 9.34 — Medullary Thyroid Carcinoma, FNA. Another feature of the tumor occasionally observed on Diff Quik stain is fine cytoplasmic vacuolization. When seen in a single dispersed cell pattern, confusion with histiocytes is not uncommon. Medullary carcinoma is also well known for rare pigment production. However, this phenomenon has rarely been reported in cytologic cases. Even the rare cases published in the literature on histopathology, pigment-laden macrophages were more numerous than pigmented tumor cells. (Diff Quik stain)

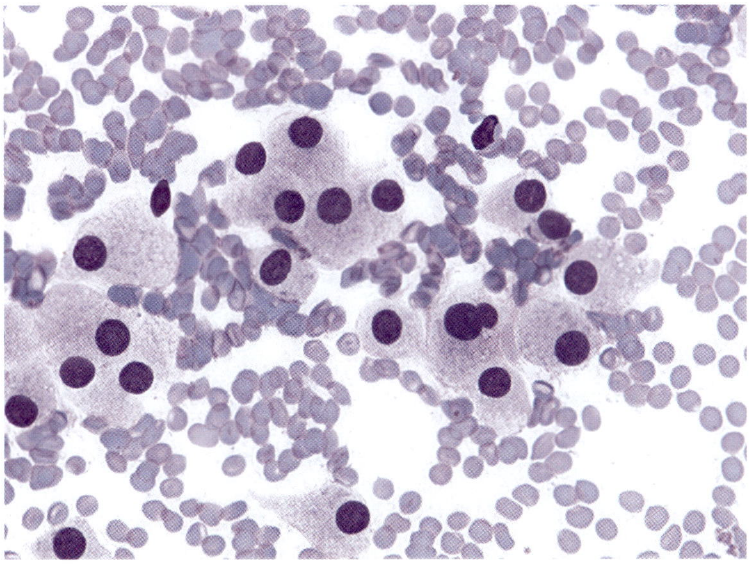

Figure 9.35 — Medullary Thyroid Carcinoma, FNA. Higher magnification beautifully depicts finely vacuolated cell cytoplasm. Differential diagnosis would include a Hürthle cell neoplasm and metastatic renal cell carcinoma. Due to the cytoplasmic vacuolization, the malignant cells often lose their cytoplasm and consequently, a large population of bare nuclei is not rare in medullary carcinomas on FNA. (Diff Quik stain)

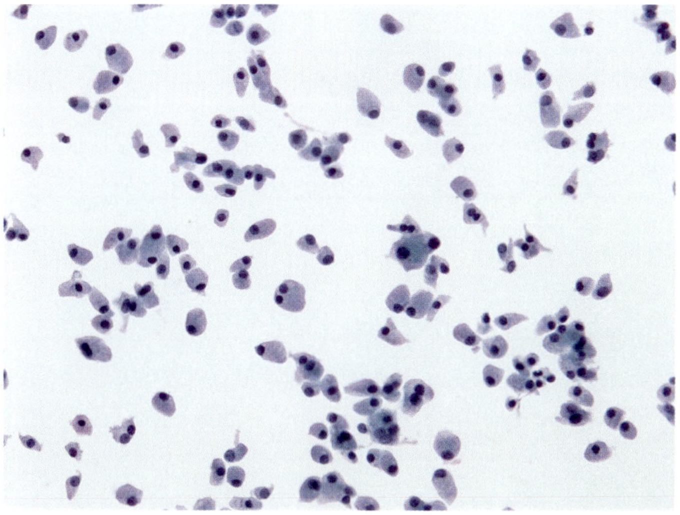

Figure 9.36 — Medullary Thyroid Carcinoma, FNA. The histiocytic appearance of medullary thyroid carcinoma cells is further enhanced on liquid-based preparation, as seen here. Cells are singly and widely dispersed and show occasional binucleation. Unlike histiocytes, the cells illustrated here show eccentrically placed nuclei and often tapering cytoplasm. (Papanicolaou stain)

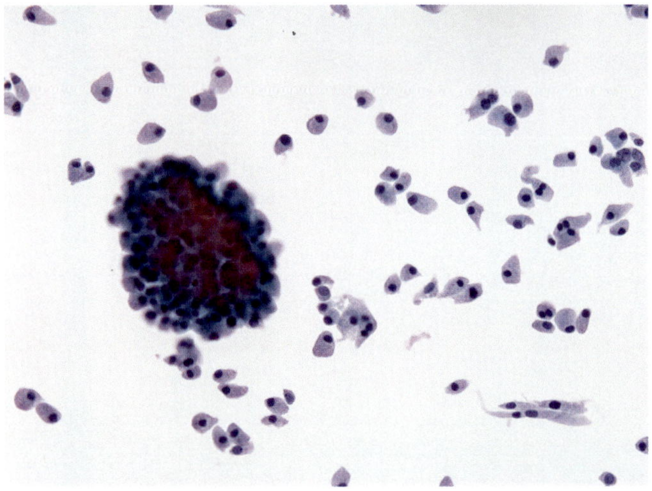

Figure 9.37 — Medullary Thyroid Carcinoma, FNA. In addition to singly dispersed cells, this liquid-based preparation displays an intact tissue fragment. Notice the elongated tumor cells with tapering cytoplasmic processes (5 o'clock) making Hürthle cell neoplasm highly unlikely in the differential diagnosis. Despite all the variations in the cytomorphologic spectrum, FNA still provides an extremely accurate interpretation of medullary carcinoma in routine clinical practice. Serum calcitonin levels and/or immunostaining further support the cytologic diagnoses. (Papanicolaou stain)

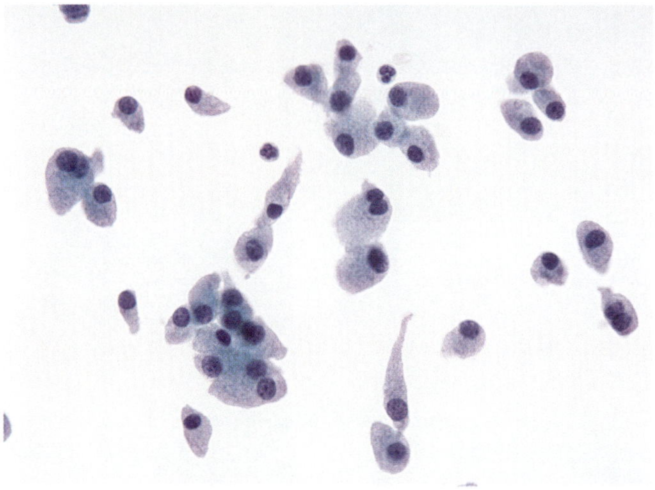

Figure 9.38 — Medullary Thyroid Carcinoma, FNA. It's not unusual for the neoplastic cells to develop long tapering cytoplasmic tails in addition to the eccentric nuclear placement in medullary carcinoma. Note binucleation in some cells as well as a prominent cytoplasmic vacuolization. Nuclei are round with a fine, dusty chromatin lacking nucleoli. (Liquid-based preparation, Papanicolaou stain)

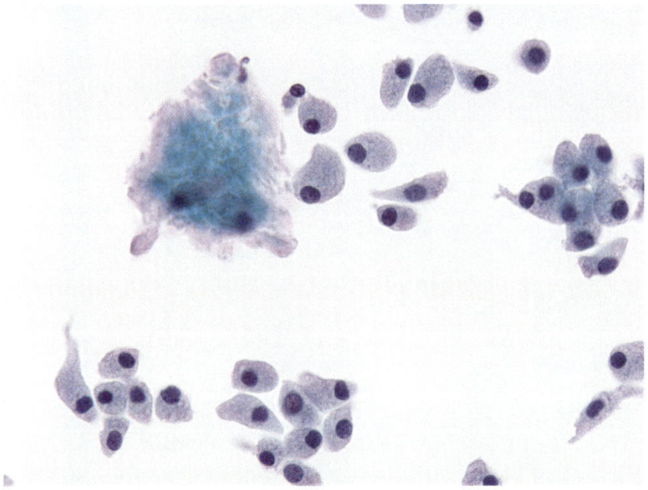

Figure 9.39 — Medullary Thyroid Carcinoma, FNA. A large deposit of amyloid is seen here associated with malignant neuroendocrine cells. Amyloid assumes a more fibrillary appearance in liquid-based preparations and needs to be accurately distinguished from colloid. The edges of amyloid material often appear much paler than the central portion which almost always displays bright green coloration. Multinucleated reactive histiocytes may or may not be present. (Papanicolaou stain)

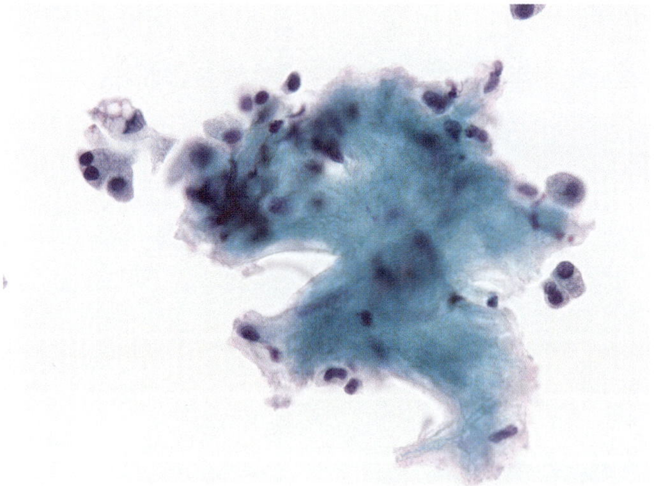

Figure 9.40 — Medullary Thyroid Carcinoma, FNA. Higher magnification of the amyloid displays its unique characteristics. Edges of the fragment in this case are focally sharply defined making a distinction from colloid much easier to accomplish. Although the fragment tends to have a somewhat lighter periphery, the classic two-tone appearance of colloid as seen in liquid-based preparations is absent. A few malignant cells with finely vacuolated cytoplasm are present in the background. Cytoplasmic granularity of these cells is much harder to appreciate on liquid-based preparations. (Papanicolaou stain)

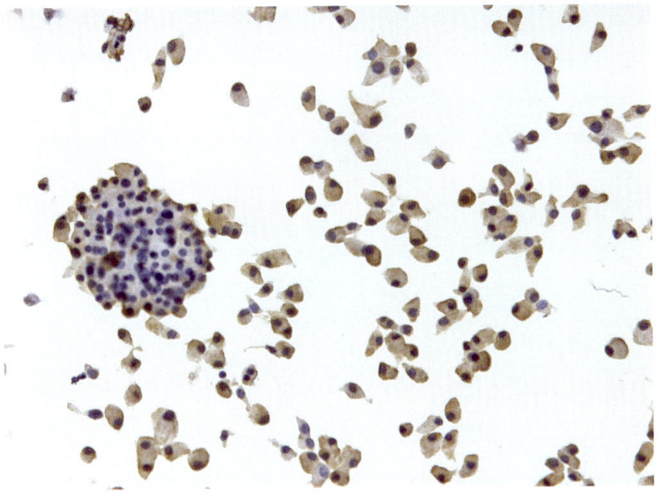

Figure 9.41 — Medullary Thyroid Carcinoma, FNA. The diagnosis of MTC can be strongly suggested by cytomorphology alone, but it is often advisable to confirm the cytologic interpretation with a Congo red stain for amyloid and/or immunoperoxidase studies using calcitonin, chromogranin, synaptophysin, and CEA. Liquid-based preparations provide ideal samples for immunostaining of the cells due to a much cleaner slide background and optimum slide fixation. This is an example of robust immunostaining with calcitonin. (Immunostain)

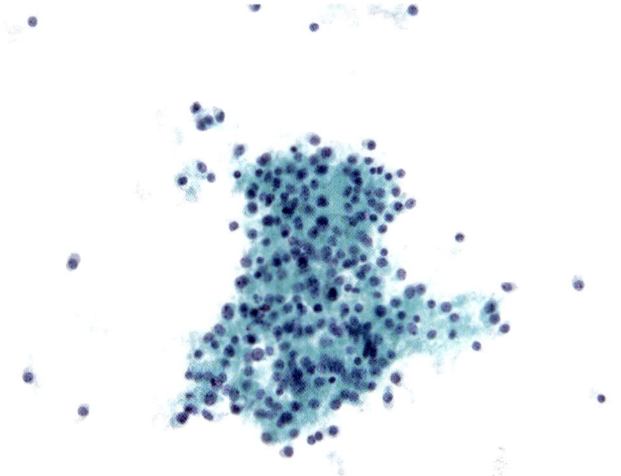

Figure 9.42 — Medullary Thyroid Carcinoma, FNA. This particular case was quite challenging on liquid-based preparation as the cells were small and uniform and resembled parathyroid tissue. Nuclei display a neuroendocrine-type chromatin pattern. Few single cells are also noted in the background, which did not show any amyloid. Immunostains are often extremely helpful and diagnostic in such cases. (Papanicolaou stain)

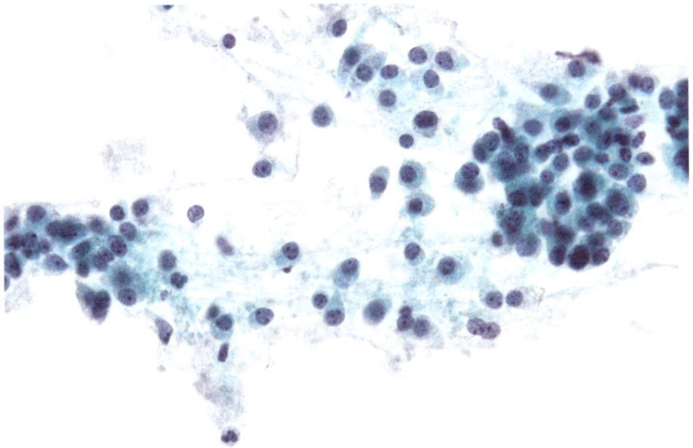

Figure 9.43 — Medullary Thyroid Carcinoma, FNA. Numerous loosely cohesive cells as well as single malignant cells highlight this field. Cells have the characteristic "plasmacytoid appearance." Nuclei have finely granular chromatin. Occasional cells display prominent nucleoli. Background contains serum and amyloid was not seen in this case. Although plasmacytoma may have similar cytomorphology on FNA, isolated thyroid plasma cell neoplasms are extremely rare and are not typically entertained in the differential diagnosis of medullary carcinoma. (Liquid-based preparation, Papanicolaou stain)

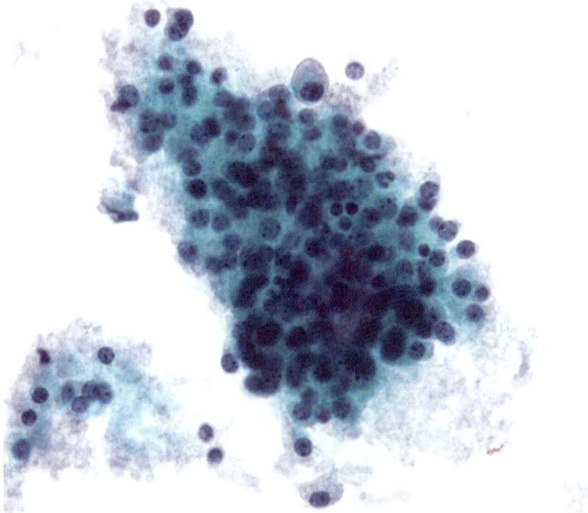

Figure 9.44 — Medullary Thyroid Carcinoma, FNA. Cytologic samples from MTC are usually moderately or highly cellular and composed of a mixture of non-cohesive cells and cell aggregates. This liquid-based preparation shows a large aggregate of malignant cells caught in the serum. Few apoptotic nuclei are visible. Mitoses and necrosis are seldom seen in FNA of these tumors. Focal anisonucleosis is also present. (Papanicolaou stain)

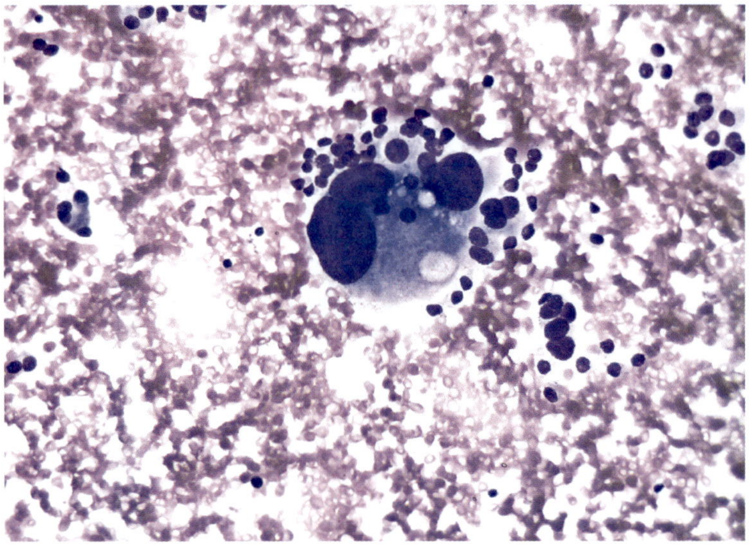

Figure 9.45 — Medullary Thyroid Carcinoma, FNA. This unusual case displayed many tumor giant cells, often with macronucleoli. This is an example of the morphologic heterogeneity that often leads to significant diagnostic challenges in the cytologic evaluation of this neoplasm. In this case, notice the huge disparity in nuclear size of the various tumor cells. Other areas in the smear showed the classic medullary carcinoma cytomorphology. (Diff Quik stain)

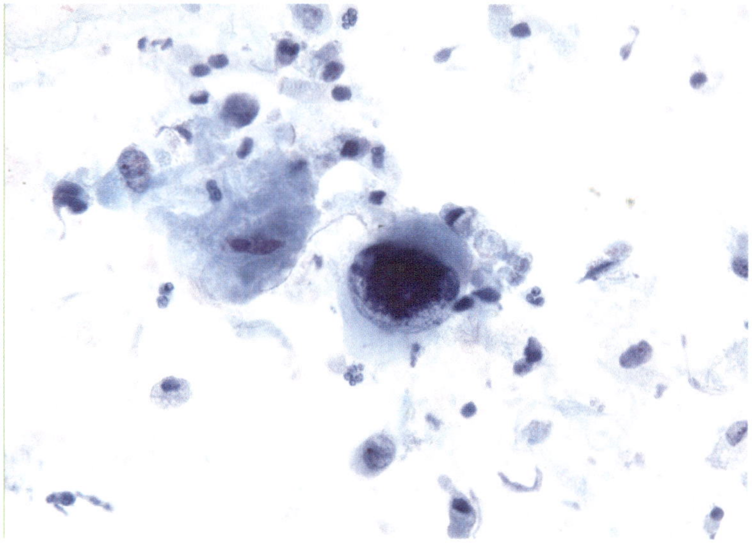

Figure 9.46 — Medullary Thyroid Carcinoma, FNA. MTC is notorious for a wide variation in the spectrum of morphologic appearances, which includes: follicular, papillary, glandular, giant cell, spindle cell, small cell, paraganglioma-like, oncocytic, clear cell, and squamous cell. The cases of medullary carcinoma with pleomorphic and bizarre tumor giant cells are often referred to as "giant cell variant" of the tumor and are quite challenging as they mimic anaplastic/undifferentiated carcinoma and metastatic tumors (melanoma, carcinoma) to the thyroid. A neuroendocrine staining pattern is retained and helps with the definitive diagnosis. (Papanicolaou stain)

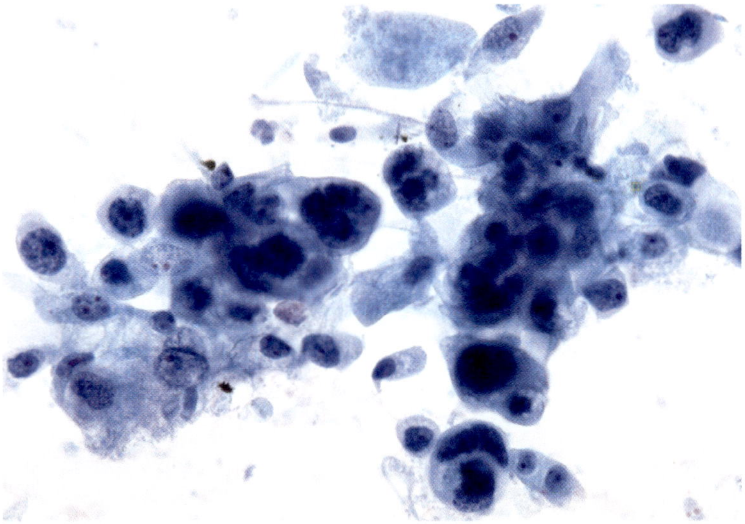

Figure 9.47 — Medullary Thyroid Carcinoma, FNA. It would be quite impossible to diagnose this particular case of the so-called "giant cell variant" of medullary carcinoma on a limited FNA sample. Cells display high-grade pleomorphic features and vary widely in size and shape. Giant cells have the most unusual and bizarre morphology. Few nuclei show prominent nucleoli. Cytoplasm shows vague granularity. Major differential diagnosis here would be with an anaplastic carcinoma and metastatic cancers to the thyroid. Immunostains are most often helpful in this rare variant of medullary carcinoma. (Papanicolaou stain)

10

Poorly Differentiated Thyroid Carcinoma

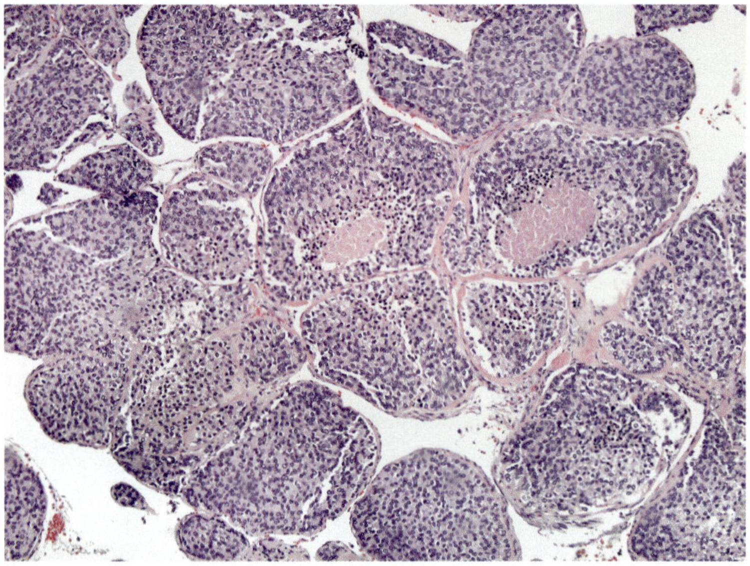

Figure 10.1a — Insular Carcinoma, Histologic Section. The hallmark feature of insular carcinoma is its insular pattern of growth characterized by round nests of cells separated by a delicate stroma with thin dilated blood vessels. The nests are usually solid, but microfollicles can sometimes be observed. This pattern can occur in pure form, but it is often encountered as a poorly differentiated component of a well differentiated papillary or follicular carcinoma. For a poorly differentiated form of thyroid carcinoma, the tumor cells are unexpectedly uniform and monotonous. Tumor necrosis within the center of the nests is a common finding. Although poorly differentiated, insular carcinomas usually retain immunoreactivity for thyroglobulin. Consequently, a panel of immunohistochemical probes that includes thyroglobulin and calcitonin can be useful in distinguishing between insular carcinoma and medullary thyroid carcinoma when dealing with a primary thyroid tumor exhibiting a nested growth pattern. (H&E stain)

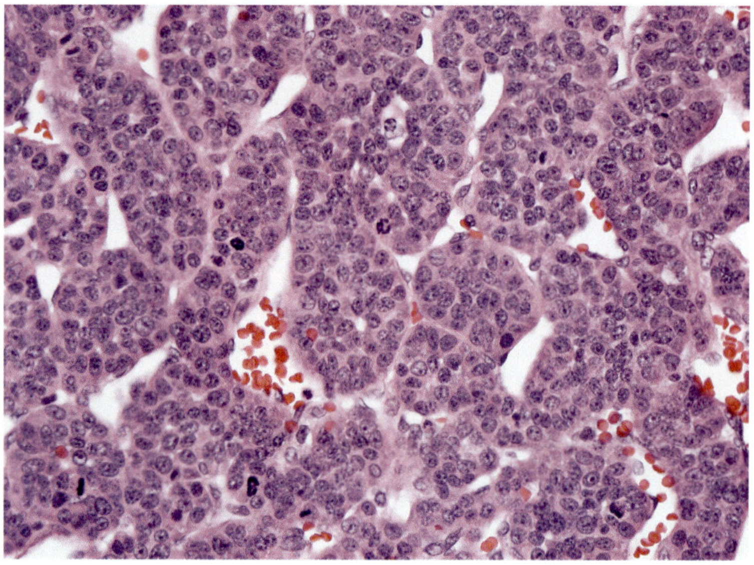

Figure 10.1b — Insular Carcinoma, Histologic Section. An insular growth pattern by itself is not sufficient for designating a tumor as poorly differentiated. In addition to insular growth, a diagnosis of insular carcinoma requires the presence of tumor necrosis and an elevated mitotic rate. At high power, mitotic figures should be easily identified. (H&E stain)

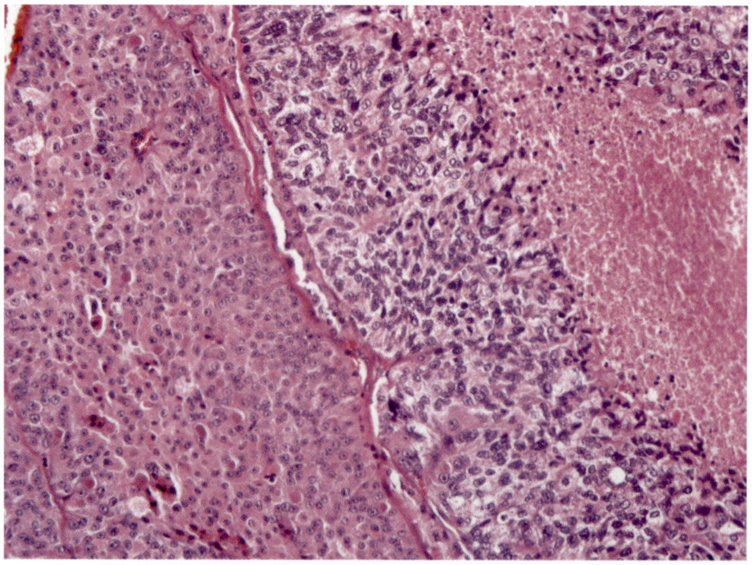

Figure 10.2 — Poorly Differentiated Hürthle Cell Carcinoma, Histologic Section. Insular carcinomas do not always occur in pure form. Instead, they sometimes are seen as a poorly differentiated component of a well differentiated papillary, follicular carcinoma or Hürthle cell carcinoma. These poorly differentiated areas exhibit solid nested growth with an elevated mitotic rate and necrosis, but their cellular features may retain some of the characteristics of the more conventional carcinoma from which they arose. In this case, there is a transition from a conventional Hürthle cell carcinoma (left) to a poorly differentiated carcinoma with necrosis (right). (H&E stain)

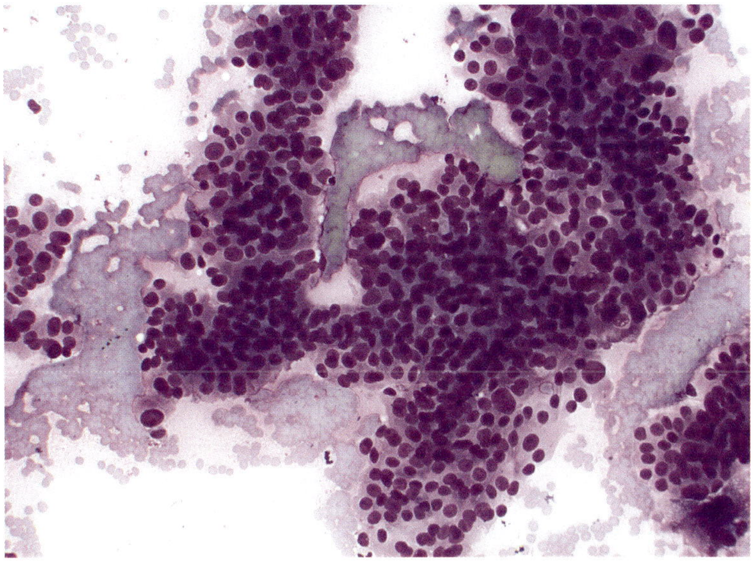

Figure 10.3a — Insular Carcinoma, Fine Needle Aspiration (FNA). The Bethesda System for Reporting Thyroid Cytopathology (TBSRTC) defines a poorly differentiated thyroid carcinoma (PDTC) as "a thyroid carcinoma of follicular cell origin characterized by an insular, solid, or trabecular growth pattern. In its pure form, PDTC lacks conventional nuclear features of papillary thyroid carcinoma and is distinguished from the latter by the presence of poorly differentiated features: mitoses, necrosis, or small convoluted nuclei." This case demonstrates a solid proliferation of malignant epithelium with uniform, mostly small sized cells with round nuclei and indistinct cytoplasm. No follicular differentiation or papillary architecture is seen. Colloid is not present. The delicate strands of stromal tissue are hard to visualize at this magnification. (Diff Quik stain)

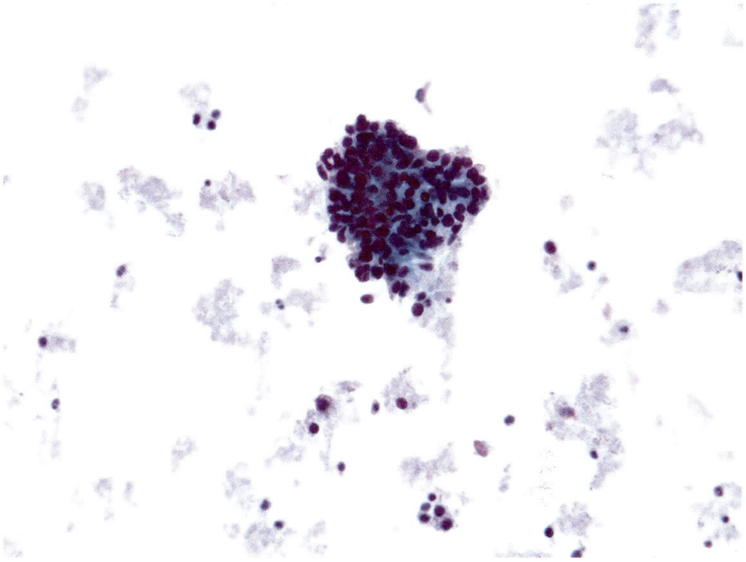

Figure 10.3b — Insular Carcinoma, FNA. This liquid-based preparation depicts the characteristic "insular" growth pattern. Cells form solid nests with uniform round dark nuclei and barely discernible stromal matrix. Occasionally an attempt at follicular differentiation may be focally apparent in some cases. Insular carcinoma has an aggressive clinical behavior intermediate between that of the well differentiated thyroid carcinomas (papillary carcinoma, follicular carcinoma, and Hürthle cell carcinoma) and undifferentiated (anaplastic) thyroid carcinoma. (Papanicolaou stain)

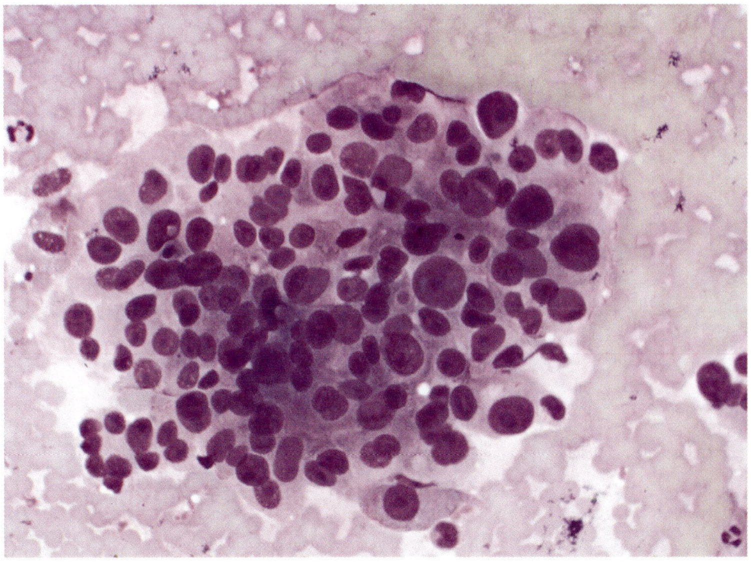

Figure 10.4 — Insular Carcinoma, FNA. Higher magnification displays some anisonucleosis with occasional cells containing macronucleoli. Cytoplasmic granularity is also observed. Most of these cases (like this one) are prospectively diagnosed as "suspicious for malignancy" and a definitive diagnosis only rendered after histopathologic examination. On FNA, insular carcinoma is extremely difficult to diagnose as such because of its rarity and also because its cytomorphologic characteristics are nonspecific and significantly overlap with those of follicular neoplasms. (Diff Quik stain)

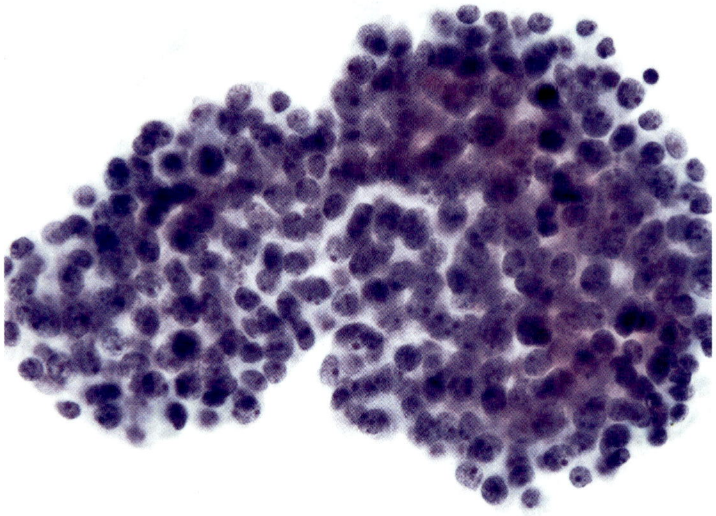

Figure 10.5 — Insular Carcinoma, FNA. A liquid-based preparation depicts cytomorphologic features similar to the previous case. Note the discreet nuclear hyperchromasia, small nucleoli and a speckled "neuroendocrine" type chromatin texture. Insular carcinoma has been consistently misdiagnosed on FNA and almost always it becomes a retrospective diagnosis after histopathologic examination of the resected tumor. (Papanicolaou stain)

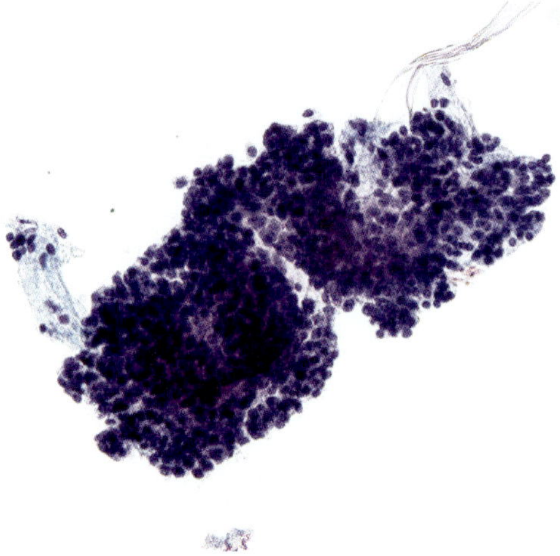

Figure 10.6 — Insular Carcinoma, FNA. Large cohesive malignant tissue fragments display an "insular" architectural pattern. Background is clean and no colloid, follicular formations or macrophages are present. Nuclear hyperchromasia gives the fragment an "over stained" look. Patients with insular carcinoma range in age from 11 to 86 years (mean age 55), and approximately two-thirds are female (Male:Female, 2.2–1). (Liquid-based Cytology, Papanicolaou stain)

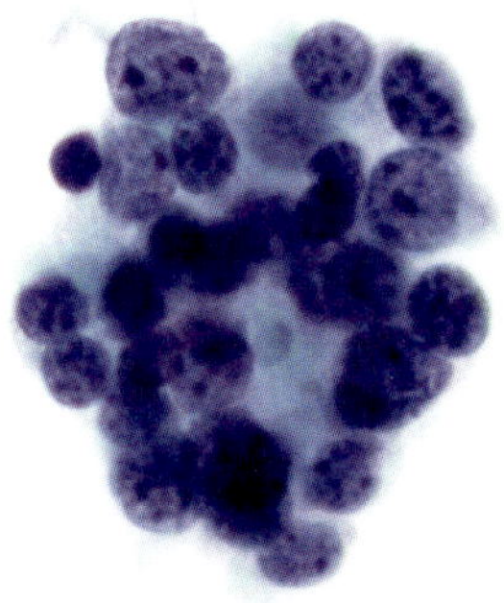

Figure 10.7 — Insular Carcinoma, FNA. Higher magnification in a case shows focal follicular differentiation. However, the pale green substance is delicate stromal tissue and not colloid. Nuclei are round and have a speckled chromatin pattern. Due to an obvious similarity with neuroendocrine-type chromatin, two of the differential diagnoses of an insular carcinoma are medullary carcinoma and metastatic small cell carcinoma. Insular carcinomas are uniformly immunoreactive with thyroglobulin. The absence of staining for calcitonin and leukocyte common antigen helps differentiate insular carcinomas from medullary carcinomas and malignant lymphomas. (Liquid-based preparation, Papanicolaou stain)

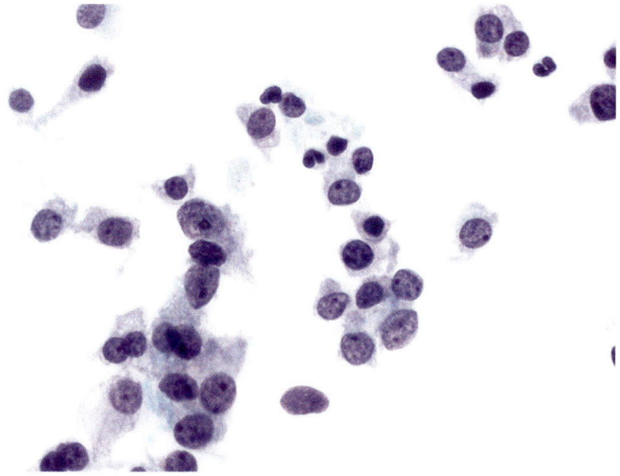

Figure 10.8 — Insular Carcinoma, FNA. This case displays a discohesive cell pattern. Cells appear epithelioid with fragile vaguely granular cytoplasm and eccentric nuclei. Nuclear chromatin is fine and dusty, thus raising the possibility of medullary carcinoma. Occasional cases of insular carcinoma in fact have been demonstrated to immunoexpress neuroendocrine markers. The most common clinical presentation is an enlarging neck mass or; dysphagia and dyspnea are common in patients with large lesions. Rarely, patients present with cervical spinal cord compression and biphasic stridor. (Papanicolaou stain)

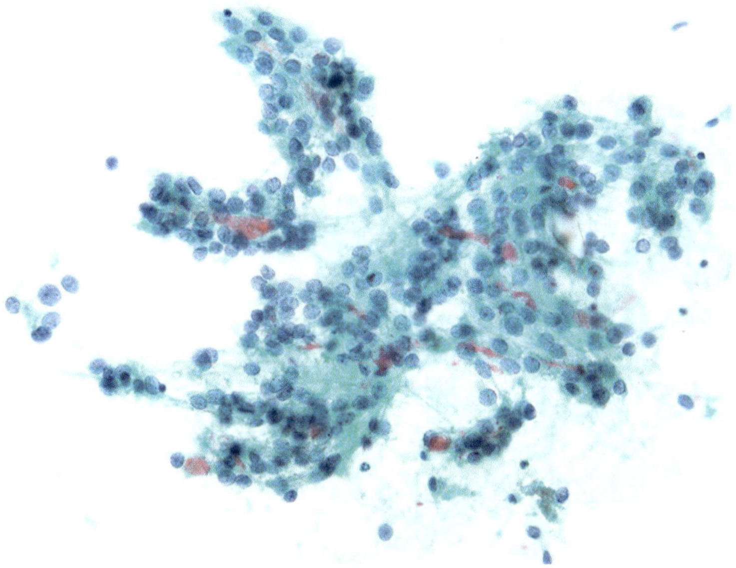

Figure 10.9 — Insular Carcinoma, FNA. This case was misdiagnosed as follicular neoplasm due to focal follicular architecture and scant colloid formation. However, on retrospective review, most of the neoplasm had a solid "insular" pattern. Also notice the fine powdery chromatin. A prospective diagnosis of an insular carcinoma on FNA is very challenging, if not impossible, even in experienced hands. At the molecular level, p53 gene, which is frequently over-expressed in anaplastic carcinoma, is uniformly absent in insular carcinoma, however, mutations of ras oncogene are found in a high percentage of insular carcinomas. (Papanicolaou stain)

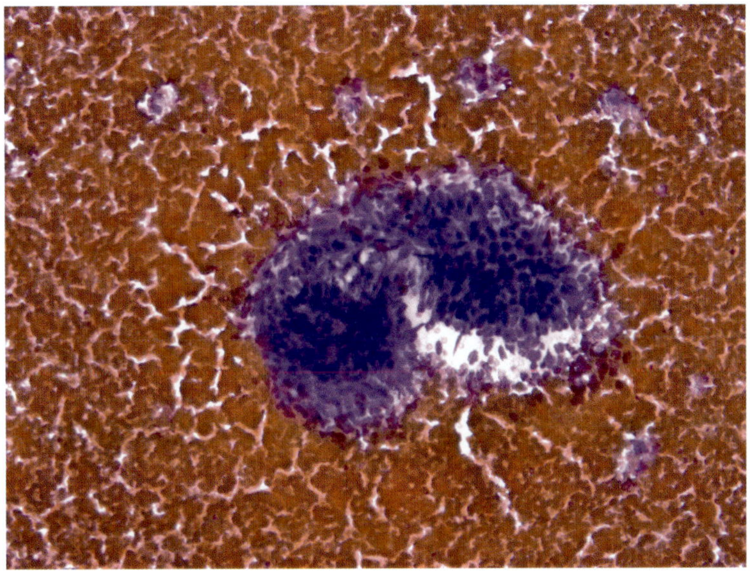

Figure 10.10a — Insular Carcinoma, FNA. This extremely bloody smear contained only rare fragments of malignant epithelium in tightly crowded, somewhat three-dimensional fragments representing the insular architectural pattern, which gives this tumor its distinct name. No single cells were present. Also there was a total absence of colloid. The most controversial point with insular carcinoma concerns prognosis. Studies have shown a rate of tumor recurrence ranging widely from 30% to 80%. Most published reports have confirmed the high aggressiveness of this tumor with a 10-year mortality rate that ranges from 13% to 41%. (Diff Quik stain)

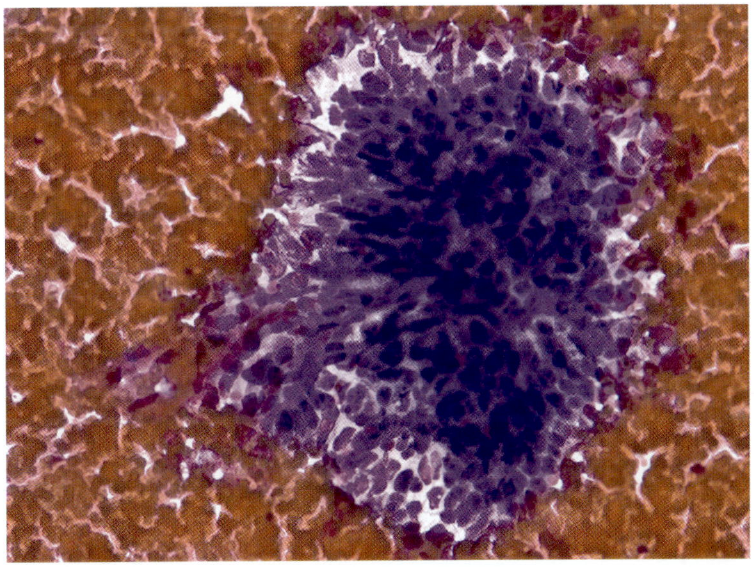

Figure 10.10b — Insular Carcinoma, FNA. At higher magnification, this case shows strong resemblance to a small cell carcinoma with mostly uniform hyperchromatic bare nuclei tightly molded against each other. Lack of single discohesive cell pattern argues against a neuroendocrine malignancy in this case. Patients with insular thyroid carcinoma have a poorer outcome compared with patients of similar age who have differentiated types of thyroid carcinoma in tumors of a similar size. Metastases to regional nodes, lungs, and bone have been reported and often result in death despite aggressive surgical, external beam therapy, and chemotherapy. (Diff Quik stain)

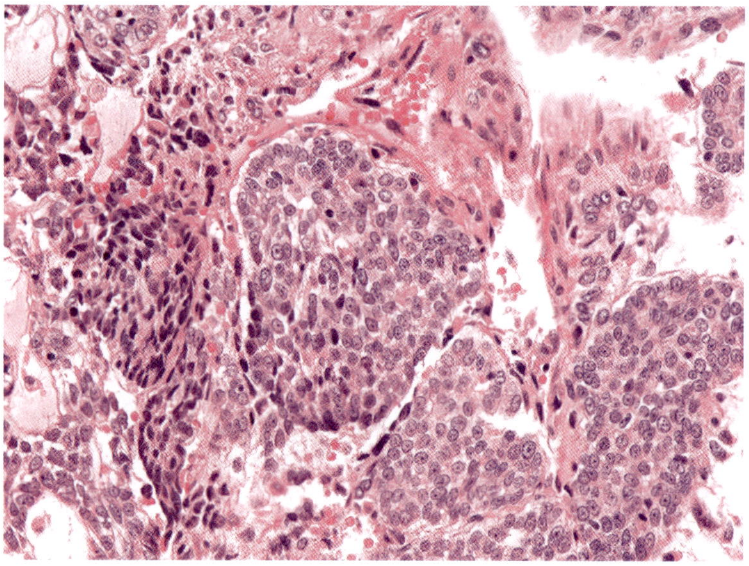

Figure 10.10c — Insular Carcinoma, Histologic Section. The resected tumor in the previous case shows nice cyto-histopathologic correlation. Note the prominent insular architectural pattern highlighting the histology in this tumor. Treatment of insular carcinoma includes total thyroidectomy and high-dose radioiodine for all patients and neck dissections for patients with lymph node disease. Papillary and follicular carcinomas have been noted within an insular carcinoma, suggesting transformation of differentiated thyroid carcinoma (DTC) into this more aggressive phenotype. (H&E stain)

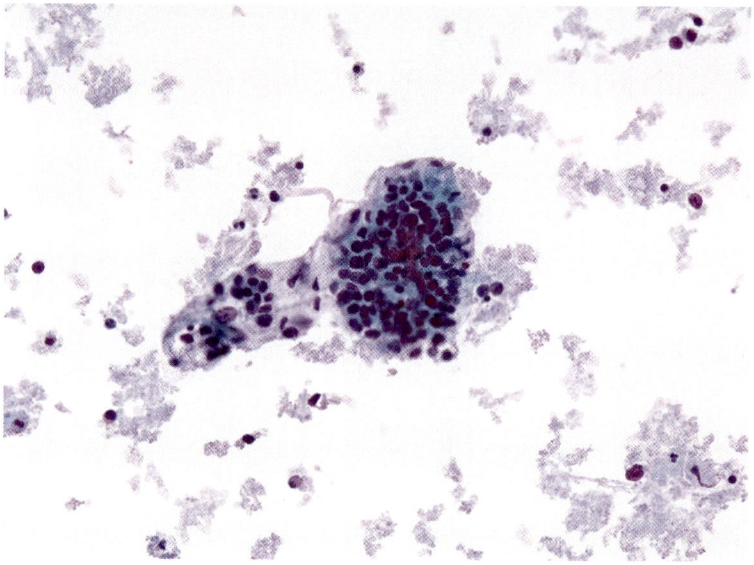

Figure 10.11 — Insular Carcinoma, FNA. A liquid-based preparation displays a partially intact tumor tissue fragment comprised of extremely monotonous hyperchromatic nuclei tightly placed against each other without follicular differentiation. Few bare nuclei are also present in the slide background. Histopathologically, a tumor is not reported as PDTC unless more than 50% of the architecture is composed of insular, solid, and/or trabecular growth patterns. (Papanicolaou stain)

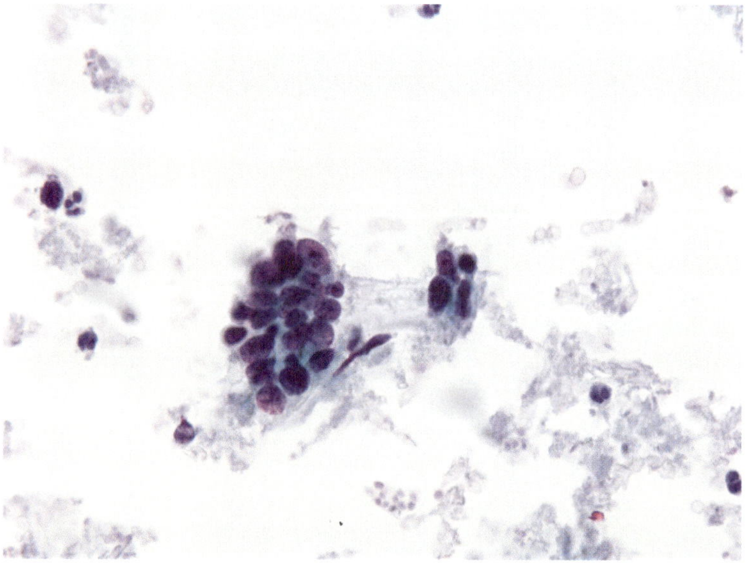

Figure 10.12a — Insular Carcinoma, FNA. Higher magnification of the previous case on liquid-based preparation displays uniform round to oval nuclei, finely granular and dark chromatin, and scant pale green matrix tissue. Insular carcinomas arise from follicular epithelial cells with distinct biologic features and often produce thyroglobulin and concentrate radioiodine and are reported to be more common in regions of iodine deficiency and endemic goiter. The rationale of radiotherapy for insular carcinoma is that most insular carcinomas and their metastatic lesions take up a large amount of iodine. (Papanicolaou stain)

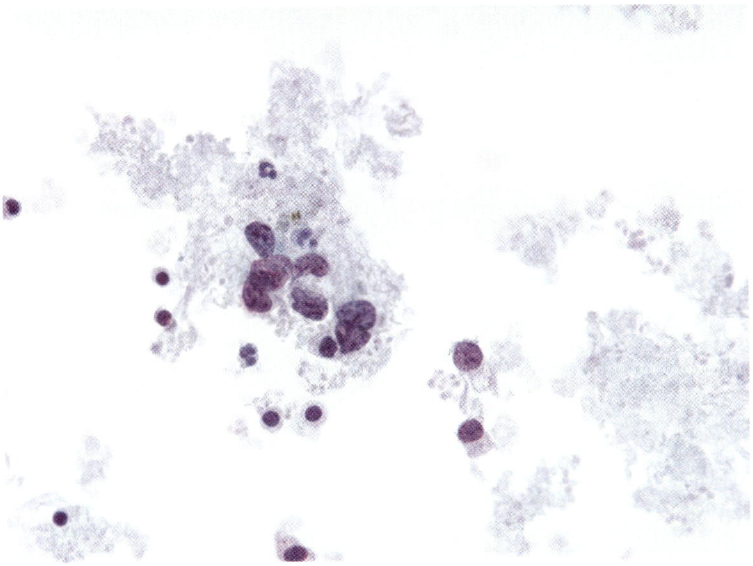

Figure 10.12b — Insular Carcinoma, FNA. Here is another high magnification view with monotonous malignant cells appearing as bare nuclei. Notice the "neuroendocrine" type chromatin. Abundant serum and few lymphocytes are present in the slide background. Published data on the FNA findings has additionally shown—most often hypercellular aspirates with a bloody background, scant colloid, and rare necrosis. The malignant cells display an architecture of either loosely cohesive solid or trabecular clusters or show insular groups measuring 0.2 to 0.4 mm in diameter. The malignant cells are typically isolated small to medium-size with scant cytoplasm, round nuclei, inconspicuous nucleoli, and high N/C ratio. The cells are characteristically monomorphic, but variable degrees of atypia can be found on higher magnification with occasional mitoses and apoptotic nuclei. (Liquid-based Cytology, Papanicolaou stain)

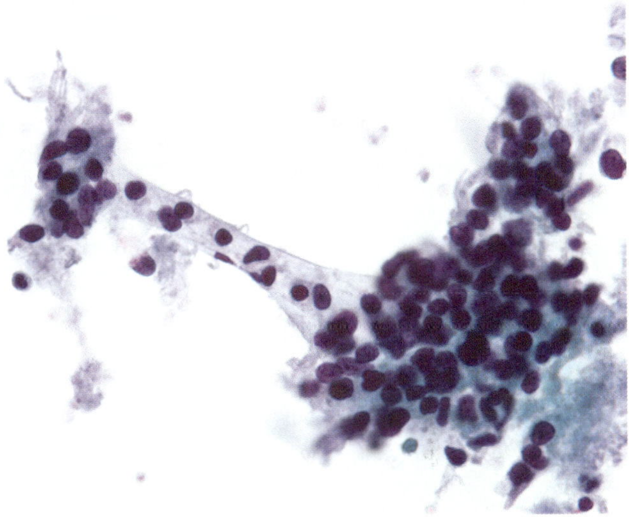

Figure 10.13 — Insular Carcinoma, FNA. Partially intact tissue fragment displays a uniform population of small cells with discreet nuclear hyperchromasia. Insular carcinoma is mostly a stroma-poor tumor. Neoplastic cells are held together by a minute amount of fine and delicate stromal tissue, which is rarely apparent in cytologic smears. Whether patients with insular carcinoma should be managed more aggressively than patients with papillary or follicular carcinoma has not been well established. Most experts have proposed aggressive management initially, including total thyroidectomy and systematic cervical lymph node dissection. Interestingly, lymph node metastasis has not been found to be a worse prognostic factor in insular carcinomas. (Liquid-based Cytology, Papanicolaou stain)

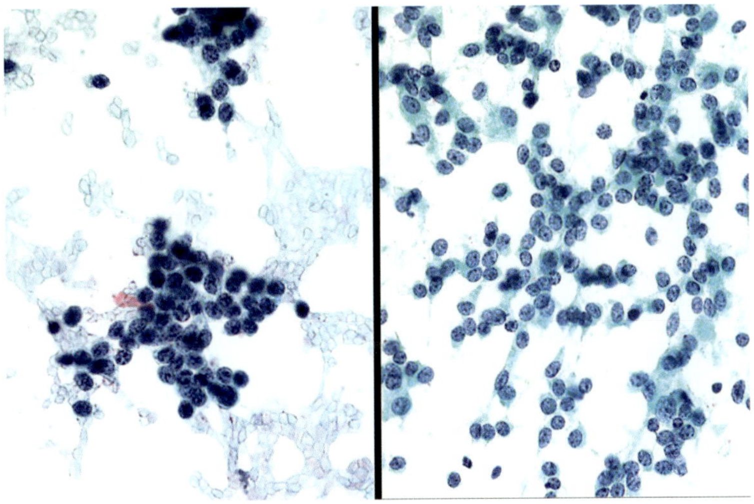

Figure 10.14 — Insular Carcinoma, FNA. These two examples of insular carcinoma bear an amazing resemblance to medullary carcinoma with mostly single cells or loose fragments of malignant epithelium displaying finely speckled chromatin and barely discernible cytoplasm. Immunostains are critical to exclude medullary carcinoma or metastases in such cases. Lack of amyloid in insular carcinoma may help in the differential diagnosis. (Papanicolaou stain)

11

Undifferentiated (Anaplastic) Carcinoma and Squamous Cell Carcinoma of the Thyroid

Armanda Tatsas

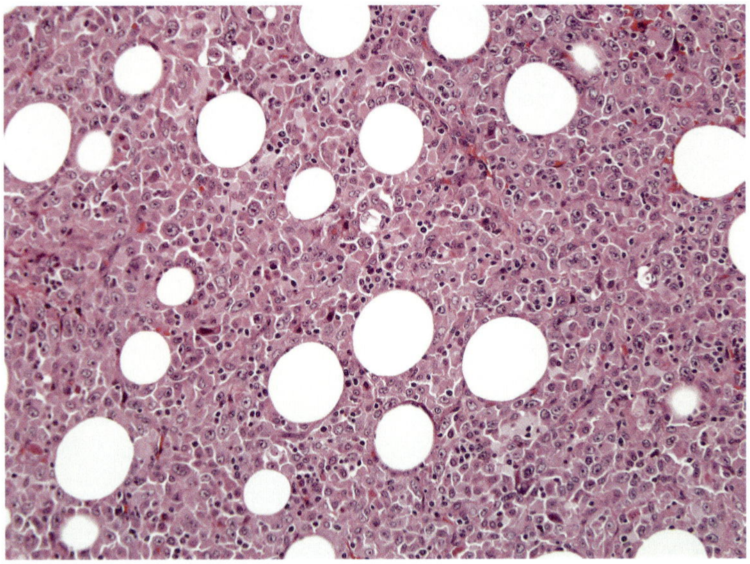

Figure 11.1 — Undifferentiated (Anaplastic) Carcinoma, Histologic Section. Undifferentiated thyroid carcinomas are high-grade carcinomas that do not demonstrate obvious follicular differentiation by routine histology or immunohistochemistry. Most undifferentiated carcinomas present with extensive local extension beyond the thyroid. Permeation of perithyroidal fat in a way that mimics malignant lymphoma is a common pattern of extrathyroidal invasion. (H&E stain)

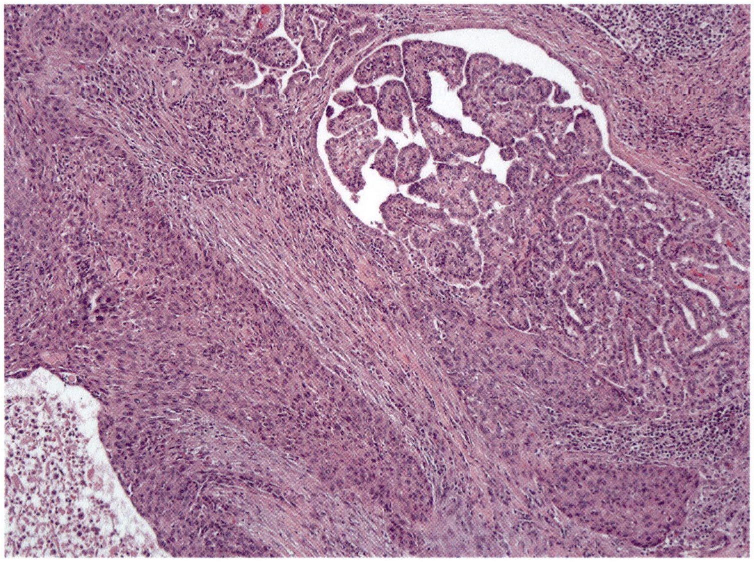

Figure 11.2a — Undifferentiated (Anaplastic) Carcinoma, Squamoid Pattern, Histologic Section. Most, if not all, undifferentiated carcinomas actually represent malignant degeneration of a preexisting well-differentiated thyroid carcinoma. Thorough microscopic examination can often uncover areas of transition from a well-differentiated to an undifferentiated carcinoma. In this case, a zone of undifferentiated carcinoma with squamoid features is arising from a papillary carcinoma. (H&E stain)

Figure 11.2b — Undifferentiated (Anaplastic) Carcinoma, Squamoid Pattern, Histologic Section. Although all undifferentiated thyroid carcinomas share high-grade cellular features and a propensity for infiltrative growth, the spectrum of microscopic features in this group of carcinomas is broad. Undifferentiated carcinomas typically demonstrate some combination of squamoid, spindle cell (sarcomatoid), and pleomorphic giant cell patterns. Shown here is an example of the squamoid pattern. These nests of cohesive epithelial cells with their glassy pink cytoplasm bear a striking resemblance to squamous cell carcinoma. Overt cytoplasmic keratinization with squamous pearl formations is only rarely encountered in undifferentiated thyroid carcinomas, and its presence should raise the possibility of secondary involvement of the thyroid by a squamous cell carcinoma of the larynx. (H&E stain)

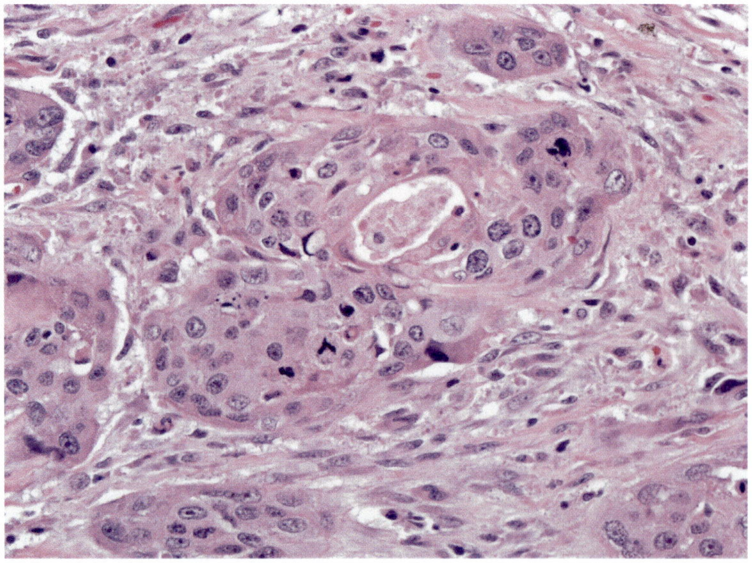

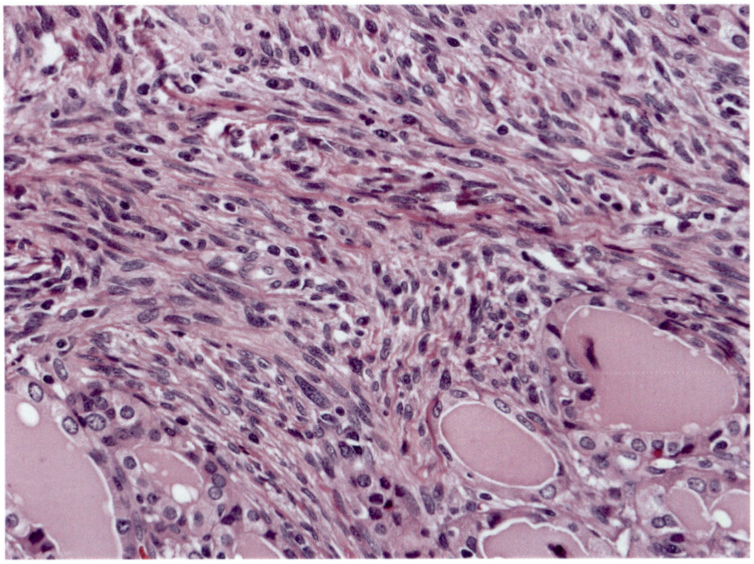

Figure 11.3 — Undifferentiated (Anaplastic) Carcinoma, Spindle Pattern, Histologic Section. This is an example of a spindle cell pattern of undifferentiated carcinoma. The thyroid follicles are overrun by malignant spindled cells. The spindled morphology resembles a mesenchymal neoplasm. Although not shown here, heterologous elements such as bone and cartilage are sometimes encountered in the spindle cell form of undifferentiated thyroid carcinoma causing further confusion with a sarcoma. Immunohistochemical stains for cytokeratin may be useful in confirming the epithelial origin of these spindled tumor cells, but not all undifferentiated thyroid carcinomas are cytokeratin positive. (H&E stain)

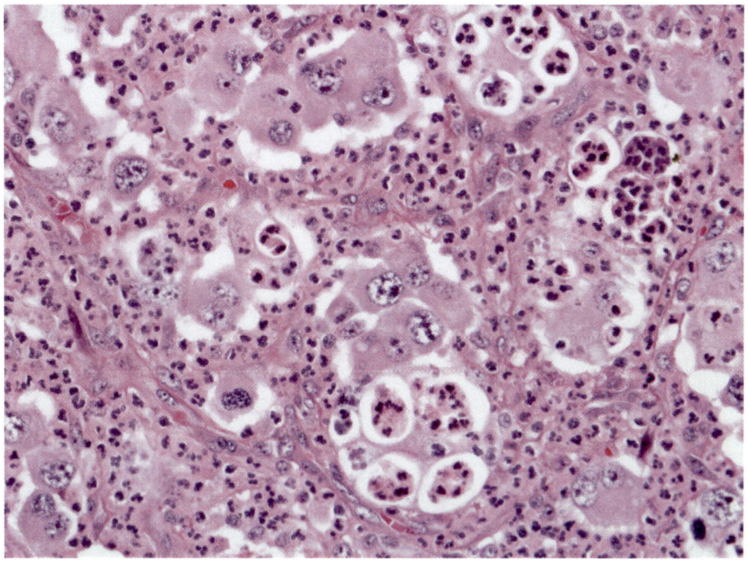

Figure 11.4a — Undifferentiated (Anaplastic) Carcinoma, Pleomorphic Giant Cell Pattern, Histologic Section. Undifferentiated carcinoma is sometimes associated with an intense infiltrate of neutrophils. Microabscesses may even form within the cytoplasm of the tumor cells. This neutrophil-rich background is usually associated with the pleomorphic giant cell pattern. (H&E stain)

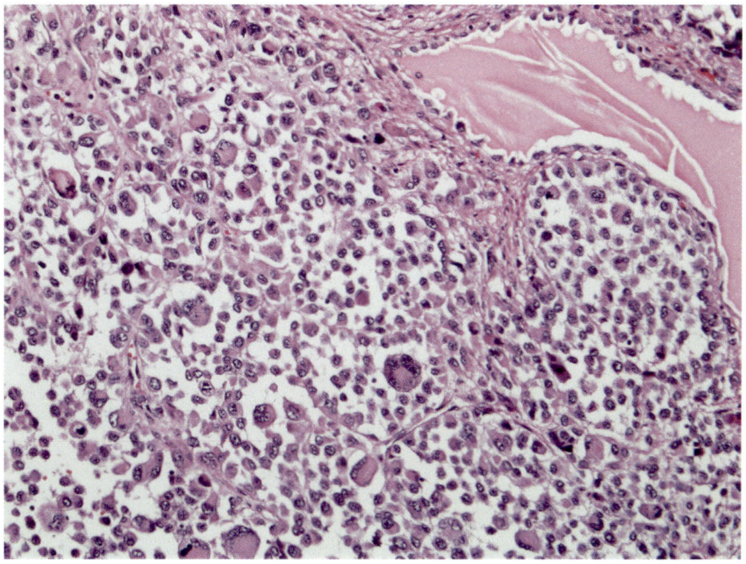

Figure 11.4b — Undifferentiated (Anaplastic) Carcinoma, Pleomorphic Giant Cell Pattern, Histologic Section. The cells that make up this pattern are rounded and highly pleomorphic. Their cytoplasm is usually deeply eosinophilic. They have one or two or several nuclei. The term "giant cell" is in reference to these multinucleated tumor cells. (H&E stain)

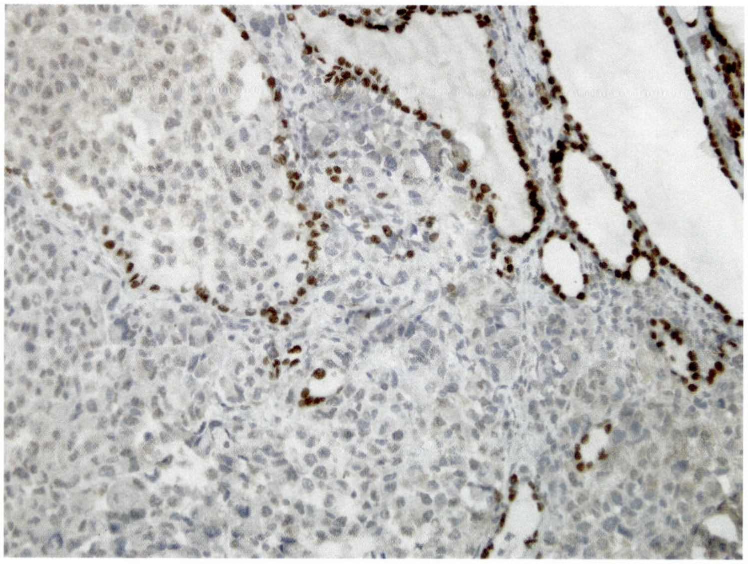

Figure 11.4c — Undifferentiated (Anaplastic) Carcinoma, Pleomorphic Giant Cell Pattern (TTF-1 Immunostain), Histologic Section. As expected for an undifferentiated thyroid carcinoma, the tumor consistently loses expression of the thyroid specific markers TTF-1 and thyroglobulin. The positive TTF-1 staining shown here is restricted to the nonneoplastic follicular epithelium. Overgrowth of the thyroid parenchyma with entrapment of TTF-1 positive thyroid follicles should not be interpreted as positive staining of the tumor. (Immunostain)

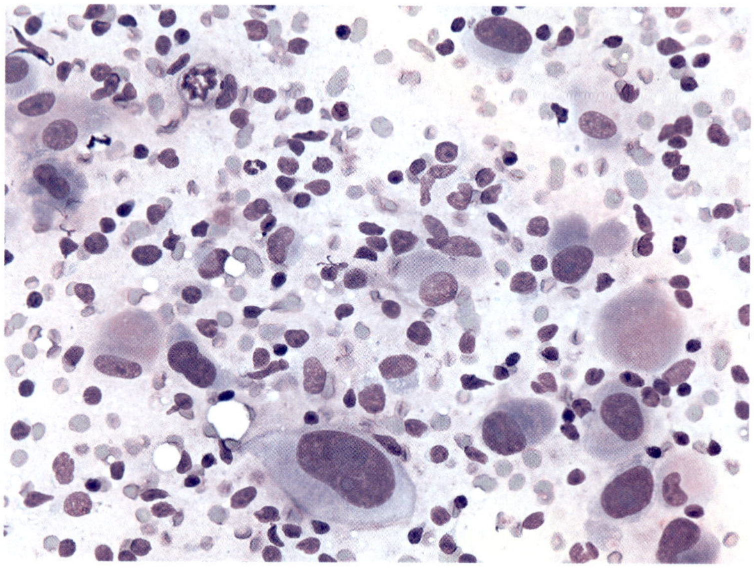

Figure 11.5a — Undifferentiated (Anaplastic) Carcinoma, Fine Needle Aspiration (FNA). Fine needle aspirates of undifferentiated thyroid carcinoma typically yield cellular smears unless there is abundant desmoplasia in the tumor, in which case aspirates may be sparsely cellular. In this case, the aspirated material shows a predominantly isolated tumor cell or single, dispersed cell population. The individual tumor cells are markedly pleomorphic, with a range of small, medium, and large tumor cells. Mitotic figures, which are not commonly encountered in thyroid aspirates, can be seen as in this case at 11 o'clock, and may have even been numerous. (Diff Quik stain)

Figure 11.5b — Undifferentiated (Anaplastic) Carcinoma, FNA. Significant pleomorphism is evident even at this magnification with mostly undifferentiated epithelioid and spindled cells. The malignant cells have large irregular nuclei, macronucleoli, and dense cytoplasm (without any evidence of cytoplasmic keratinization). A bizarre giant cell is seen at the 3 o'clock position. The background is relatively clean in this liquid-based preparation although foci of granular debris can be observed in some areas. (Papanicolaou stain)

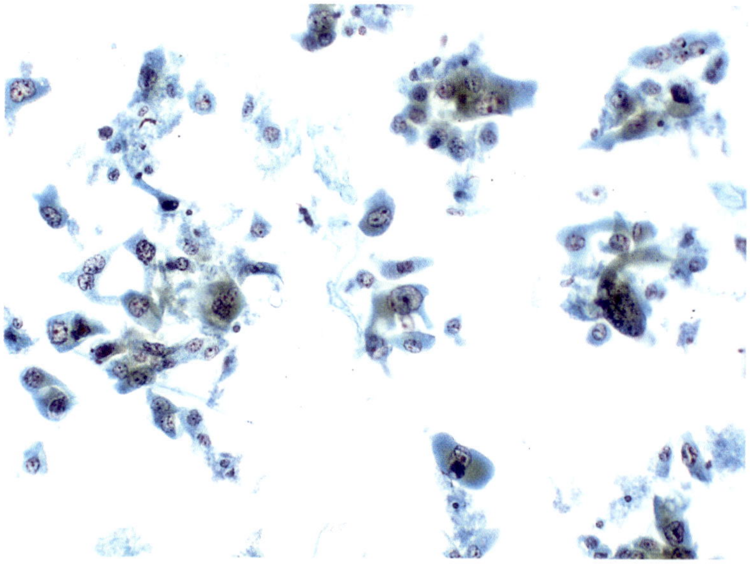

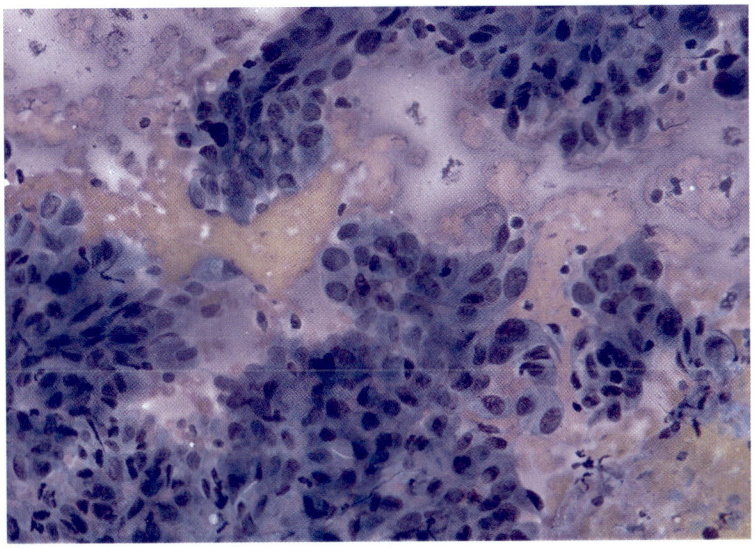

Figure 11.6a — Undifferentiated (Anaplastic) Carcinoma, FNA. Cohesive tissue fragments of malignant cells are seen. Cells are densely packed and overlapping and overall cellularity is markedly increased. Typically no distinct architectural patterns are present in undifferentiated carcinoma, although papillary or follicular architecture may be observed in the background when a better differentiated component of the tumor is present. (Diff Quik stain)

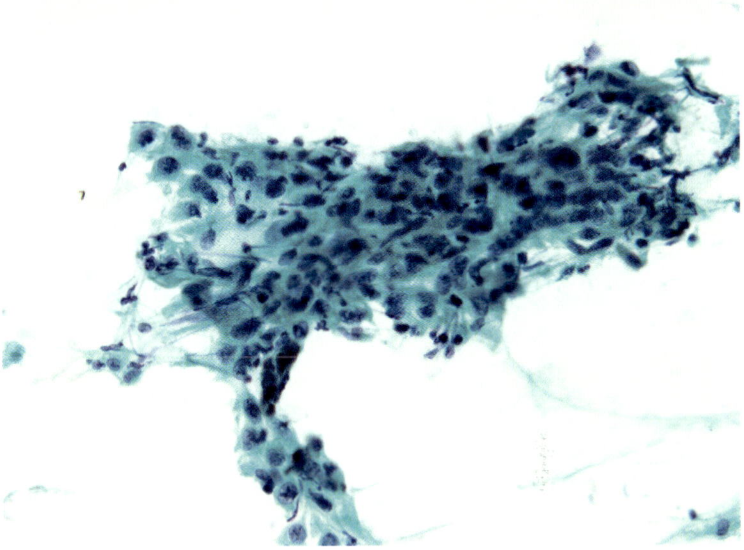

Figure 11.6b — Undifferentiated (Anaplastic) Carcinoma, FNA. A syncytium of undifferentiated malignant cells is depicted in this case. Cytoplasm is dense with distinct opacity; however, no obvious keratinization is evident. Anaplastic thyroid carcinoma (ATC) represents 2% to 5% of all thyroid malignancies; however, it accounts for possibly >50% of thyroid cancer mortality. ATC incidence peaks at the sixth to seventh decade of life, with more than 90% of patients being older than 50 years. (Papanicolaou stain)

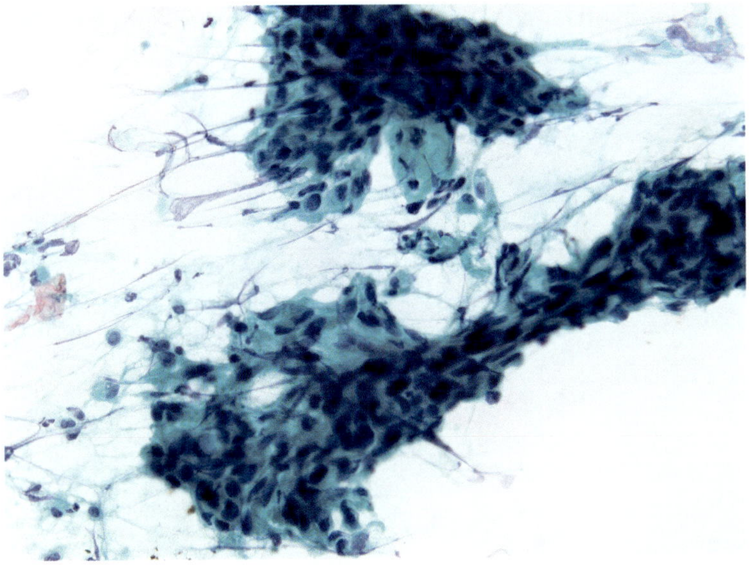

Figure 11.6c — Undifferentiated (Anaplastic) Carcinoma, FNA. Another field demonstrates highly pleomorphic malignant epithelial cells in a syncytial architecture. There is some suggestion of cellular whorling (3 o'clock) and dense green cytoplasmic opacity. Background inflammatory cells display crush artifact. The role of surgery in the treatment of ATC has been controversial. Most studies that discuss surgery as a treatment option refer to thyroidectomy only for intrathyroidal ATC and report that extrathyroidal extension represents unresectable disease. (Papanicolaou stain)

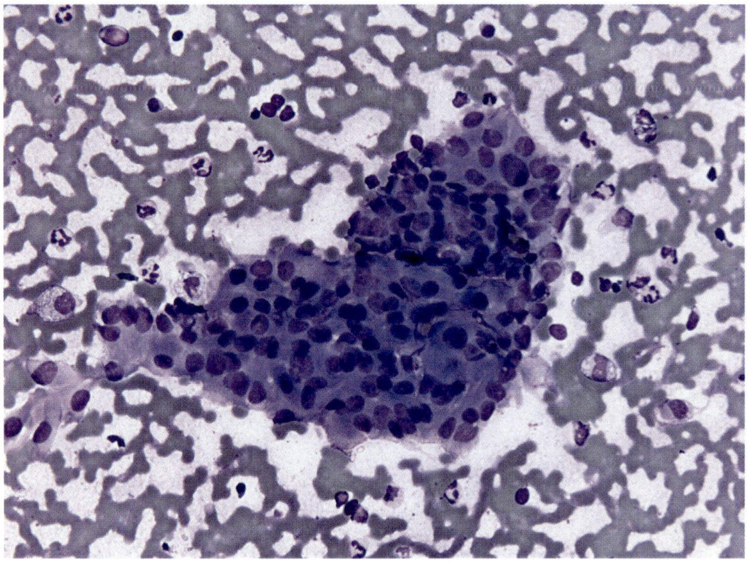

Figure 11.6d — Undifferentiated (Anaplastic) Carcinoma, FNA. This case illustrates a large sheet of malignant cells with round to oval nuclei and significantly less pleomorphism with only focal anisonucleosis. Cytoplasm displays focal basophilic granularity. This case was diagnosed as "suspicious for malignancy" as the typical high-grade features of an anaplastic carcinoma were not overtly present. Scattered background inflammatory cells suggest necrosis. (Diff Quik stain)

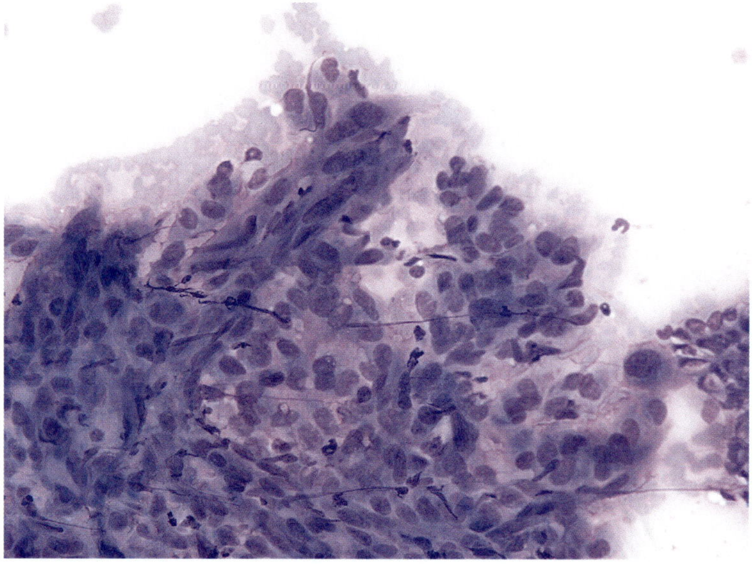

Figure 11.7a — Undifferentiated (Anaplastic) Carcinoma, FNA. The tumor fragment seen here shows traversing vessels surrounded by densely packed, hyperchromatic neoplastic nuclei with increased nuclear to cytoplasmic ratio. The neoplastic cells are pleomorphic and epithelioid to spindle shaped. Single, dispersed cells seen here adjacent to the tissue fragment have an epithelioid appearance with ample granular cytoplasm. (Diff Quik stain)

Figure 11.7b — Undifferentiated (Anaplastic) Carcinoma, FNA. Extreme pleomorphism highlights this case. A peculiar fine cytoplasmic vacuolization is seen as well as few cells display densely opaque green cytoplasm. Cells have eccentrically placed nuclei as well as occasional binucleation. Any high-grade metastatic malignancy to the thyroid gland would be in the differential diagnosis in this case. Background shows extensive necrosis, which is highly unusual in well-differentiated thyroid cancers. (Papanicolaou stain)

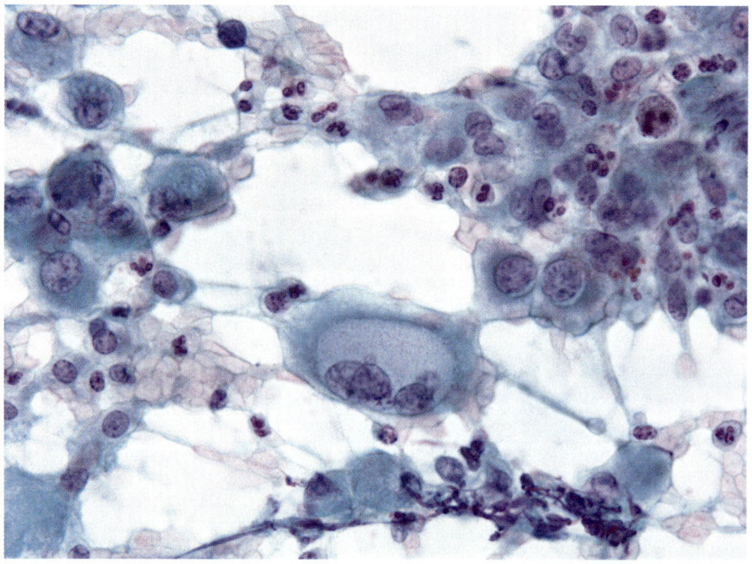

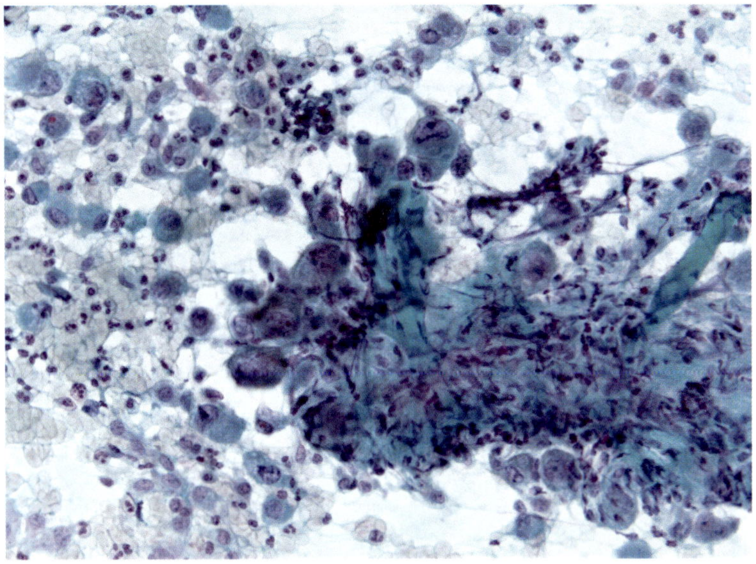

Figure 11.7c — Undifferentiated (Anaplastic) Carcinoma, FNA. Markedly pleomorphic carcinoma cells are seen associated with extensive necrosis. "Cherry red" macronucleoli are present in some cells. There is focal fibrosis and vascular proliferation. About 25% to 50% of patients with ATC also have a previous or concurrent history of well-differentiated thyroid cancer (papillary or follicular carcinoma). (Papanicolaou stain)

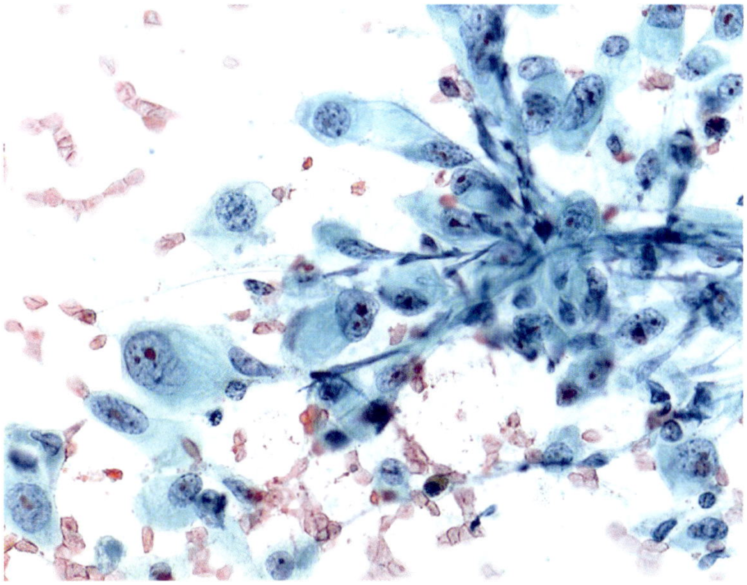

Figure 11.8a — Undifferentiated (Anaplastic) Carcinoma, FNA. The neoplastic cells in this cluster have eccentric nuclei with abundant cytoplasm that ranges from pale and vacuolated to dense and cyanophilic. The nuclei are enlarged and have irregular nuclear membranes, coarse chromatin and prominent nucleoli. Focal marked nuclear atypia can be seen in cyst lining cells, or in follicular cells following radiation therapy, including radio-iodine therapy. The cellularity and extent of nuclear atypia distinguish undifferentiated carcinoma from these benign lesions. (Papanicolaou stain)

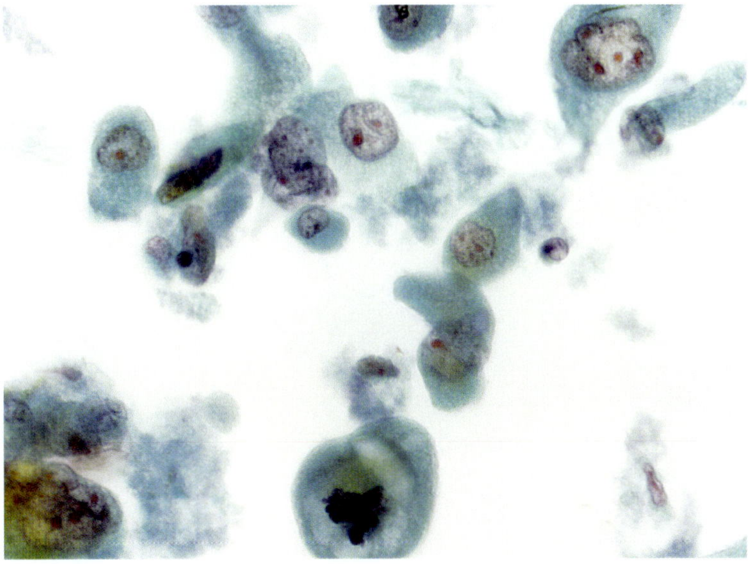

Figure 11.8b — Undifferentiated (Anaplastic) Carcinoma, FNA. The liquid-based preparation shows bizarre pleomorphic cells. Note the deeply convoluted nuclear envelopes, open chromatin, and macronucleoli. Mitotic figures, apoptotic bodies, and granular necrosis are often present in these cases (as seen here). A definitive diagnosis of a primary thyroid malignancy needs careful exclusion of metastases to the thyroid and occasionally needs confirmatory immunostaining. (Papanicolaou stain)

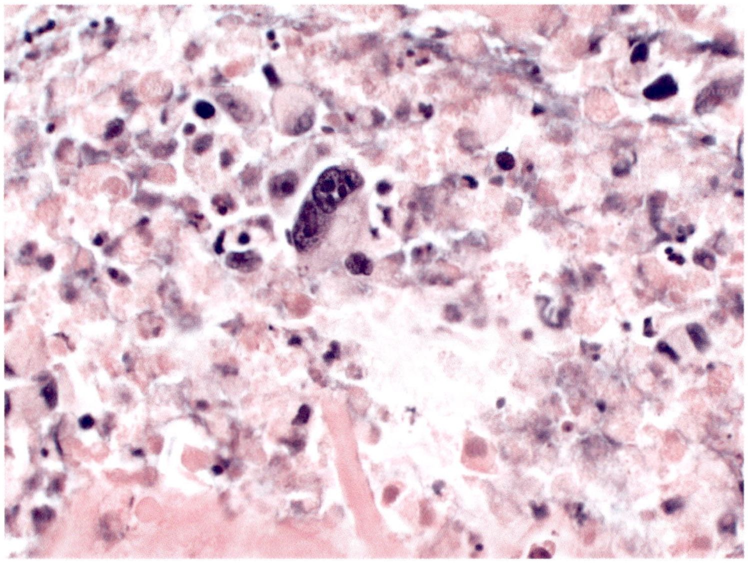

Figure 11.8c — Undifferentiated (Anaplastic) Carcinoma, FNA. Extensive necrosis is quite apparent in the cell block section and only rare viable cells are observed. An interpretation of high-grade malignancy is easy to render in such cases, however, the diagnosis of a primary undifferentiated carcinoma should only be made after careful exclusion of metastasis to the thyroid gland by review of clinical history and immunostaining. (Cell block section, H&E stain)

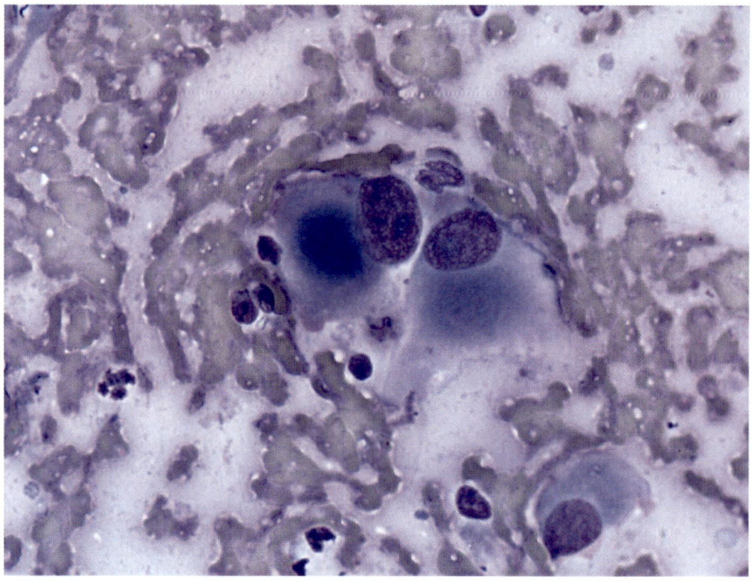

Figure 11.9 — Undifferentiated (Anaplastic) Carcinoma, Rhabdoid Variant, FNA. The rare rhabdoid variant of undifferentiated carcinoma is shown here. On Diff Quik staining, the tumor cells have an area of dense, deep blue cytoplasm (a cytoplasmic inclusion) surrounded by voluminous pale blue cytoplasm. The nuclei are enlarged, ovoid, and hyperchromatic with prominent nucleoli. These cells can resemble Hürthle cells, as both have eccentric nuclei with prominent nucleoli, but Hürthle cells have more granular cytoplasm and round nuclei. (Diff Quik stain)

Figure 11.10 — Undifferentiated (Anaplastic) Carcinoma, Pleomorphic Giant Cell Type, FNA. Two malignant multinucleated giant cells are seen in this image. These giant cells must be distinguished from benign multinucleated histiocytes. The key features indicating that these giant cells are malignant are the enlarged nuclei with irregularly distributed, coarse chromatin, and multiple macronucleoli. Benign histiocytes are seen at 12 and 3 o'clock for comparison. The pleomorphic giant cell pattern of undifferentiated carcinoma often presents with a neutrophil-rich background, as in this case. (Papanicolaou stain)

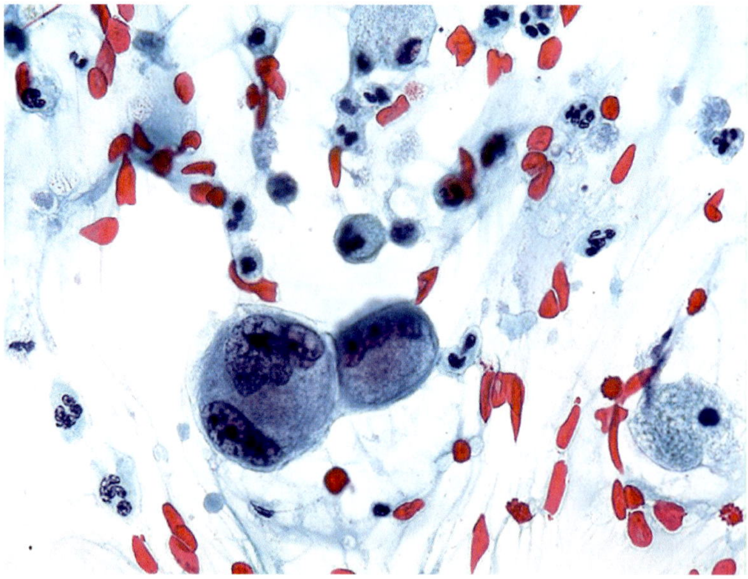

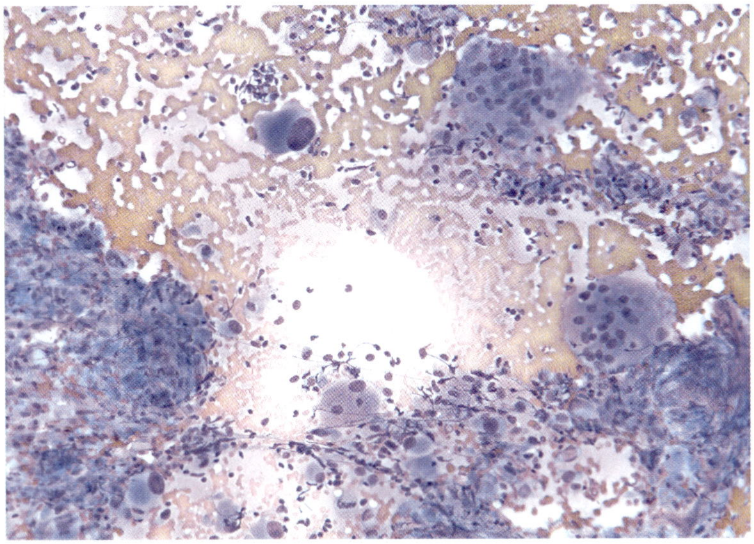

Figure 11.11 — Undifferentiated (Anaplastic) Carcinoma, FNA. Benign-appearing osteoclast-like giant cells are commonly encountered. In this case, they are interspersed with single epithelioid and rhabdoid tumor cells. The single, dispersed tumor cells, as seen here have a plasmacytoid appearance, thus medullary carcinoma is considered in the differential diagnosis. The clinical history can aid in the diagnosis as patients with undifferentiated carcinoma are typically over age 60 and present with a rapidly enlarging, locally invasive neck mass. Patients with medullary carcinoma may have a family history of multiple endocrine neoplasia (MEN) syndrome and serum calcitonin is typically elevated. (Diff Quik stain)

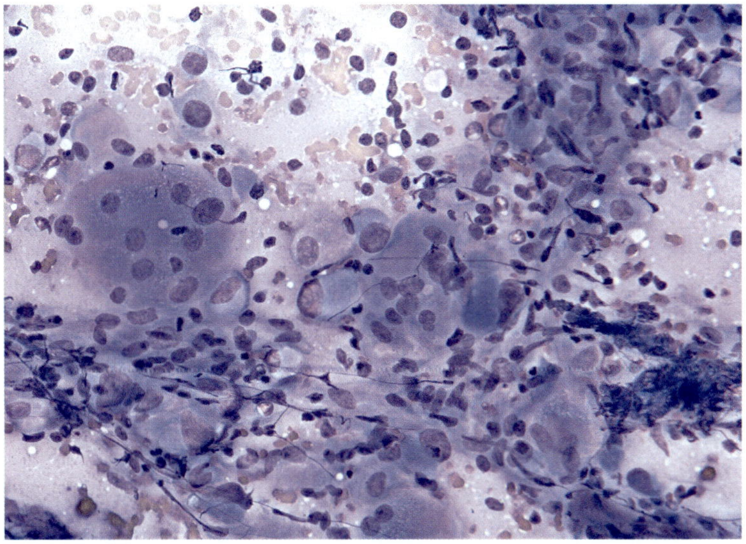

Figure 11.12 — Undifferentiated (Anaplastic) Carcinoma, FNA. This loose aggregate of neoplastic cells is comprised of epithelioid cells with large, oval-shaped eccentric nuclei and abundant cytoplasm which ranges from vacuolated to dense. Few spindle-shaped cells and scattered lymphocytes, as well as bare nuclei of varying sizes are seen in the background. If a predominantly single-cell population is present, a large cell lymphoma enters the differential diagnosis, but the presence of abundant cytoplasm makes that diagnosis less likely. (Diff Quik stain)

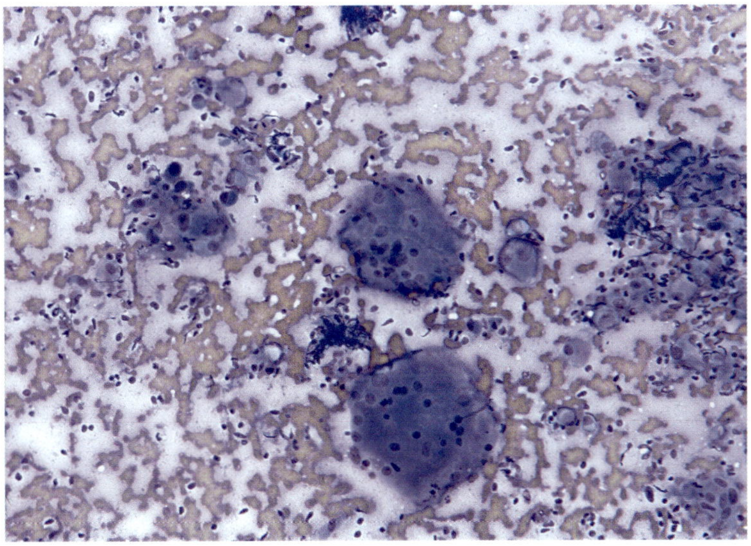

Figure 11.13 — Undifferentiated (Anaplastic) Carcinoma, FNA. Two osteoclast-like giant cells showing numerous small, round to oval nuclei are seen in the center of this image. Scattered isolated neoplastic cells of widely varied sizes are seen in the background, most of which have a plasmacytoid appearance. Inflammatory cells and bare neoplastic nuclei are dispersed throughout the aspirate. (Diff Quik stain)

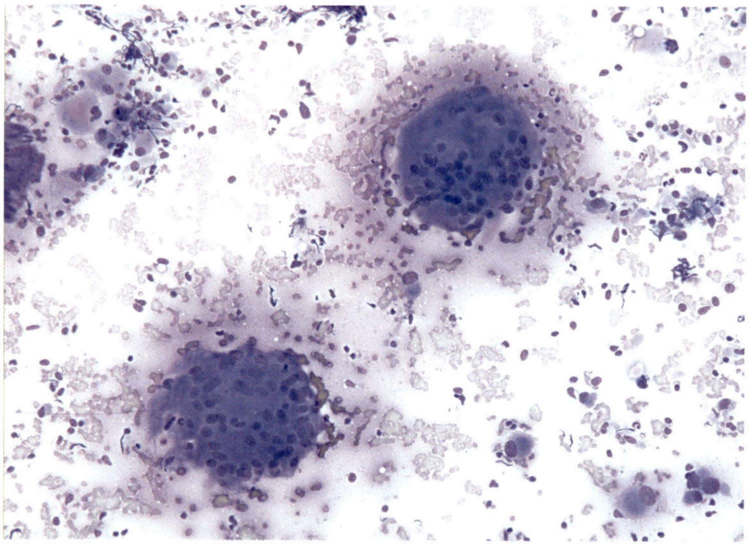

Figure 11.14 — Undifferentiated (Anaplastic) Carcinoma, FNA. The osteoclast-like giant cells seen here are occasionally found in undifferentiated carcinoma, and are distinct from the malignant pleomorphic giant cells which can also be seen. These osteoclast-like giant cells are benign-appearing and may raise the differential of a benign or reactive process such as subacute or granulomatous thyroiditis. However, numerous pleomorphic tumor cells seen throughout the aspirate make the diagnosis of malignancy apparent. (Diff Quik stain)

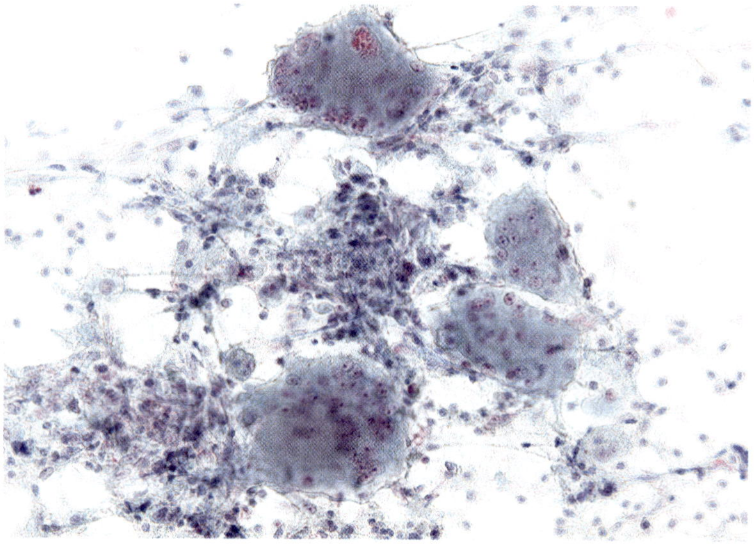

Figure 11.15a — Undifferentiated (Anaplastic) Carcinoma, FNA. Numerous multinucleated giant cells of the osteoclast type are noted. Multiple small, round to oval nuclei with occasional nucleoli are distributed throughout the cytoplasm. Blood and inflammatory debris can be seen in the background. In the presence of numerous benign-appearing giant cells, benign entities such as subacute or granulomatous thyroiditis are considered in the differential diagnosis. (Papanicolaou stain)

Figure 11.15b — Undifferentiated (Anaplastic) Carcinoma, FNA. A single large osteoclast-like giant cell is seen associated with abundant background mixed inflammatory cells and histiocytes. Mononucleated malignant epithelial cells form a loose syncytium at 11 o'clock of the field. ATC is a disease more common in women with a female/male ratio of 5 to 1. ATC remains an aggressive and lethal disease with a dismal prognosis despite numerous treatment regimens. The median survival in the vast majority of published studies ranges between 3 and 9 months. (Diff Quik stain)

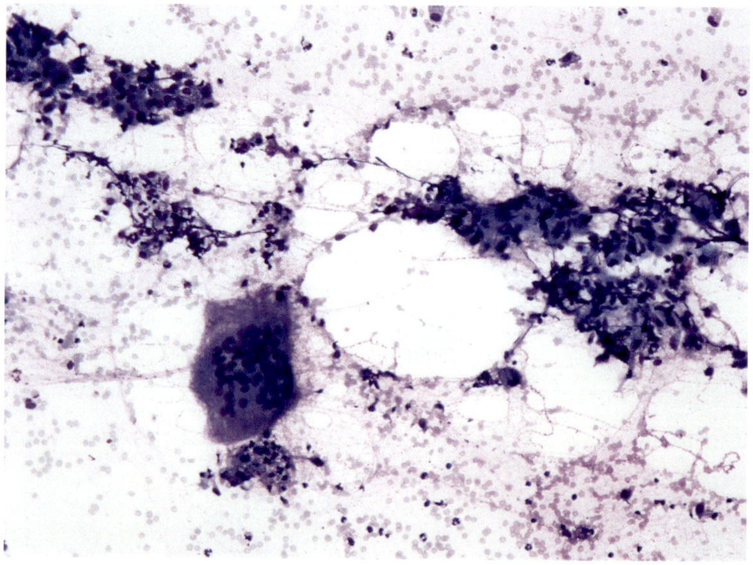

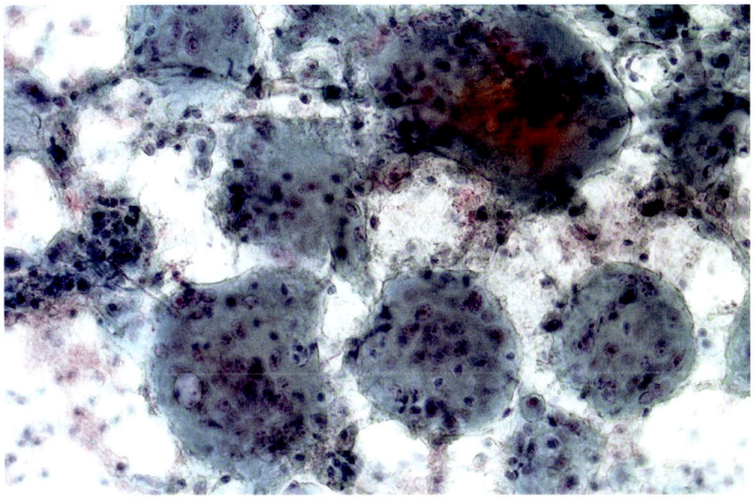

Figure 11.16 — Undifferentiated (Anaplastic) Carcinoma, FNA. ATC clinically presents as a rapidly growing mass in the neck, associated with dyspnea, dysphagia, and vocal cord paralysis. It is usually locally advanced and often metastatic at initial presentation. Around 20% to 50% of patients present with distant metastases, most often pulmonary, and another 25% develop new metastasis during the rapid course of the disease. This case shows numerous osteoclast-like giant cells, representing reactive histiocytes. The malignant cell population is small and mostly seen as high N/C ratio cells in the background, either as single cells or loose aggregates. (Papanicolaou stain)

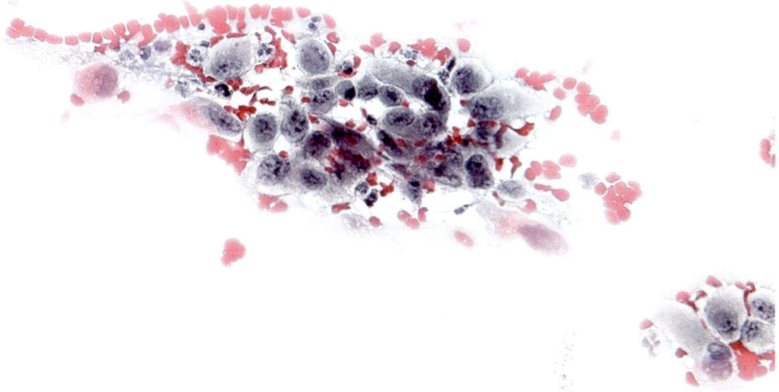

Figure 11.17 — Undifferentiated (Anaplastic) Carcinoma, FNA. A group of single tumor cells with malignant features is seen. The neoplastic cells show coarse, clumped chromatin, irregular nuclear membranes, and occasional macronucleoli. The cytoplasm is vacuolated to coarsely granular. A bloody background, as seen here, is common in undifferentiated carcinoma. Mortality in ATC is often caused by tracheal and esophageal invasion (reflection of the local aggressiveness of the tumor) and obstruction, as well as by consequences of metastatic disease. (Papanicolaou stain)

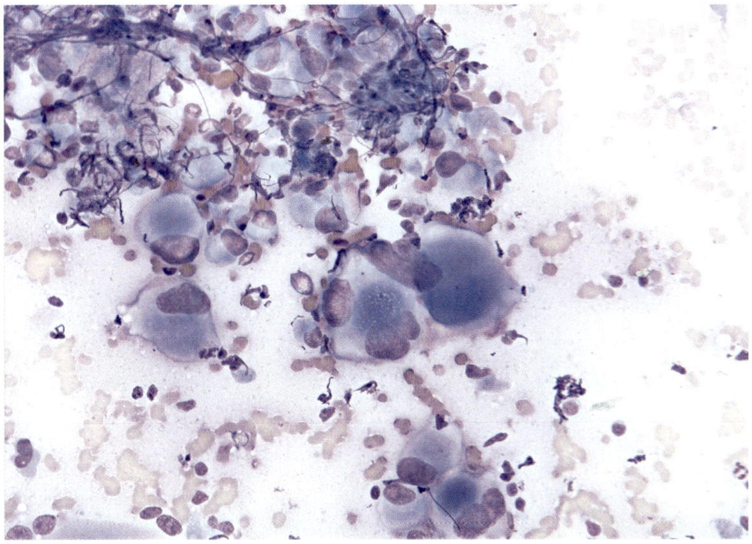

Figure 11.18 — Undifferentiated (Anaplastic) Carcinoma, FNA. Single neoplastic cells with marked pleomorphism are present in this field. Some show rhabdoid features with a cytoplasmic inclusion. The smaller neoplastic cells in the background have a plasmacytoid appearance reminiscent of medullary carcinoma, but the larger, markedly atypical neoplastic cells indicate an undifferentiated malignancy. (Diff Quik stain)

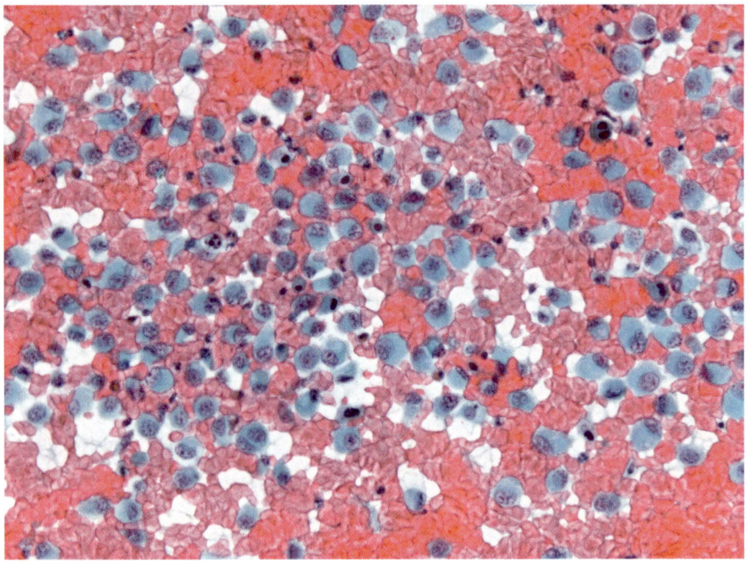

Figure 11.19a — Undifferentiated (Anaplastic) Carcinoma, FNA. A dispersed population of malignant cells is seen with a prominent "rhabdoid" phenotype. Notice the eccentric nuclei and dense green opaque cytoplasm. The patient had a previous history of head and neck malignant melanoma and this FNA was initially misdiagnosed as "metastatic malignant neoplasm consistent with previous history of melanoma." Resection showed anaplastic carcinoma. (Papanicolaou stain)

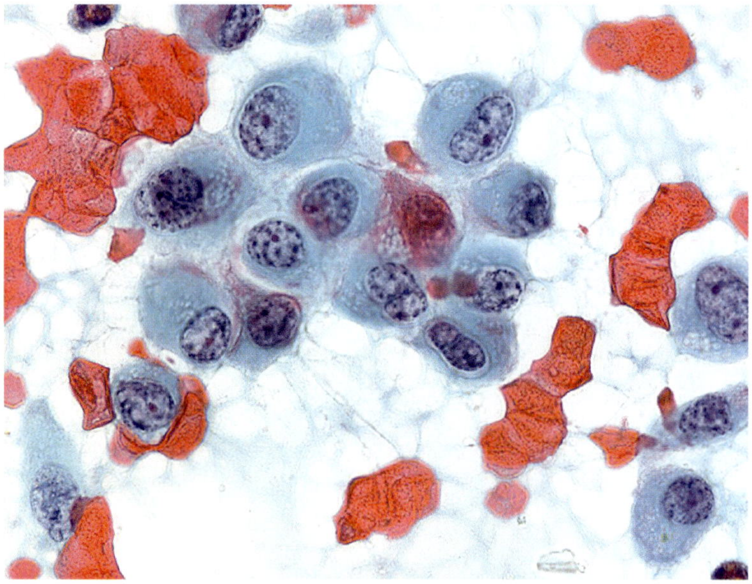

Figure 11.19b — Undifferentiated (Anaplastic) Carcinoma, FNA. Higher magnification beautifully displays the rhabdoid-like morphology. Cells have eccentric nuclei, densely opaque green cytoplasm and macronucleoli. In general, there are three main morphologic subtypes typically described in ATC (squamoid, spindle cell, and giant cell). Interestingly, they all present with similar biological and clinical features and the same dismal prognosis. The coexistence of both well-differentiated thyroid carcinoma and ATC has been reported, with the prognosis being determined by the ATC component. (Papanicolaou stain)

Figure 11.20 — Undifferentiated (Anaplastic) Carcinoma, Spindle Pattern, FNA. A cohesive fragment of neoplastic spindle cells is seen. The nuclei are hyperchromatic and oval-shaped with occasional marked pleomorphism. Metastatic malignant melanoma and sarcoma, including fibrosarcoma and undifferentiated pleomorphic sarcoma (UPS), are diagnostic considerations. Adequate sampling of the tumor and thorough review of clinical and radiographic findings are essential to make the correct diagnosis as undifferentiated carcinoma is essentially a diagnosis of exclusion. (Diff Quik stain)

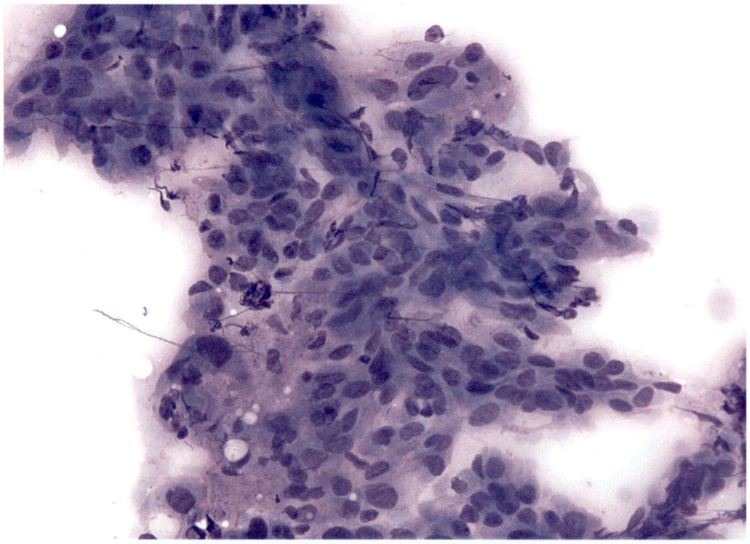

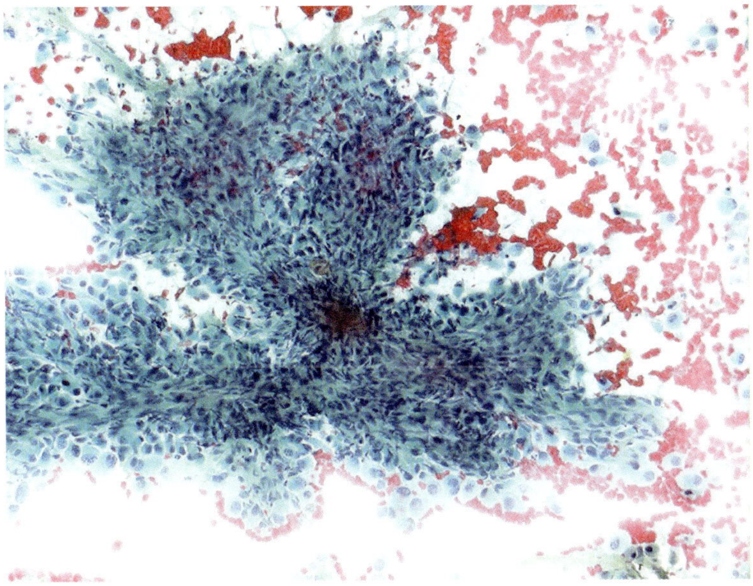

Figure 11.21 — Undifferentiated (Anaplastic) Carcinoma, FNA. This is a cellular aspirate with a large tissue fragment comprised of spindle and epithelioid cells in a bloody background. Other primary thyroid neoplasms such as a Hürthle cell neoplasm and papillary carcinoma would be included in the differential diagnosis on low power. Examination at higher power is necessary to appreciate the marked atypia of the neoplastic cells. (Papanicolaou stain)

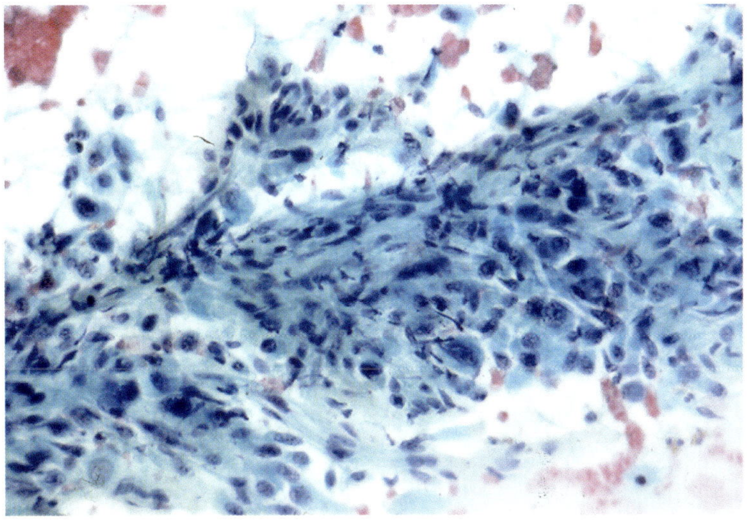

Figure 11.22 — Undifferentiated (Anaplastic) Carcinoma, FNA. At high power, malignant nuclear features are evident. This tissue fragment has numerous, densely packed spindle cells. Given the marked atypia, the differential diagnosis includes metastatic carcinoma, such as poorly differentiated squamous cell carcinoma or sarcomatoid renal cell carcinoma, metastatic malignant melanoma, and sarcoma. (Papanicolaou stain)

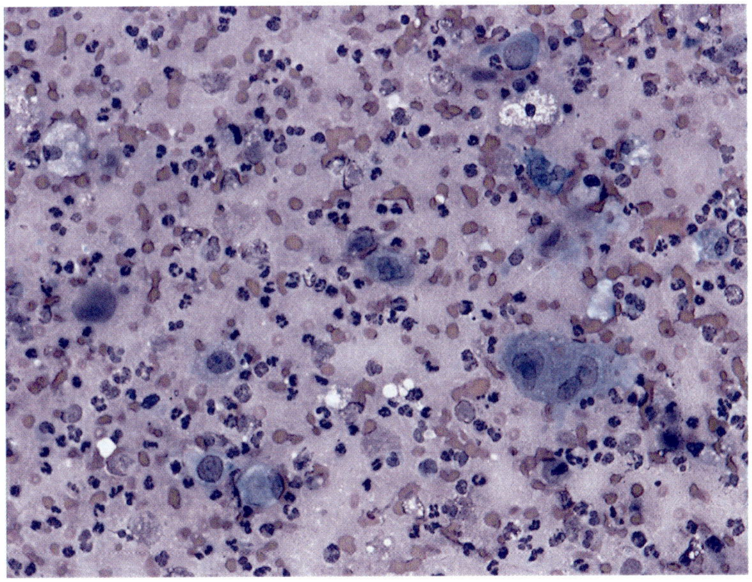

Figure 11.23 — Undifferentiated (Anaplastic) Carcinoma, FNA. Although the diagnosis of undifferentiated carcinoma is usually clear-cut, the presence of abundant acute inflammation in the background can obscure the malignant cells and the tumor can be mistaken for an abscess. Both can present as a rapidly enlarging and tender thyroid mass. In this case, scattered single tumor cells are admixed with acute inflammatory cells. Careful examination at medium to high power is essential to appreciate the marked atypia of the neoplastic cells, which may be mistaken for histiocytes on low magnification. (Diff Quik stain)

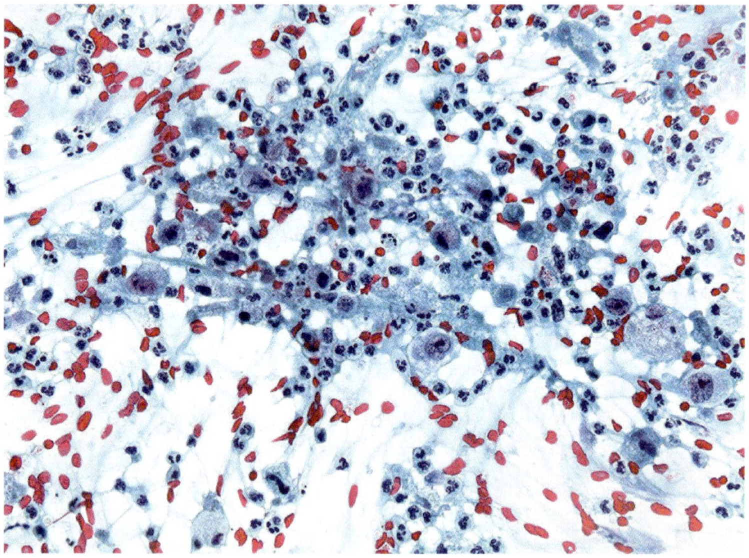

Figure 11.24a — Undifferentiated (Anaplastic) Carcinoma, FNA. A necrotic or inflammatory background is commonly encountered. Note the acute inflammation intimately admixed with neoplastic cells showing marked nuclear atypia. The neoplastic cells are readily distinguished from benign histiocytes by the presence of nuclear hyperchromasia, coarse chromatin, and prominent nucleoli. (Papanicolaou stain)

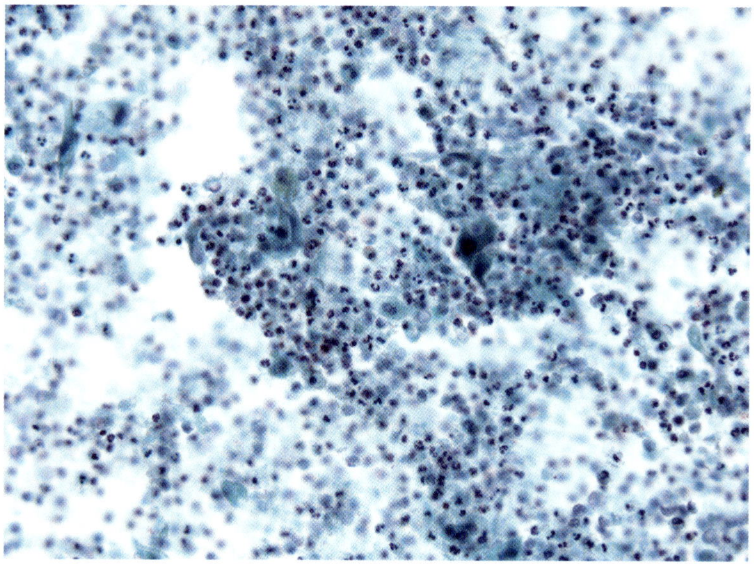

Figure 11.24b — Undifferentiated (Anaplastic) Carcinoma, FNA. This case was even harder to diagnose as viable tumor cells were far and few and were heavily obscured by the dense inflammatory exudate. These cases clinically and cytopathologically, may mimic an enlarging neck abscess and on gross examination, the aspirate often appears as pale yellow "pus-like" material. (Papanicolaou stain)

Figure 11.24c — Undifferentiated (Anaplastic) Carcinoma, FNA. A similar case with extensive acute inflammatory exudate did disclose rare fragments of overtly malignant epithelium. ATC is known to have an abscess-like appearance on FNA. The most reliable immunoperoxidase marker is pan-keratin, positive in 50% to 100% of the cases. Thyroglobulin and TTF-1 are most often negative (as would be a variety of metastatic tumors in the thyroid) making the differential diagnosis of ATC particularly challenging. (Papanicolaou stain)

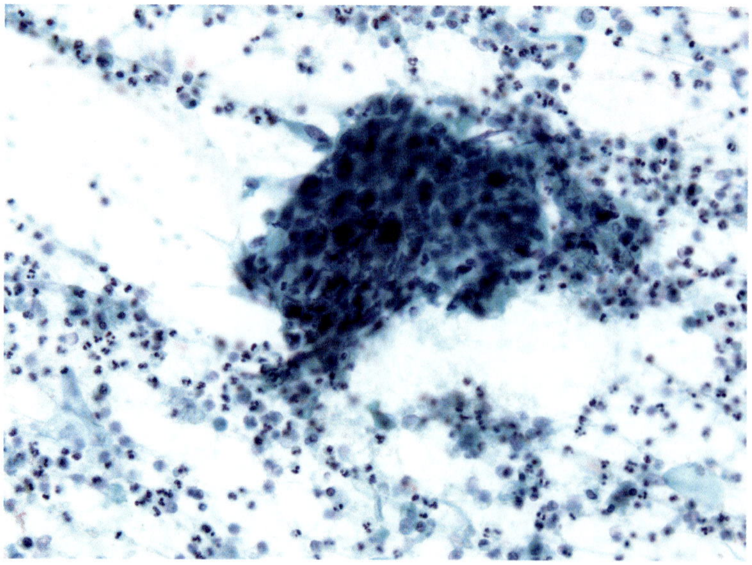

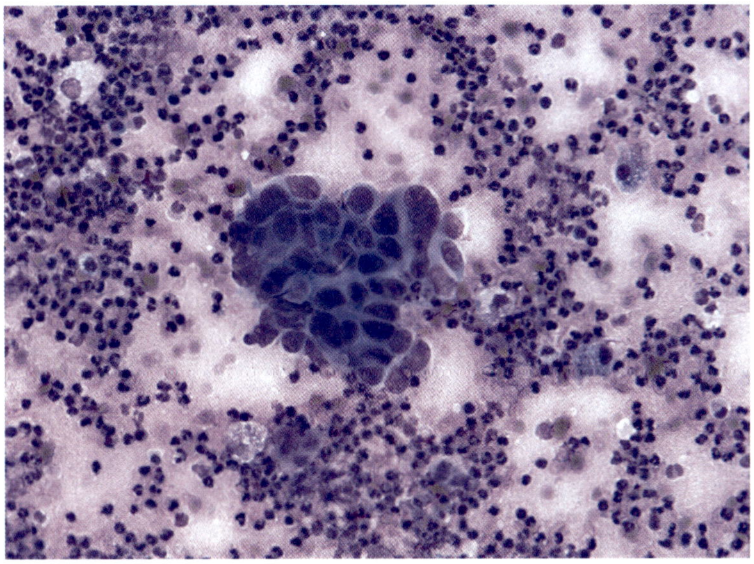

Figure 11.24d — Undifferentiated (Anaplastic) Carcinoma, FNA. Here is another example of extensively necrotic and inflamed carcinoma with only one rare fragment of viable tumor seen in the entire aspirate. Notice the background rich in neutrophils and few scattered histiocytes. Such cases need a careful screening to locate the rare viable malignant cells which are pivotal for an accurate diagnosis. (Diff Quik stain)

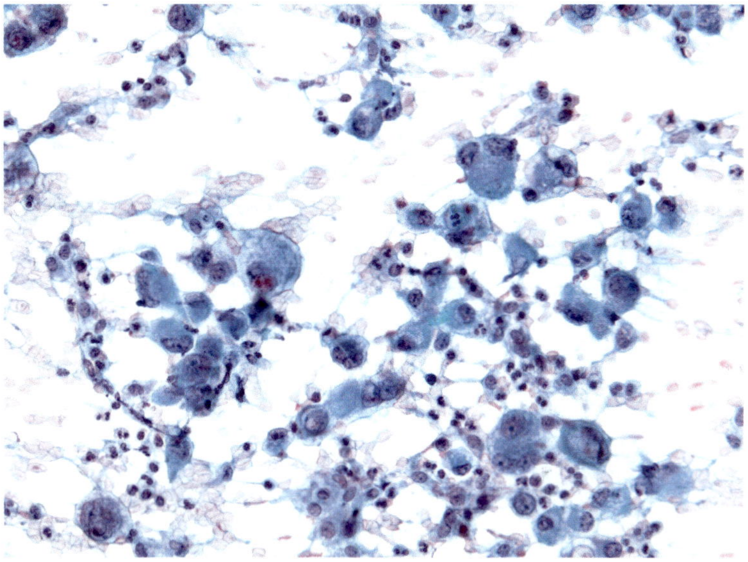

Figure 11.24e — Undifferentiated (Anaplastic) Carcinoma, FNA. Most of the malignant cells in this case with extensive inflammatory background have a histiocytic appearance with finely vacuolated cytoplasm. However, an enlarged nucleus with macronucleolus supports the diagnosis of a high-grade cancer. Nuclear pleomorphism in ATC can be striking with giant, bizarre, hyperchromatic forms identified. (Papanicolaou stain)

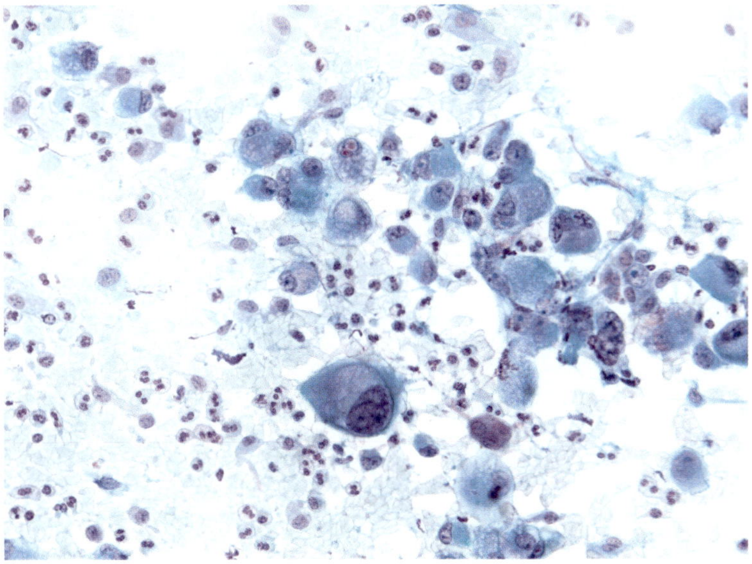

Figure 11.24f — Undifferentiated (Anaplastic) Carcinoma, FNA. Another field from the previous case displays malignant cells in an inflamed and necrotic background. Note the extreme nuclear pleomorphism and finely vacuolated "histiocyte-like" cytoplasm. Neutrophilic infiltration of tumor cell cytoplasm has also been reported. (Papanicolaou stain)

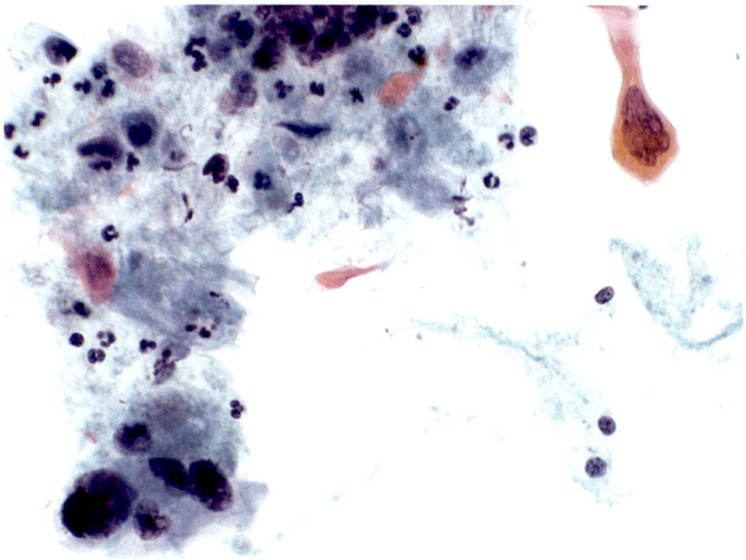

Figure 11.25 — Undifferentiated (Anaplastic) Carcinoma, FNA. Although this case shows pleomorphic malignant features and extensive necrosis common to all previous examples, there is obvious squamous differentiation present in the form of cytoplasmic orangeophilia. A significant number of patients with ATC have foci of co-existing well-differentiated thyroid carcinoma; papillary carcinoma (most often), follicular carcinoma, Hürthle cell carcinoma, insular carcinoma or medullary carcinoma, which may result in mixed cytologic features on FNA of such cases. Therefore, thorough sampling on FNA is imperative so that the most biologically significant component of the tumor (ie, ATC) is adequately sampled. (Papanicolaou stain)

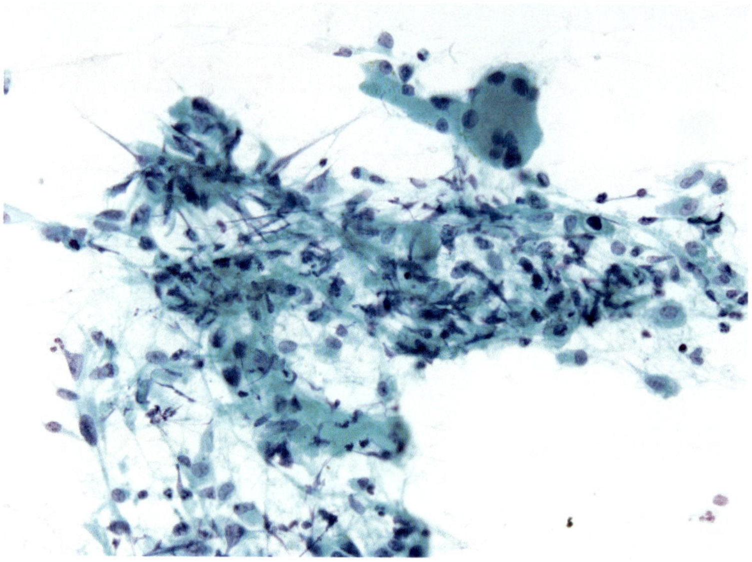

Figure 11.26a — Undifferentiated (Anaplastic) Carcinoma, FNA. A fragment of skeletal muscle is seen (1 o'clock) associated with a population of malignant pleomorphic epithelioid and spindle cells. The presence of skeletal muscle fragments, when intermixed with malignant cells often indicate extra thyroidal extension by the carcinoma and is often helpful in a definitive diagnosis in borderline cases. (Papanicolaou stain)

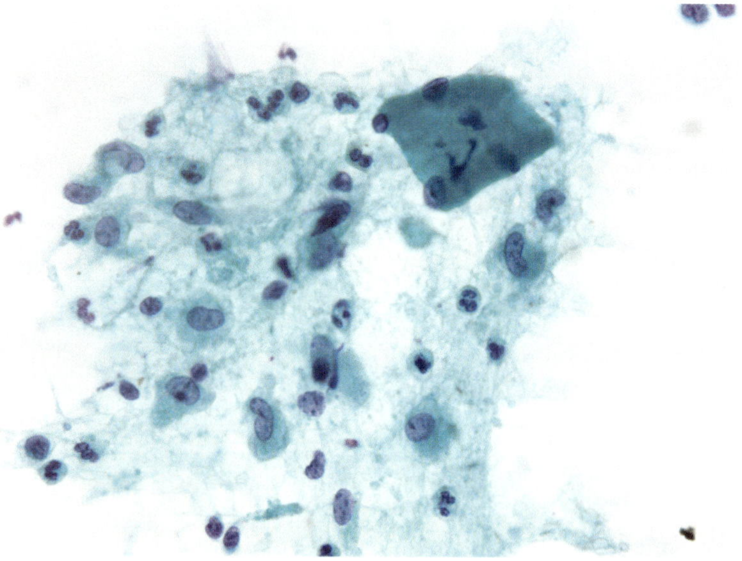

Figure 11.26b — Undifferentiated (Anaplastic) Carcinoma, FNA. This case also illustrates pleomorphic malignant epithelioid cells and juxtaposed skeletal muscle fragment indicating extra thyroidal extension of the thyroid cancer into the surrounding neck fibromuscular soft tissues. Immunohistochemical studies of molecular markers in ATC have displayed frequent and strong overexpression of beta-catenin, cyclin D1, and EGFR. These findings support the development of clinical trials with agents such as cetuximab and small-molecule tyrosine kinase inhibitors. (Papanicolaou stain)

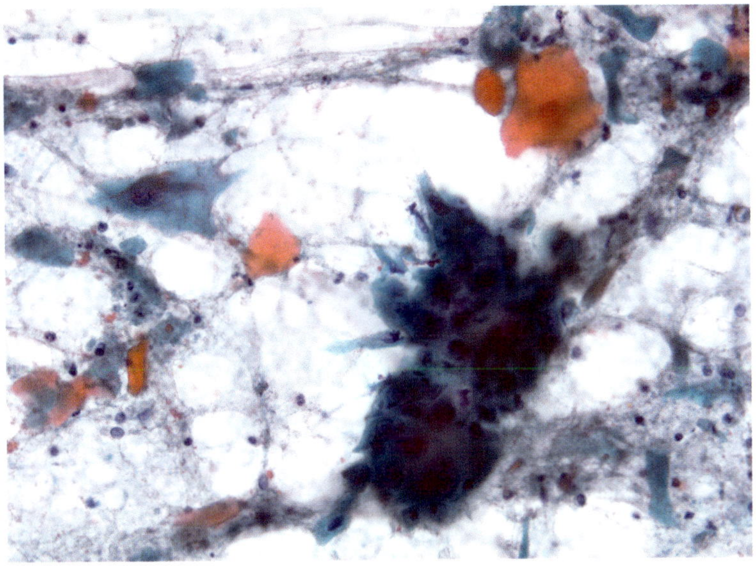

Figure 11.27a — Squamous Cell Carcinoma, FNA. Primary squamous cell carcinoma (SQCC) of the thyroid gland is a rare tumor accounting for about 0.2% to 1.1% of all thyroid cancers. As part of the differential diagnosis, metastases or direct extension from an extra-thyroidal primary tumor should always be considered first and adequately ruled out. Heavily keratinized and orangeophilic cytoplasmic fragments of the malignant cells are observed in this case. Background suggests tumor necrosis. Primary SQCC of the thyroid cannot be morphologically distinguished from a metastatic or locally invasive head and neck carcinoma involving the thyroid gland. (Papanicolaou stain)

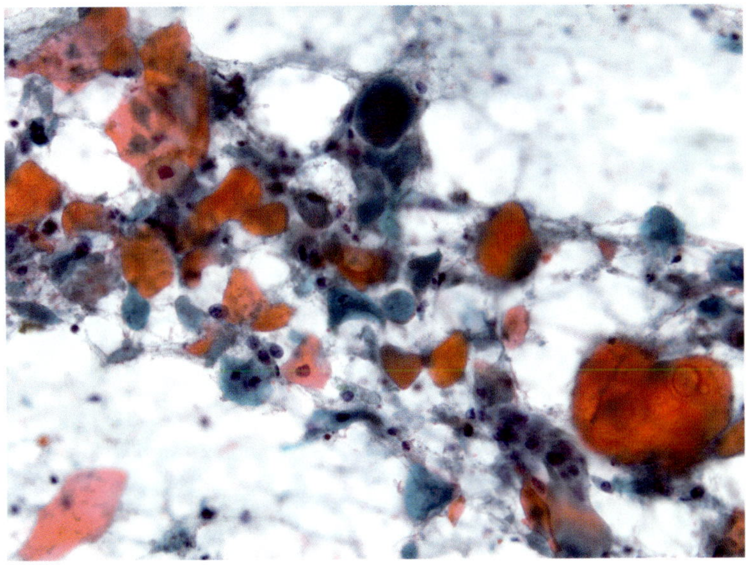

Figure 11.27b — Squamous Cell Carcinoma, FNA. This case demonstrates keratinizing malignant squamous cells which are admixed with necrotic debris. Primary SQCC of the thyroid usually presents during the fifth to sixth decade of life and occurs more commonly in women than men. Typical positive stains are cytokeratins (100%), thyroglobulin (63%), TTF-1 (38%), p53, and Ki-67. Treatment of primary thyroid squamous cell carcinoma is multimodal, with surgery and radiotherapy showing potential benefit. Prognosis is generally very poor because of the rapid growth and metastasis of the tumor, with a low median survival. (Papanicolaou stain)

12

Rare Primary Carcinomas and Mesenchymal Neoplasms

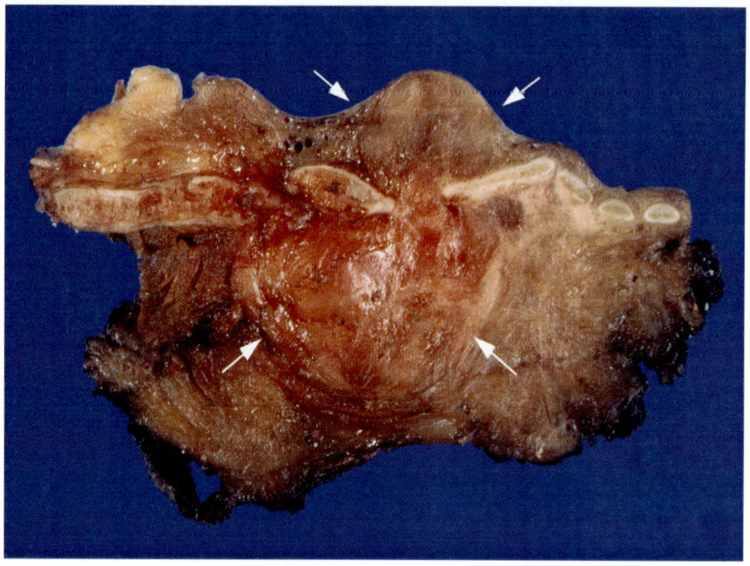

Figure 12.1 — Paraganglioma of the Thyroid, Gross Appearance. Paragangliomas can, on rare occasions, arise within the thyroid parenchyma presumably from displaced laryngeal paraganglia. They typically arise from the periphery of the thyroid near the thyroid capsule. Their invasive front is generally broad and pushing. This paraganglioma (outlined by arrows) is centered in the left lobe of the thyroid, but it extends beyond the thyroid and into the trachea. When it comes to paragangliomas of the thyroid, extension of tumor beyond the thyroid is not predictive of metastatic spread or fatal outcome. Thyroid paragangliomas tend to behave in a benign fashion even when they exhibit aggressive local extension. (Papanicolaou, low power)

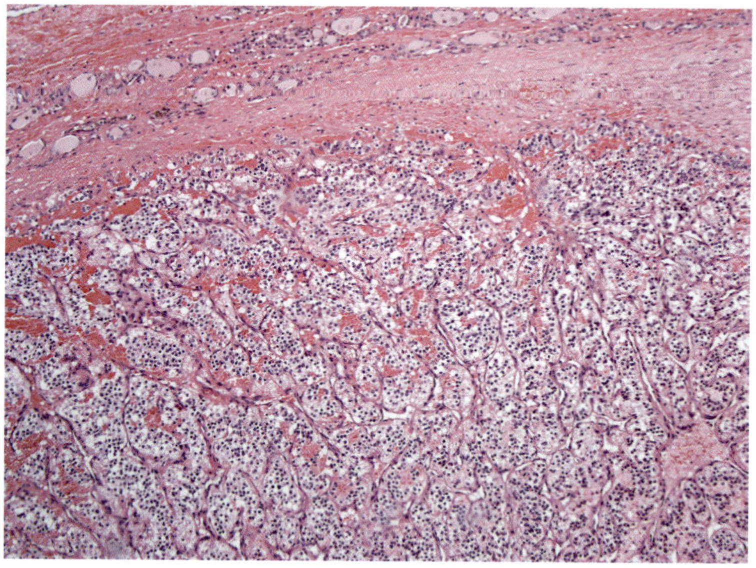

Figure 12.2a — Paraganglioma, Histologic Section. The histologic appearance of thyroid paragangliomas is no different from paragangliomas arising from more common head and neck sites such as the carotid body. The tumor cells are arranged in a prominent nested pattern, and the nests are separated by a delicate stroma with thin-walled vessels. (H&E stain)

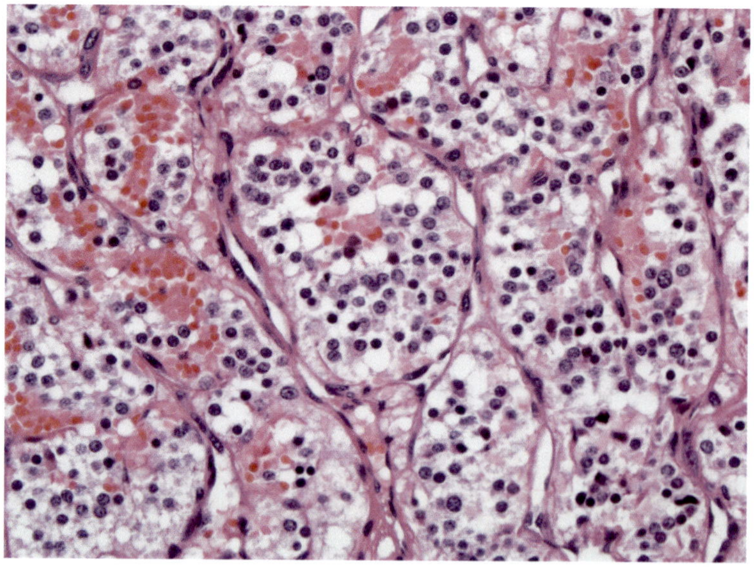

Figure 12.2b — Paraganglioma, Histologic Section. The tumor cells have round to oval vesicular nuclei and occasional small nucleoli. The cellular features together with the nested pattern of growth may cause confusion with medullary thyroid carcinoma. A battery of immunohistochemical stains can be very useful in distinguishing between medullary carcinoma and paraganglioma. (H&E stain)

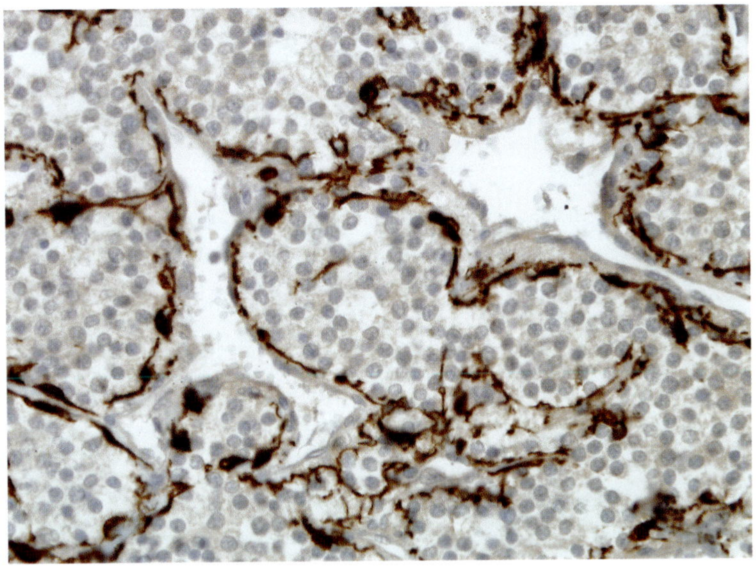

Figure 12.2c — Paraganglioma (S100 Protein Immunostain), Histologic Section. Both medullary carcinomas and thyroid paragangliomas are generally positive for chromogranin, but thyroid paragangliomas also demonstrate S-100 staining in sustentacular cells compressed at the periphery of the cell nests; and they lack staining for cytokeratin, carcinoembryonic antigen (CEA), and calcitonin. (Immunostain)

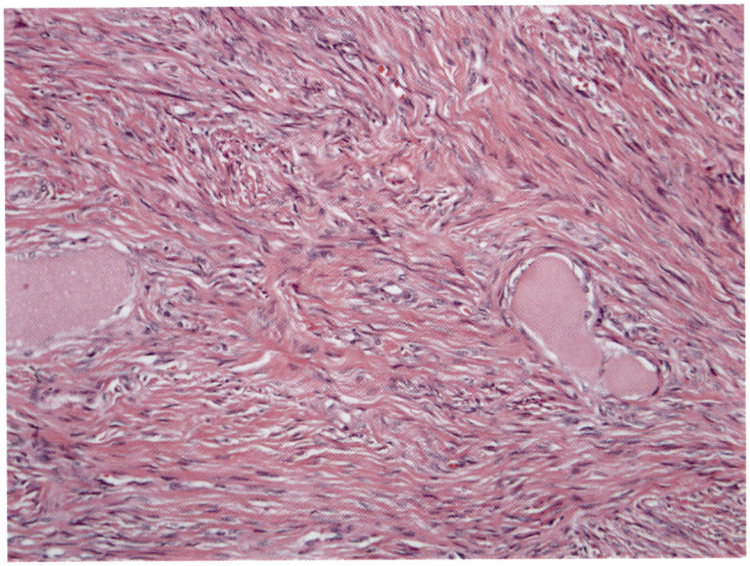

Figure 12.3a — Solitary Fibrous Tumor (SFT) of the Thyroid, Histologic Section. Solitary fibrous tumors usually arise in mesothelial-lined sites such as the pleural surface of the lung, but they can sometimes arise in sites entirely unassociated with a mesothelial lining such as the thyroid. Histologically, they are characterized by the proliferation of spindled to plump cells within a fibrocollagenous background. Here, a proliferation of cytologically bland spindled cells entraps thyroid follicles. Common morphologic findings of SFT include a haphazard or storiform arrangement of the tumor cells, alternating zones of hypocellularity and hypercellularity, and a lace-like deposition of intercellular collagen. Most solitary fibrous tumors of the thyroid are benign and should not be confused with the sarcomatoid variant of anaplastic carcinoma. (H&E stain)

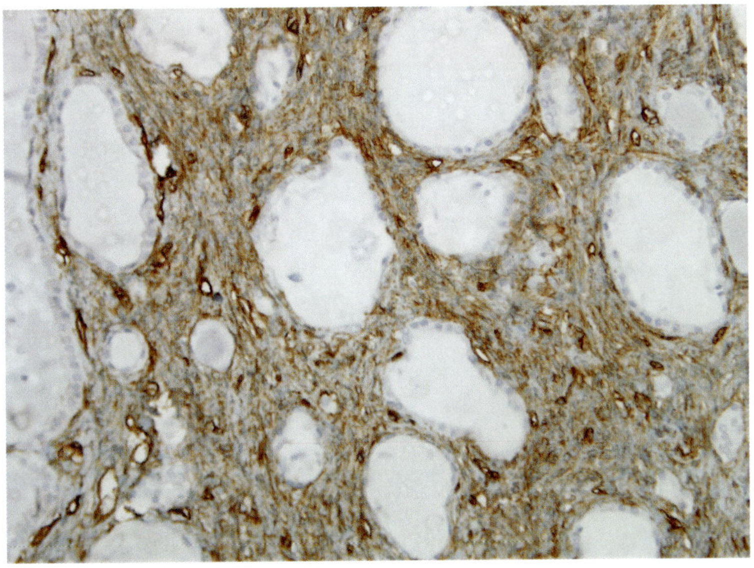

Figure 12.3b — Solitary Fibrous Tumor of the Thyroid (CD34 Immunostain), Histologic Section. CD34 tends to be strongly expressed in SFT, irrespective of tumor site. Thus CD34 immunoreactivity is an important confirmatory finding, particularly for those SFTs arising in extra pleural locations like the thyroid. (Immunostain)

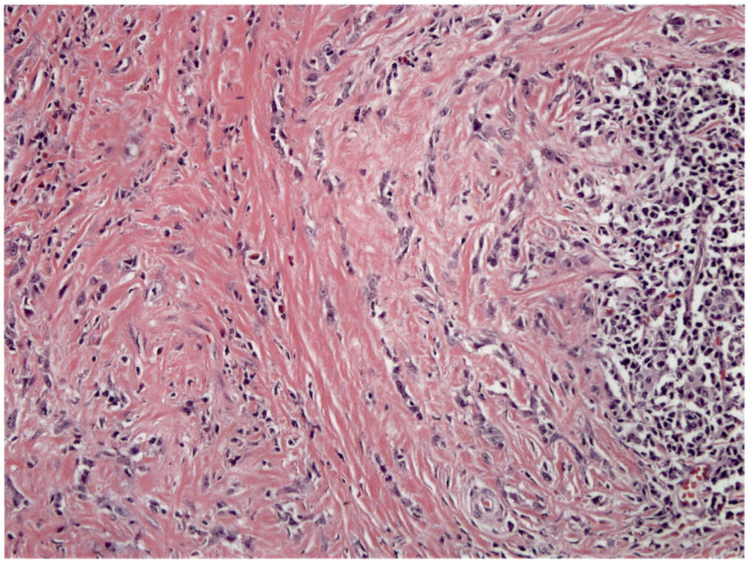

Figure 12.4 — Sclerosing Mucoepidermoid Carcinoma With Eosinophilia, Histologic Section. Sclerosing mucoepidermoid carcinoma is a rare low-grade neoplasm of the thyroid that arises in a background of fibrosing Hashimoto thyroiditis. Indeed, the tumor likely takes origin from the metaplastic follicles of Hashimoto thyroiditis. The tumor is seen as irregular strands of cells in a fibrotic background. Cellular atypia is not striking. The tumor cells have a somewhat squamoid appearance, but overt squamous differentiation may be a focal finding. Glandular differentiation is not well developed, but focal mucin deposition may be demonstrated by special stains. The stroma is dense and hyalinized and peppered with an inflammatory infiltrate of lymphocytes and eosinophils. (H&E stain)

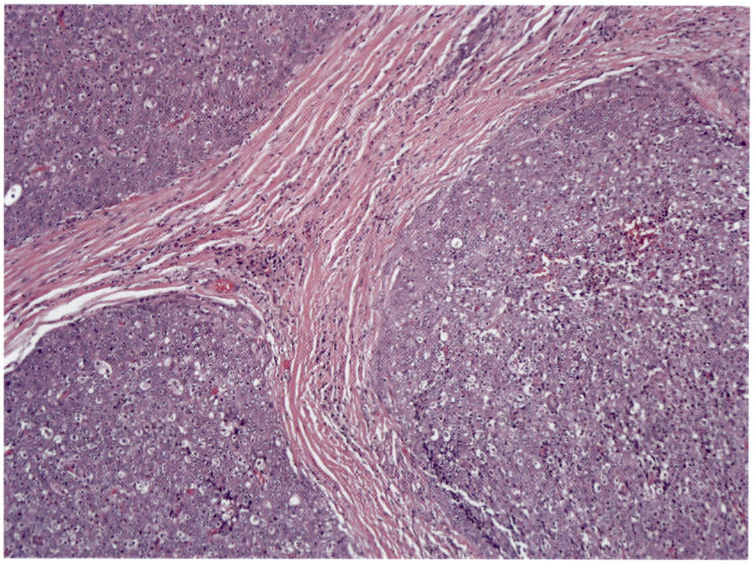

Figure 12.5a — Carcinoma Showing Thymus-Like Differentiation (CASTLE), Histologic Section. Carcinoma showing thymus-like differentiation (CASTLE) is a rare intrathyroidal carcinoma that is likely derived from ectopically displaced thymic tissue. Not surprisingly, its morphologic features are highly reminiscent of thymic neoplasms. In this case, the thyroid follicles have been replaced by a solid mass. The tumor grows as expansile lobules separated by fibrous septae. (H&E stain)

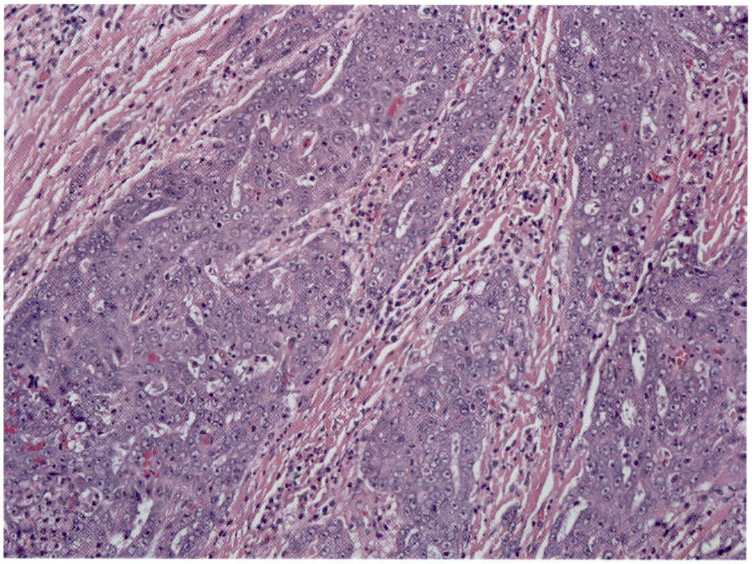

Figure 12.5b — Carcinoma Showing Thymus-Like Differentiation (CASTLE), Histologic Section. At higher magnification, the tumor cells show lymphoepithelial features including syncytial cytoplasm, vesicular nuclei, and prominent nucleoli. The mitotic count is generally low. Like thymic carcinomas, the tumor cells of CASTLE are usually immunoreactive for CD5 — a finding that helps in the distinction of CASTLE from undifferentiated thyroid carcinoma. (H&E stain)

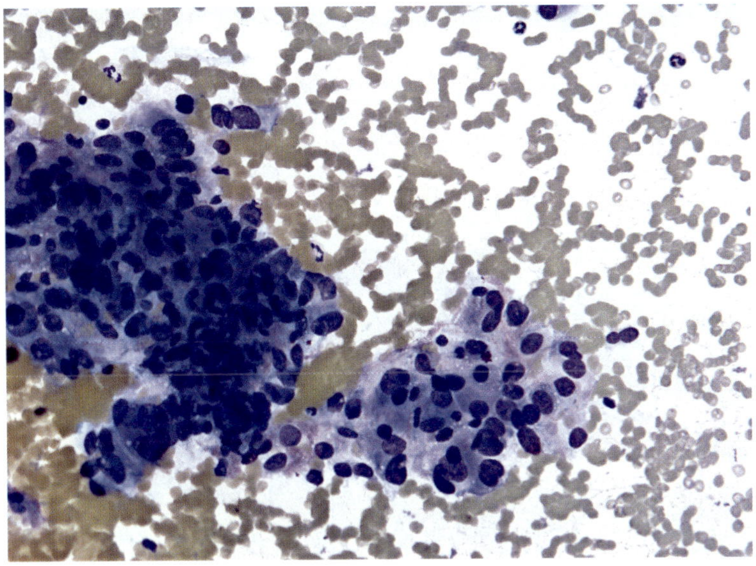

Figure 12.6a — Paraganglioma, Fine Needle Aspiration (FNA). Paragangliomas are relatively rare tumors, accounting for only about 0.3% of all neoplasms. Most paragangliomas are benign with only 10% to 20% tumors possess metastatic potential. This case depicts fragments of pleomorphic epithelioid cells with pale blue granular cytoplasm. Few naked nuclei are also present. No native thyroid follicular epithelium and colloid is observed. Cytologic diagnosis of thyroid paraganglioma is exceedingly difficult with most cases called "suspicious for malignancy." Medullary thyroid carcinoma and hyalinizing trabecular neoplasm top the list of differential diagnosis. (Diff Quik stain)

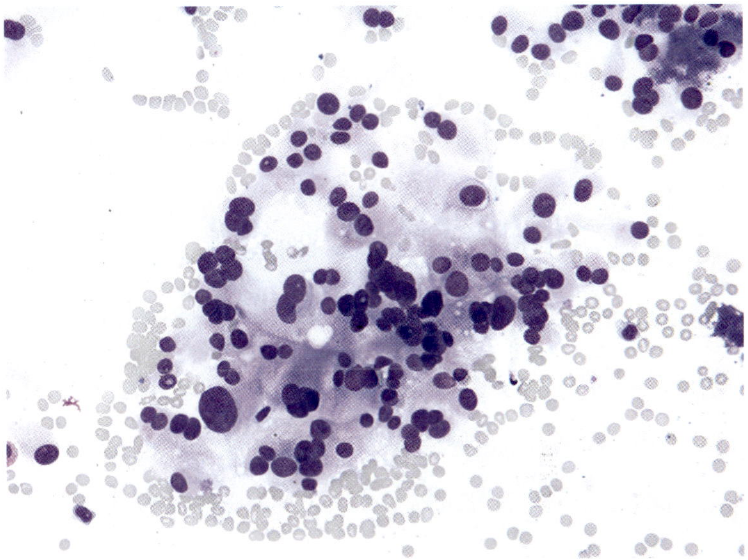

Figure 12.6b — Paraganglioma, FNA. Cells in this case have more rounded "epithelioid" appearance with fragile and wispy finely granular cytoplasm. Anisonucleosis is prominent with neoplastic cells varying markedly in size. Few bare nuclei are also noted as well as few intranuclear inclusions. A medullary carcinoma has to be excluded with immunostains such as calcitonin and CEA. Paragangliomas of the head and neck account for 0.012% of all head and neck tumors, with the carotid body and *glomus jugulare* accounting for more than 80% of the cases. Thyroid is an extremely rare site and hence such tumor in the thyroid most often becomes a difficult diagnostic issue, both for the clinician and the pathologist. With rare exceptions, thyroid paragangliomas are functionally silent. (Diff Quik stain)

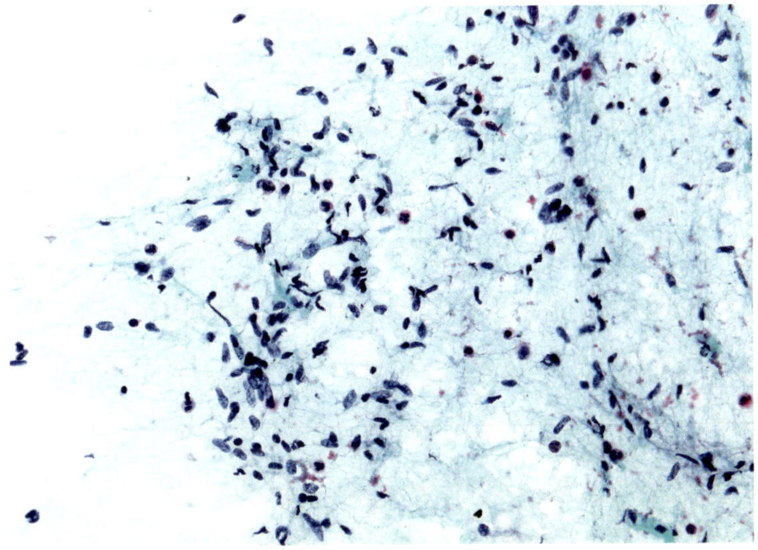

Figure 12.7 — Solitary Fibrous Tumor, FNA. The patternless pattern of the neoplastic cells is nicely depicted here. Cells have short spindled nuclei that vary in their length and appearance and have no discernible cytoplasm. Only rare shreds of pale green collagenized stroma are noticed. Vascular proliferation was minimal. No native thyroid epithelium or colloid was seen. Major differential diagnoses in this case would be with spindle cell medullary carcinoma, paraganglioma, spindle epithelial tumor with thymus-like differentiation (SETTLE), and nerve sheath tumor. (Papanicolaou stain)

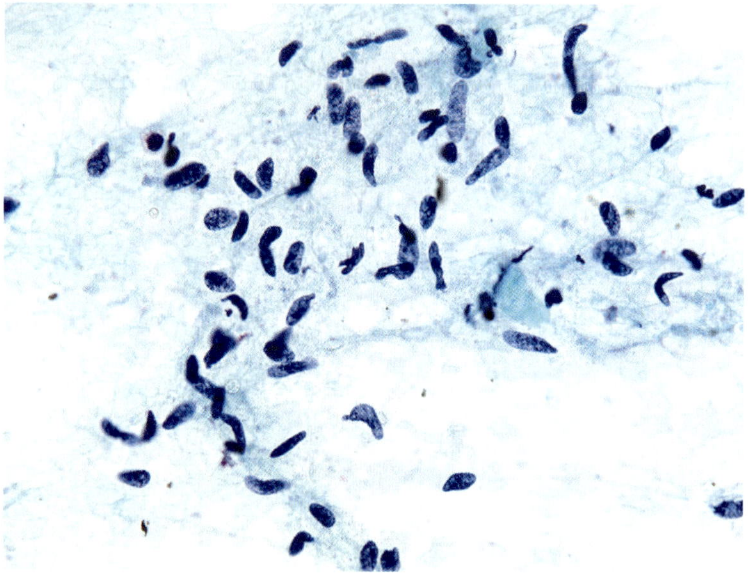

Figure 12.8 — Solitary Fibrous Tumor, FNA. Some authors have suggested that SFTs originate from mesenchymal (totipotent) thyroid capsule cells, a relationship of the tumor with the capsule has never been well-documented. Hence, the origin of primary thyroid SFT remains obscure. This case displays a haphazard pattern of neoplastic cells. Cells have mostly naked nuclei that have oval to short spindled morphology. Solitary fibrous tumor (SFT) is a relatively rare tumor that was originally described in the pleura. Primary thyroid SFT is rare. (Papanicolaou stain)

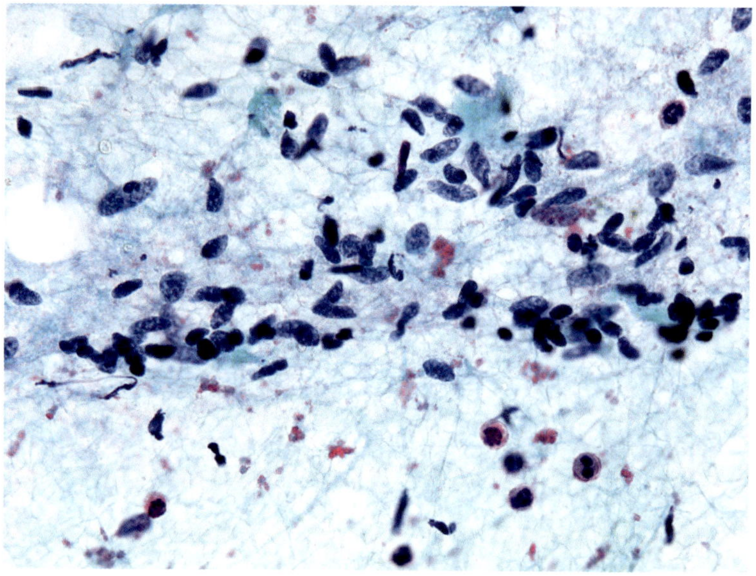

Figure 12.9 — Solitary Fibrous Tumor, FNA. Numerous bare nuclei of malignant cells are shown here with short spindled to fusiform morphology. No distinct architectural pattern is seen. Differential diagnosis would include medullary thyroid carcinoma, paraganglioma, hyalinizing trabecular neoplasm, and other benign and malignant mesenchymal tumors (such as nerve sheath tumor). In recent years, SFTs have been increasingly described in many extrapleural sites such as the lung, mediastinum, pericardium, peritoneum, upper respiratory tract, liver, thyroid, nasal and paranasal sinuses, parotid and salivary glands, and spine and other soft tissue. (Papanicolaou stain)

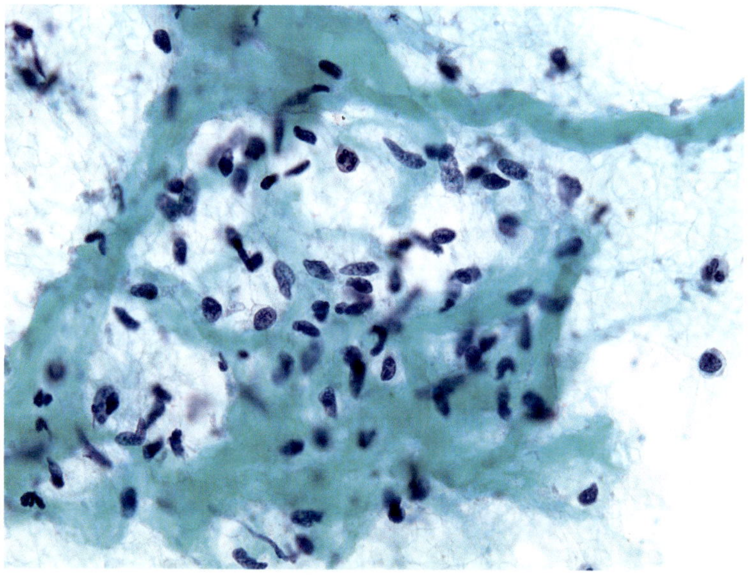

Figure 12.10 — Solitary Fibrous Tumor, FNA. Numerous fusiform and spindled neoplastic cell nuclei are associated with large shreds of collagenized stroma. Differential diagnosis would include medullary thyroid carcinoma with amyloid deposition. Immunoperoxidase stains are helpful in the differential diagnosis and are supportive of the cytomorphologic findings. Solitary fibrous tumors are typically positive for CD34, BCL2, and CD99, and negative for desmin, cytokeratins, vascular marker, S-100 protein, and smooth muscle markers. (Papanicolaou stain)

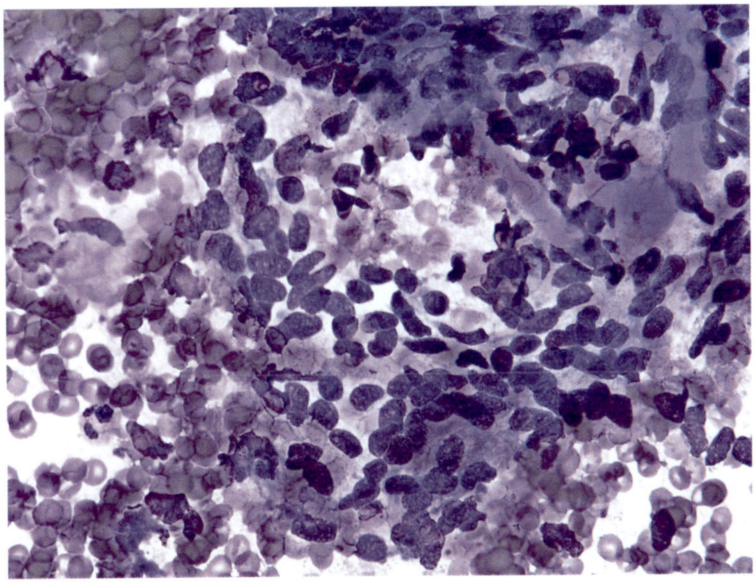

Figure 12.11 — Solitary Fibrous Tumor, FNA. Higher magnification depicts neoplastic cells with oval to fusiform nuclei in a vague fascicular pattern. Small amount of loose stromal matrix is also noted appearing as pale magenta material. Incomplete resection of benign SFT results in a higher recurrence rate and carries potential for malignant transformation. Malignant SFT may metastasize and may result in mortality. Rarely, papillary carcinoma has been observed to harbor an exuberant nodular fasciitis-like stroma, giving rise to a spindle cell proliferation resembling a mesenchymal neoplasm, such as an SFT. (Papanicolaou stain)

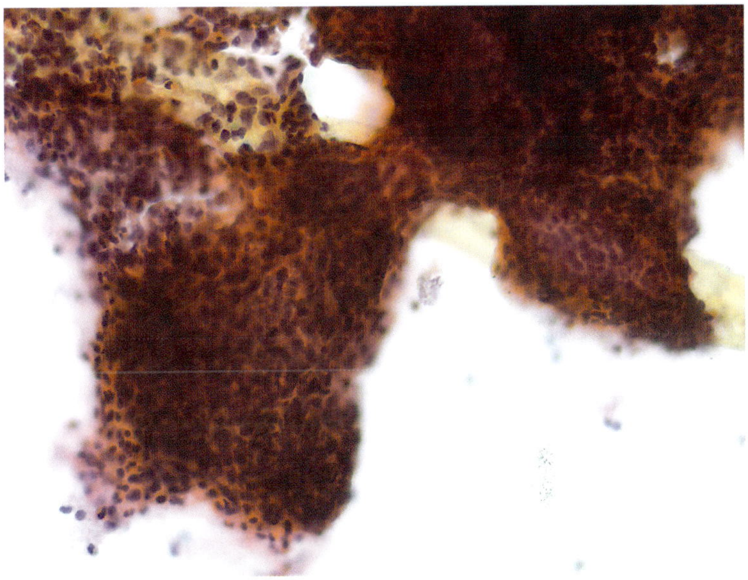

Figure 12.12 — Sclerosing Mucoepidermoid Carcinoma With Eosinophilia, FNA. Sclerosing mucoepidermoid carcinoma with eosinophilia (SMECE) is a distinctive low-grade carcinoma of the thyroid gland generally occurring in a background of Hashimoto thyroiditis. Low magnification in this case displays large syncytial fragments of malignant squamous cells interspersed with numerous eosinophils. Mucin-producing epithelial cells are not observed here. There is no thyroid follicular epithelium or colloid present. Mucoepidermoid carcinoma is most commonly encountered in salivary glands but can also occur at other anatomic sites such as bronchus, trachea, esophagus, breast, pancreas, and thyroid gland. SMECE occurs in adults between 35 and 71 years of age. (Papanicolaou stain)

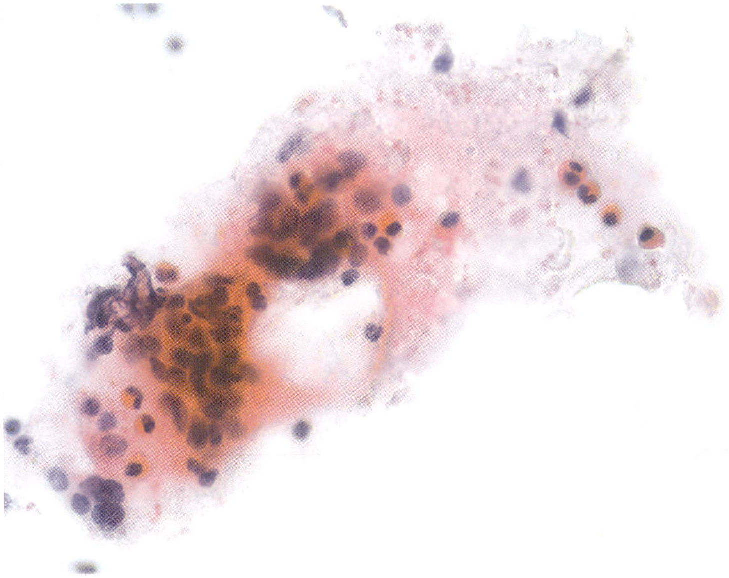

Figure 12.13 — Sclerosing Mucoepidermoid Carcinoma With Eosinophilia, FNA. The overall prognosis of SMECE is represented by an indolent behavior. SMECE can give rise to regional nodal metastases but rarely spreads beyond the neck. It displays a slow growing pattern and even in the presence of extra-thyroidal extension, is often associated with prolonged survival. Rare cases of lung and other distant metastases are reported. This particular field beautifully illustrates the main cytologic characteristics of SMECE, that is, malignant squamous cells, abundant eosinophils and mucin. Mucin-producing epithelium is rarely observed in the cytology of this tumor. (Papanicolaou stain)

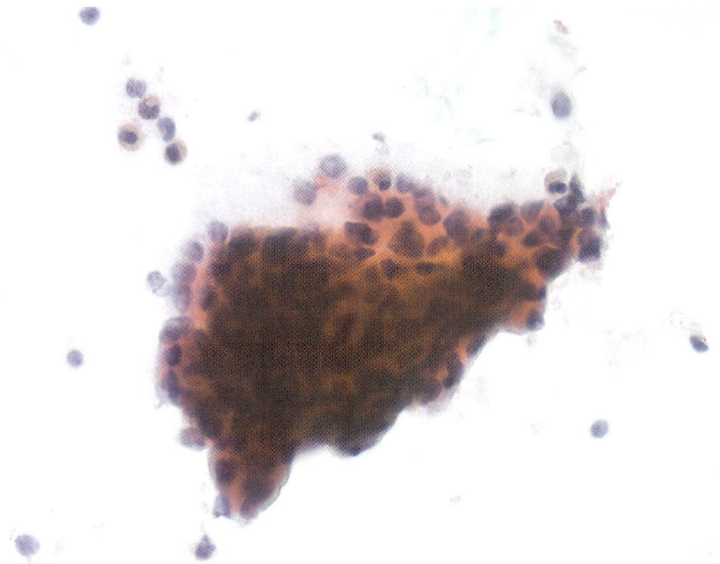

Figure 12.14 — Sclerosing Mucoepidermoid Carcinoma With Eosinophilia, FNA. SMECE should be differentiated from other thyroid tumors that can show foci of squamous differentiation as well as from the primary squamous carcinoma of thyroid. The differential diagnosis therefore would include tumors with areas of squamous change such as papillary carcinoma and its variants (squamous metaplasia is a common event in papillary carcinoma, having been reported in 20% to 40% of the cases), medullary carcinoma, carcinoma with thymus-like differentiation, and anaplastic carcinoma. This smear displays malignant epidermoid cells forming a tight syncytium. Numerous eosinophils are noted in the smear background. (Papanicolaou stain)

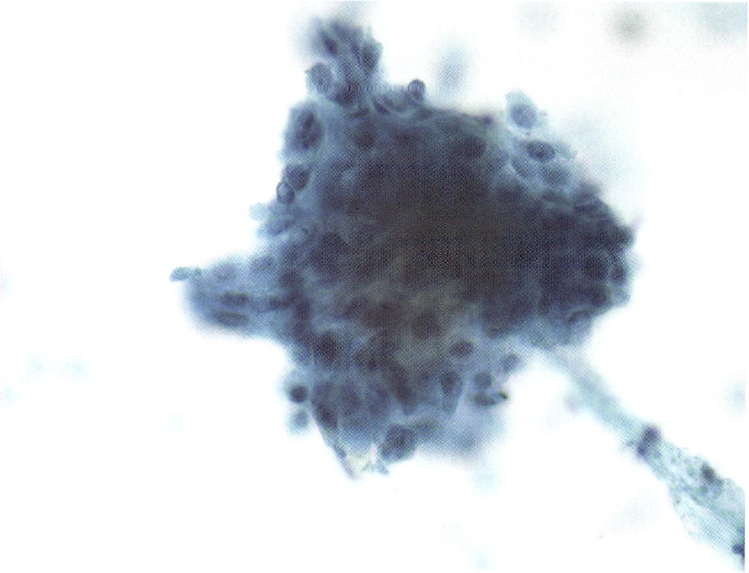

Figure 12.15 — Sclerosing Mucoepidermoid Carcinoma With Eosinophilia, FNA. SMECE is overwhelmingly a tumor of women (female:male ratio, 17:1). It is a tumor of adults and occurs in patients between 35 and 71 years of age. This smear displays a fragment of malignant nonkeratinized squamous cells. One differential diagnosis here would be a nodular tumor-like squamous metaplasia associated with Hashimoto thyroiditis, which is a rare benign occurrence that can potentially resemble a mucoepidermoid carcinoma. (Papanicolaou stain)

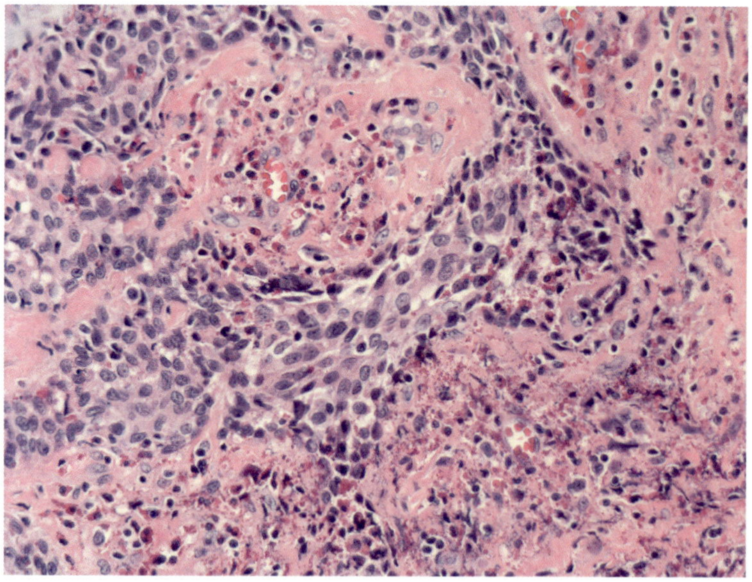

Figure 12.16 — Sclerosing Mucoepidermoid Carcinoma With Eosinophilia, Histologic Section. The most common presenting symptom of SMECE is a painless neck mass or cold nodule on thyroid scan. Symptoms secondary to locoregional extension such as hoarseness have been described. High magnification in this case displays a nice cytohistologic correlation with the FNA seen in the previous case. Nests of malignant nonkeratinized squamous cells are seen interspersed with a fibrotic stroma containing innumerable eosinophils. (H&E stain)

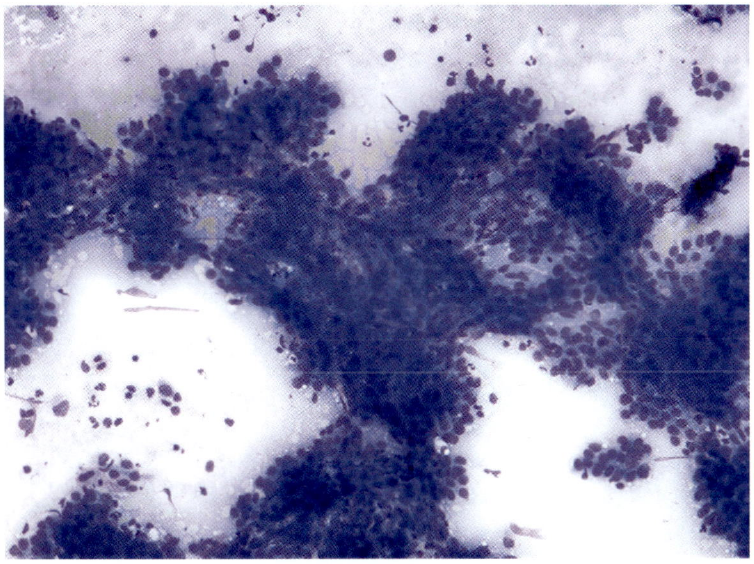

Figure 12.17 — Carcinoma Showing Thymus-Like Differentiation (CASTLE), FNA. Carcinoma showing thymus-like differentiation (CASTLE) is a rare neoplasm located in the thyroid and adjacent soft tissues which histologically resembles thymic carcinoma. Low magnification in this case displays large syncytia of a high-grade carcinoma. Malignant cells form predominantly cohesive fragments with only rare dispersed cells. Lymphocytes were observed interspersed in most fields. No native thyroid tissue was present. CASTLE typically affects middle-aged adults, shows a slight female predominance (Male:Female, 1:1.3), and most often involves the lower poles of the thyroid gland. (Diff Quik stain)

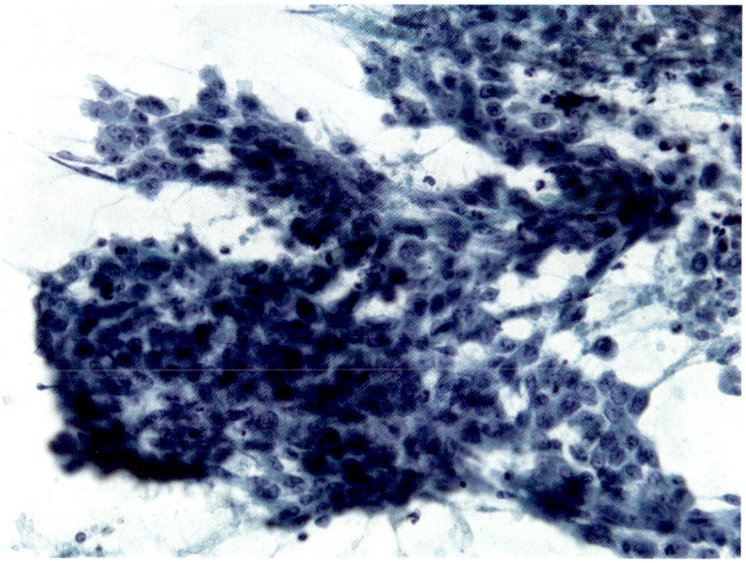

Figure 12.18 — Carcinoma Showing Thymus-Like Differentiation (CASTLE), FNA. CASTLE is postulated to arise from either ectopic thymic tissue in the neck, from remnants of the thymopharyngeal duct or from ultimobranchial body remnants within the thyroid gland. This case shows a large syncytium of malignant epithelial cells with numerous mitoses and karyorrhexis. No follicular architecture or colloid was apparent in the entire case and no keratinization was observed. Possibility of metastatic carcinoma needs to be excluded before considering a primary thyroid malignancy in such cases. (Papanicolaou stain)

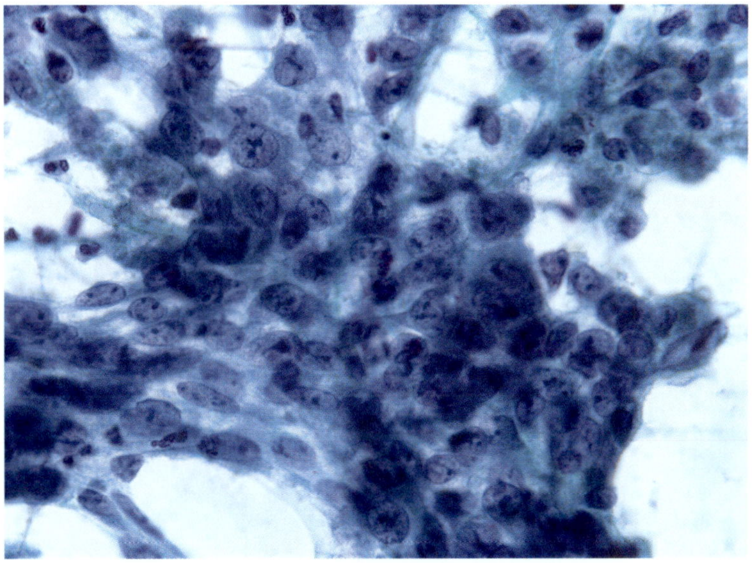

Figure 12.19 — Carcinoma Showing Thymus-Like Differentiation (CASTLE), FNA. High magnification illustrates markedly enlarged nuclei with open "vesicular" chromatin and macronucleoli. Cells have fused cytoplasmic borders creating a syncytial architecture. Few karyorrhectic nuclei are also noted. Prognostically, it is important to exclude metastatic nasopharyngeal or squamous cell carcinoma to the thyroid gland, due to their far worse prognoses compared to CASTLE. (Papanicolaou stain)

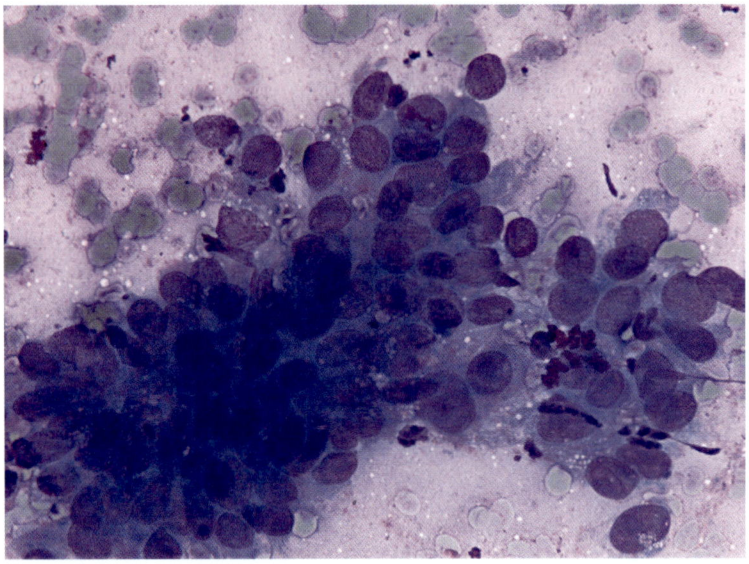

Figure 12.20 — Carcinoma Showing Thymus-Like Differentiation (CASTLE), FNA. A syncytium of malignant cells seen at high magnification. Cells have markedly enlarged round nuclei with macronucleoli. Cytoplasmic boundaries are indistinct and cells have high N/C ratios. Differentiating thymic from thyroidal origin is supported by immunoreactivity for markers associated with thymic carcinoma such as CD5, bcl-2, and mcl-1 and negativity for TTF-1 (Diff Quik stain)

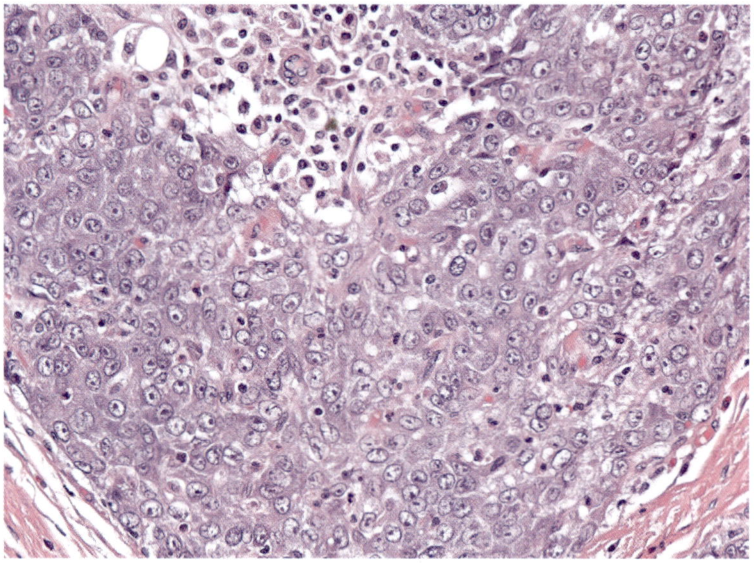

Figure 12.21 — Carcinoma Showing Thymus-Like Differentiation (CASTLE), Histologic Section. This is higher magnification of a syncytium of malignant cells showing large nuclei with open vesicular chromatin and macronucleoli, correlating beautifully with the FNA morphology seen in the corresponding FNA (Figure 12.20). It's common to find abundant necrosis and karyorrhexis in this tumor. The histopathology of CASTLE is characterized by well-defined lobulated architecture, expansive growth pattern, poorly differentiated malignant cells in sheets and nests intermixed with small lymphocytes, fibrous bands separating tumor lobules, whorl formation similar to Hassall's corpuscles and increased pleomorphism of nuclei when compared to the conventional thymoma. (H&E stain)

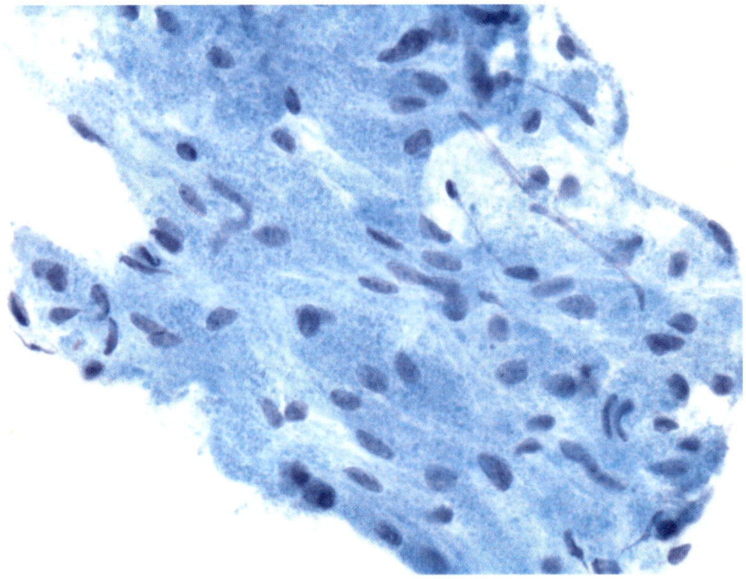

Figure 12.22 — Granular Cell Tumor, FNA. Primary thyroid granular cell tumor is extremely rare. The main morphologic feature of this tumor is the granularity of the cytoplasm which is caused by a massive accumulation of lysosomes. These neoplastic cells have voluminous markedly granular cytoplasm with uniform round to oval to elongated nuclei. Cells have low N/C ratios. Cytoplasmic granules have a bright green appearance on Papanicolaou stain. Some lesions display prominent vascularity and hence a metastatic renal cell carcinoma should always be excluded in these cases. (Papanicolaou stain)

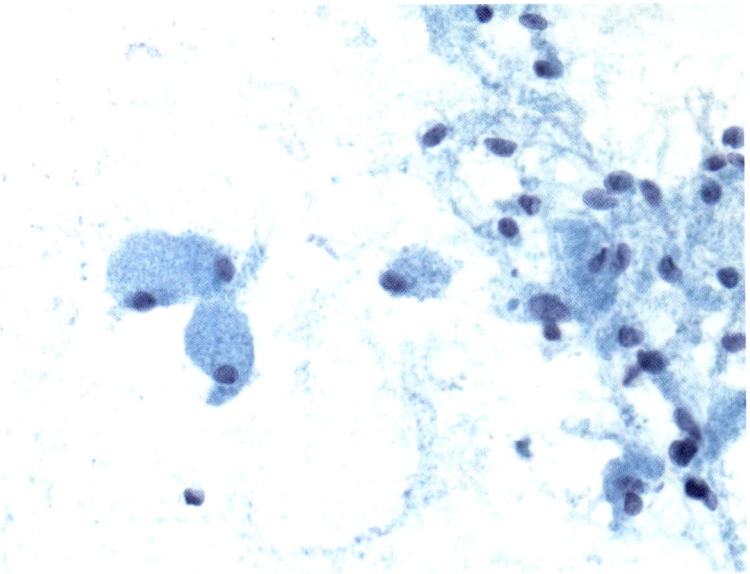

Figure 12.23 — Granular Cell Tumor, FNA. This tumor can occur in virtually any anatomic location with roughly one half of the lesions found in the head and neck. A differential diagnosis of thyroid granular cell tumor includes more frequent thyroid lesions containing abundant cytoplasmic granules such as Hürthle cell neoplasms, lesions with abundant macrophages, reparative lesions and metastatic renal cell carcinoma. Note the round to elongated uniform nuclei. Abundant free granules are also noted in the smear background. (Papanicolaou stain)

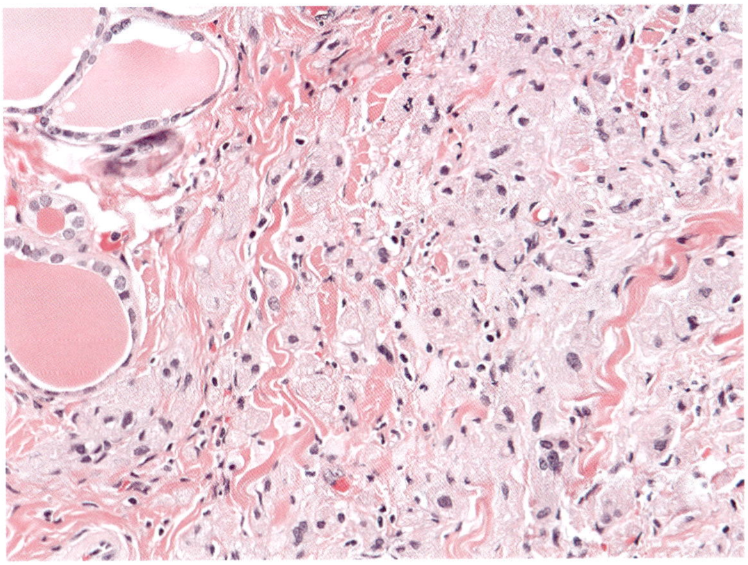

Figure 12.24 — Granular Cell Tumor, Histologic Section. The tongue is the most common site of occurrence of granular cell tumor with primary thyroid tumors being extremely rare with only a handful reported in the English literature. Although most investigators currently favor a Schwann cell derivation based on immunohistochemical and electron microscopic findings, the histogenesis of granular cell tumor has been a source of controversy. Histologically, granular cell tumor is composed of strands and fascicles of large cells with distinct cell borders containing abundant granular cytoplasm. Features of malignancy include spindle cell morphology, necrosis, prominent nucleoli, increased nuclear to cytoplasmic ratio, nuclear pleomorphism, and increased mitotic rate. Normal thyroid tissue is noted on the left. This case was associated with focal extra-thyroidal extension. (H&E stain)

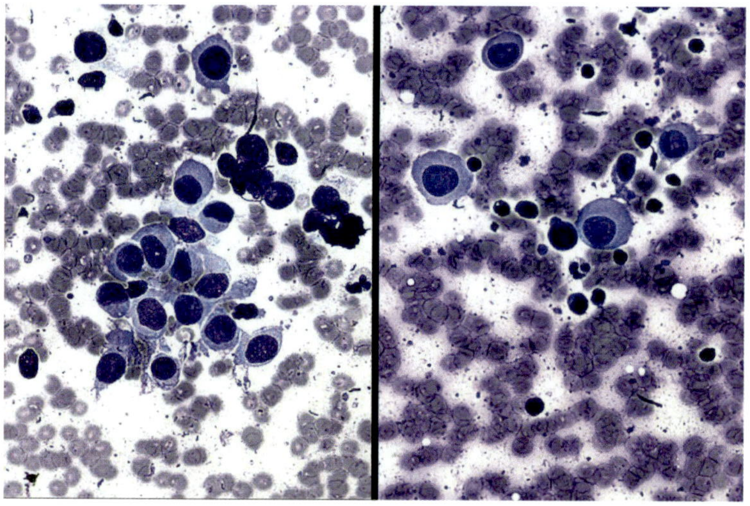

Figure 12.25 — Langerhans Cell Histiocytosis, FNA. Primary involvement of the thyroid gland by Langerhans cell histiocytosis (LCH) is exceedingly rare. LCH is a group of idiopathic disorders characterized by the cellular infiltrate with characteristics similar to bone marrow–derived Langerhans cells. LCH results from the clonal proliferation of immunophenotypically and functionally immature, morphologically rounded LCH cells along with eosinophils, macrophages, lymphocytes, and occasionally, multinucleated giant cells. This case, which was originally called "atypical thyroid lesion" was especially challenging as the reniform/grooved nuclei were not clearly apparent and only a few eosinophils were noted. (Diff Quik stain)

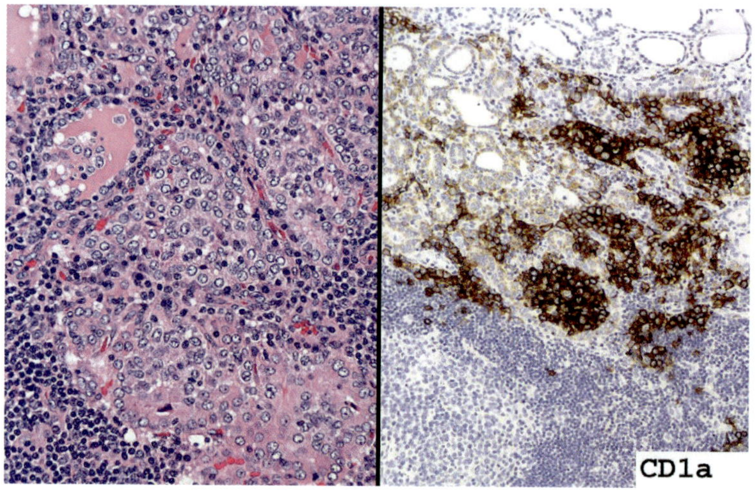

Figure 12.26 — Langerhans Cell Histiocytosis, Histologic Section. LCH is usually a sporadic and nonhereditary condition but familial clustering has been noted in limited number of cases. LCH cells have been found to express markers of both resting epidermal Langerhans cells (CD1a) as well as activated Langerhans cells (including CD54 and CD58). The histologic section of the thyroid shows an almost complete replacement of the parenchyma by a diffuse mononuclear cell infiltrate interspersed with a nest of large atypical histiocytic cells with abundant granular pink cytoplasm and grooved nuclei. Only rare thyroid tissue is visible. Numerous eosinophils are present as well. The histiocytic cells strongly immunoexpress CD1a. (H&E and immunostain)

13

Metastatic and Secondary Cancers

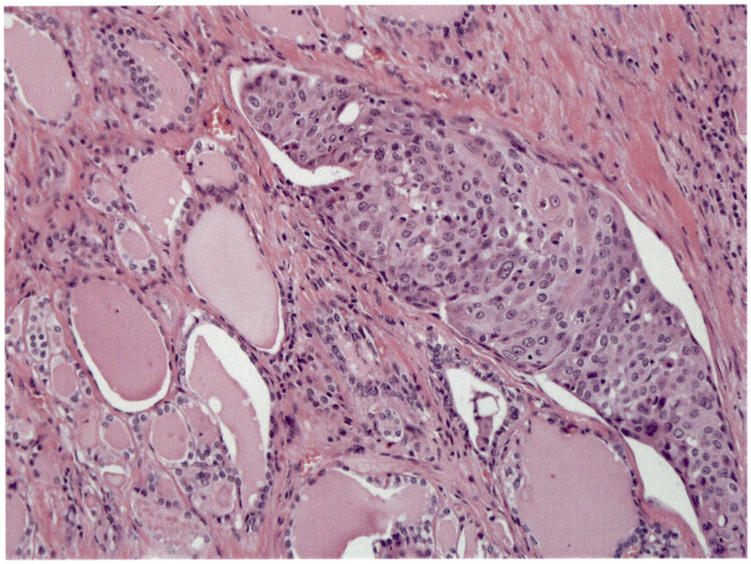

Figure 13.1 — Squamous Cell Carcinoma of the Larynx With Secondary Extension into the Thyroid, Histologic Section. The thyroid gland can be secondarily involved via direct local extension from a squamous cell carcinoma of the larynx. Nests of focally keratinizing squamous cell carcinoma infiltrate between thyroid follicles. The differential diagnosis would include a squamoid variant of anaplastic carcinoma as well as a rare primary squamous cell carcinoma of the thyroid. This differential diagnosis is usually quite easily resolved on clinical grounds. (H&E stain)

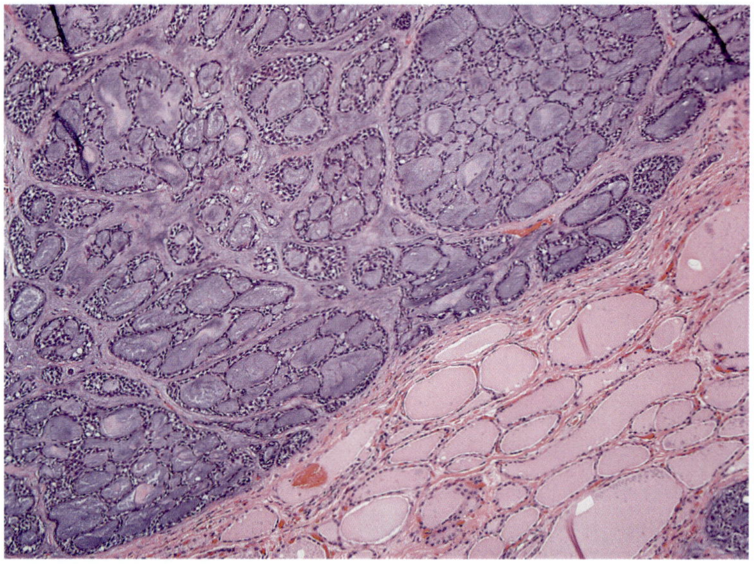

Figure 13.2 — Adenoid Cystic Carcinoma of the Trachea With Secondary Extension into the Thyroid, Histologic Section. The thyroid can also be secondarily involved by carcinomas arising from the seromucinous glands lining the respiratory tract. In this case, an adenoid cystic carcinoma of the trachea directly infiltrates the thyroid parenchyma. The tumor displays a cribriform architecture. The cribriform spaces are filled with a basophilic mucoid material. (H&E stain)

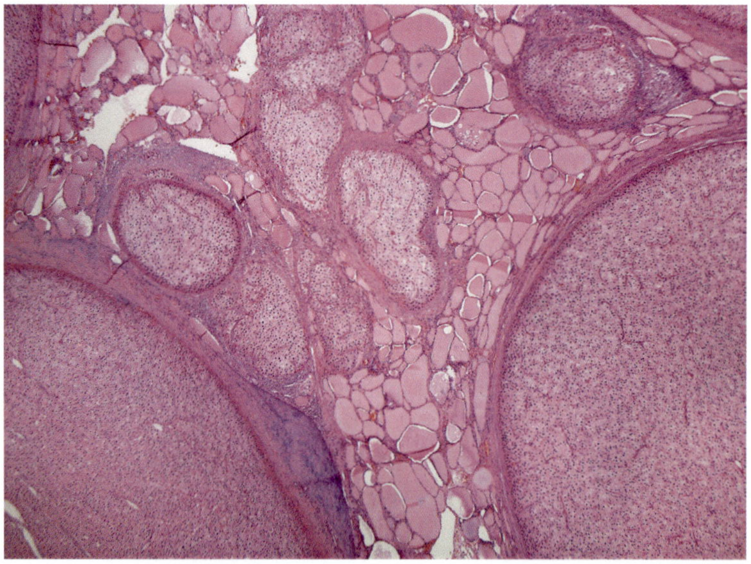

Figure 13.3 — Parathyroid Carcinoma With Secondary Extension into the Thyroid, Histologic Section. The parathyroid gland is often located in the capsule of the thyroid and is sometimes even embedded within the thyroid parenchyma (ie, intrathyroidal parathyroid). Not surprisingly, the thyroid gland is a common site of secondary involvement for the rare parathyroid carcinoma. In this case, the parathyroid carcinoma has invaded through the capsule of the parathyroid to infiltrate the thyroid parenchyma in a multinodular fashion. The malignant nature of the carcinoma may not be apparent at the cellular level. Here the tumor cells show minimal variation in size and shape, and mitotic figures are not readily identified. (H&E stain)

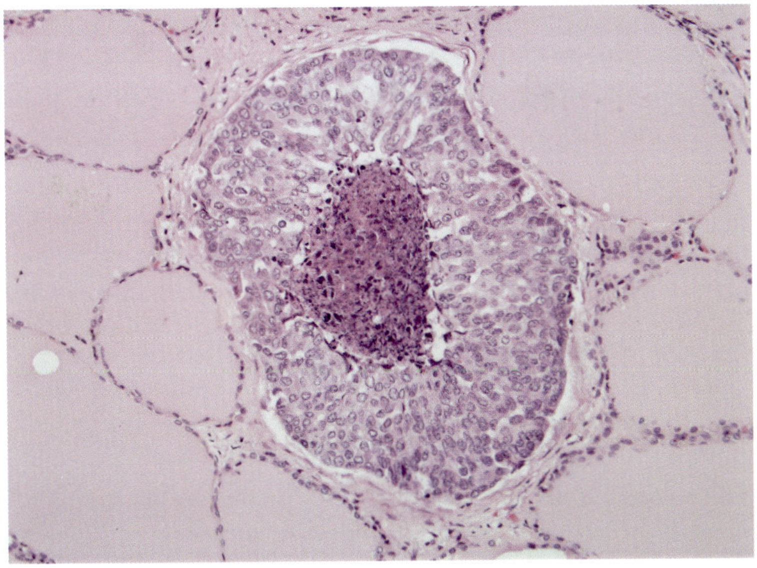

Figure 13.4 — Metastatic Breast Carcinoma, Histologic Section. Involvement of the thyroid by metastatic carcinoma is usually seen in the context of widely disseminated metastatic spread. In this case, the thyroid is involved by widely disseminated breast carcinoma. Thyroid metastases are usually multifocal rather than solitary lesions. The pattern of thyroid involvement shown here is typical of metastatic spread. The metastatic implants are usually distributed within interstitial lymphatics, often without directly invading the thyroid follicles. (H&E stain)

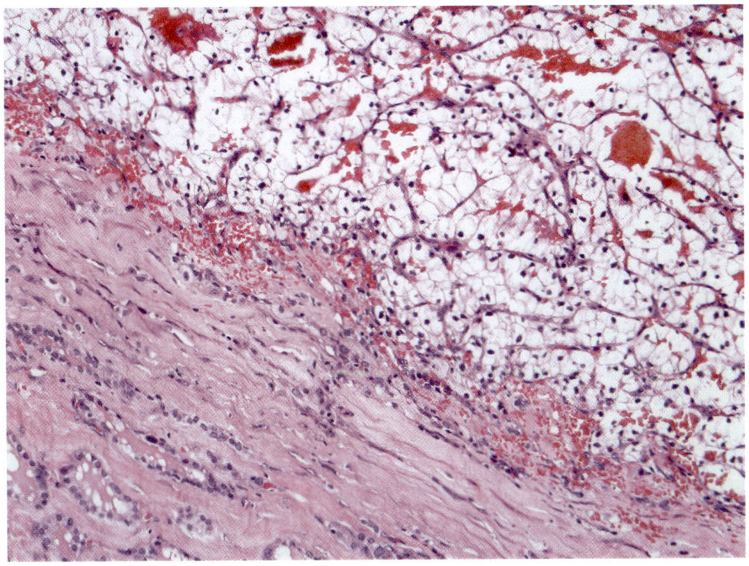

Figure 13.5 — Metastatic Renal Cell Carcinoma, Histologic Section. In metastatic renal cell carcinoma, the thyroid gland is sometimes targeted as a solitary site in the absence of widely disseminated spread to other organs. The recognition of its kidney origin may be confounded by the tendency of renal cell carcinomas to be locally silent and to disseminate long after removal of the primary tumor. At the histologic level, confusion between metastatic renal cell carcinoma and a primary thyroid neoplasm is heightened by overlapping morphologic features. In particular, the distinction between metastatic renal cell carcinoma and a Hürthle cell neoplasm with prominent clear cell change can be challenging. Morphologic features that support kidney origin include the water-clear quality of the cytoplasm, a prominent vascularity including delicate and dilated vascular channels, and central luminal spaces packed with red blood cells. Immunohistochemical studies including thyroid (eg, TTF-1 and thyroglobulin) and renal (eg, RCC) markers are useful if diagnostic uncertainty persists. (H&E stain)

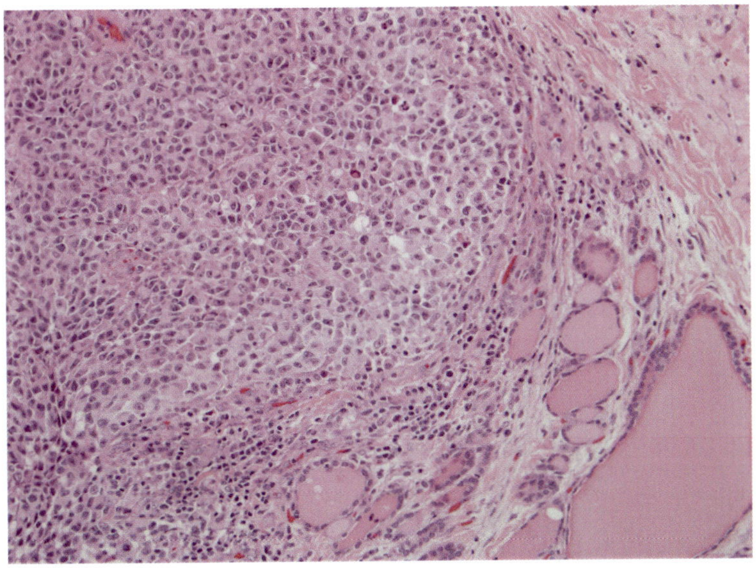

Figure 13.6 — Metastatic Melanoma, Histologic Section. Metastatic melanoma is another tumor that can initially present as an enlarging thyroid mass. In this case the melanoma cells have a somewhat plasmacytoid appearance with eccentrically placed nuclei and prominent nucleoli, but the morphologic findings can be highly variable. Melanin pigmentation is often not evident (ie, amelanotic melanoma) such that the diagnosis may require immunohistochemical documentation of melanocytic differentiation. (H&E stain)

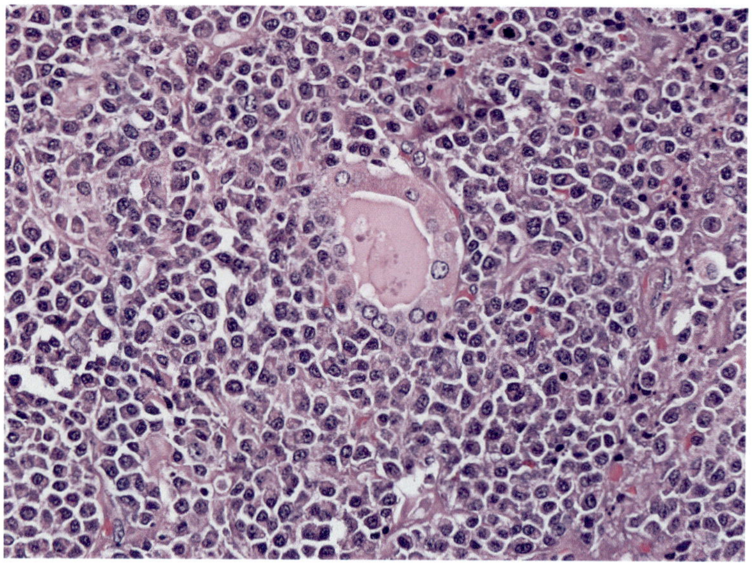

Figure 13.7a — Plasmacytoma, Histologic Section. The thyroid parenchyma is effaced by dense infiltration of mature appearing plasma cells with eccentric nuclei, coarse chromatin, pinpoint nucleoli, and abundant amphophilic cytoplasm. Although most plasma cell tumors in the thyroid are localized findings (ie, plasmacytomas), the thyroid gland can be involved as part of a systemic process (myeloma). (H&E stain)

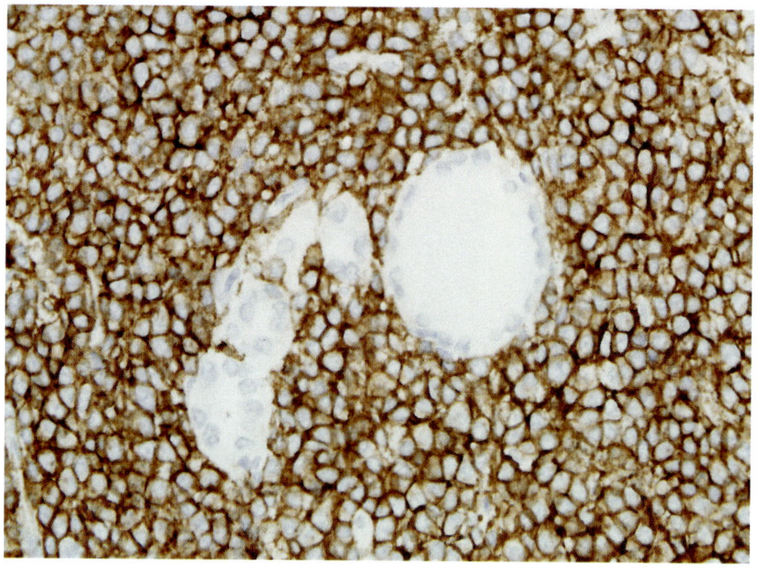

Figure 13.7b — Plasmacytoma (Kappa Immunostain), Histologic Section. The monoclonal nature of this plasma cell infiltrate is confirmed by immunoglobulin light chain restriction. (Immunostain)

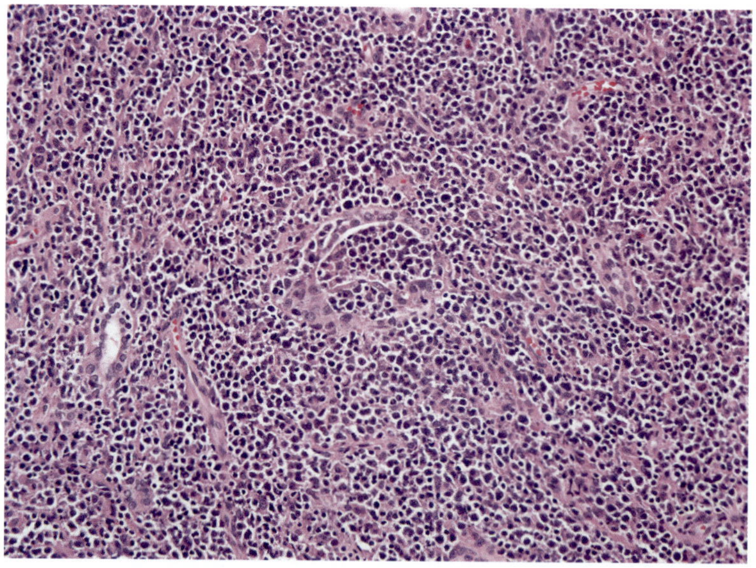

Figure 13.8a — Low Grade B-Cell Lymphoma of Mucosa-Associated Lymphoid Tissue (MALT), Histologic Section. MALT lymphomas of the thyroid invariably arise in a background of autoimmune thyroiditis. In this field, the normal architecture of the thyroid is effaced by an atypical lymphoid infiltrate composed of a mixed population of lymphoid cells including small mature lymphocytes, monocytoid cells, and plasma cells. Unlike most cases of autoimmune thyroiditis where the lymphocytes permeate between the thyroid follicles, thyroid lymphomas often invade the follicular epithelium and accumulate within the follicular spaces. (H&E stain)

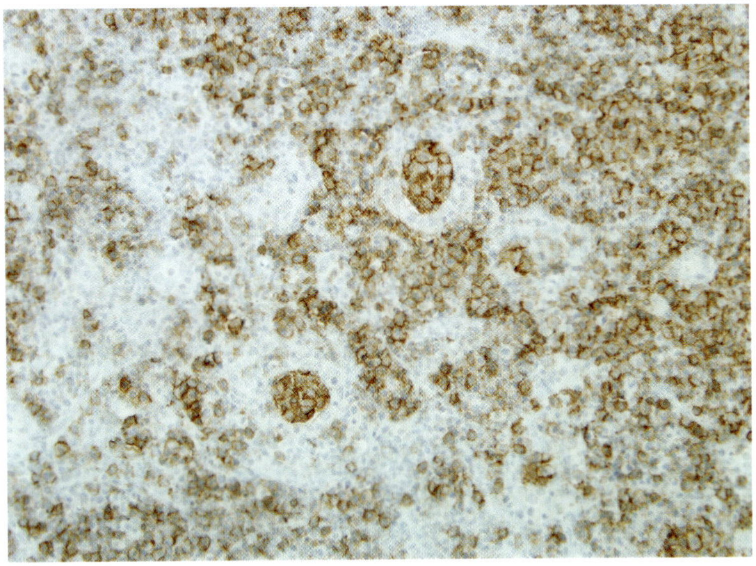

Figure 13.8b — Low Grade B-Cell Lymphoma of Mucosa-Associated Lymphoid Tissue (MALT) (CD20 Immunostain), Histologic Section. This CD20 stain shows that the dense lymphoid infiltrate is distributed both in and around the follicles. The accumulation of lymphoid cells within the thyroid follicles, sometimes referred to as "lymphoepithelial lesions," tends to be a particularly well developed feature of MALT lymphomas of the thyroid. (Immunostain)

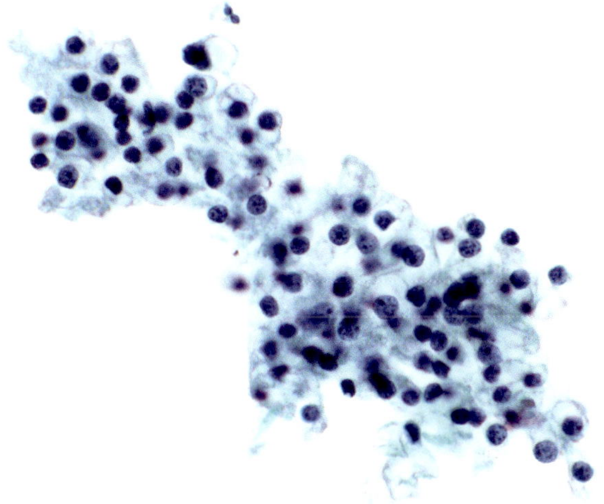

Figure 13.9 — Metastatic Renal Cell Carcinoma, Fine Needle Aspiration (FNA). A large group of cells with abundant clear cytoplasm and relatively minimal nuclear atypia is present. The differential diagnosis includes clear cell follicular neoplasms as well as parathyroid neoplasms. Renal cell carcinoma must always be considered with any clear cell neoplasm since the renal primary may be occult or delayed metastasis may occur after many years. The most common primary sites of metastases to the thyroid are cancers of the lung, breast, skin (especially melanoma), colon, and kidney. However, recent surgical data have shown that metastatic renal cell carcinoma now accounts for most of the metastases seen in the thyroid gland. (Liquid based preparation, Papanicolaou stain)

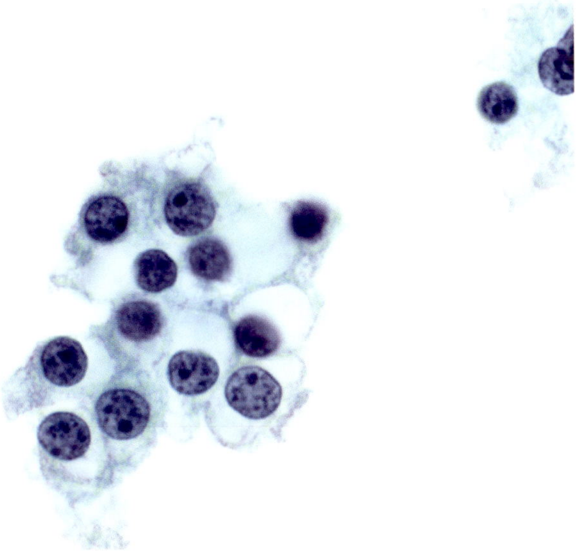

Figure 13.10 — Metastatic Renal Cell Carcinoma, FNA. In other groups, the presence of enlarged nuclei with a prominent nucleolus is evident. The abundant clear cytoplasm in renal cell carcinoma tends to have less granularity than is seen in a follicular neoplasm with clear cell change. The most common primary sites for origin of metastases to the thyroid are lung, breast, skin (especially melanoma), colon, and kidney. (Liquid based preparation, Papanicolaou stain)

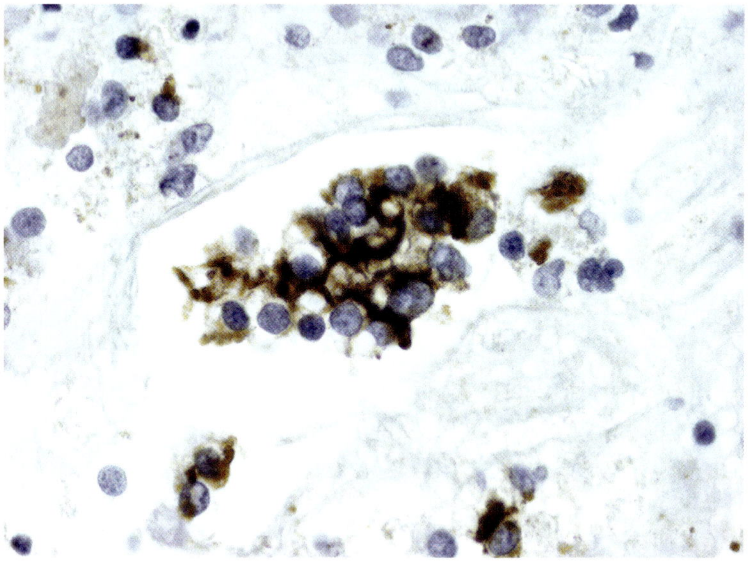

Figure 13.11 — Metastatic Renal Cell Carcinoma, FNA. Marker studies are necessary to establish whether a clear cell neoplasm is primary or metastatic. RCC immunoreactivity shown here supports the diagnosis of metastatic renal cell carcinoma. TTF-1 and thyroglobulin are negative in renal cell carcinoma. Thyroglobulin may be challenging to interpret in limited material as it may only be expressed focally in clear cell follicular neoplasms and may also be extruded from admixed follicular cells potentially resulting in a false positive interpretation (immunodiffusion). (RCC immunolabeling, cell block section)

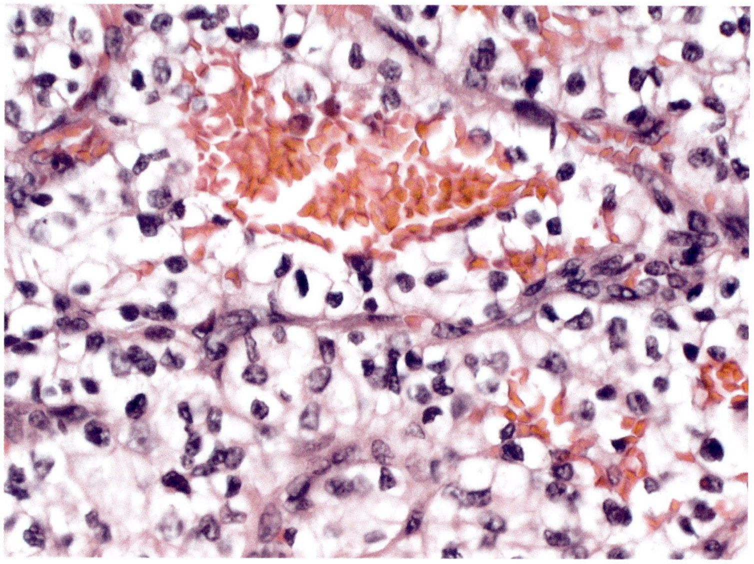

Figure 13.12 — Metastatic Renal Cell Carcinoma, Histologic Section. In the resected metastasis, classic features of renal cell carcinoma are present. The cells are polygonal with abundant clear cytoplasm, a prominent vascular network, and "blood lakes" within glandular lumina. Metastatic carcinomas characteristically present as either multiple small discrete nodules, a solitary large nodule or with diffuse involvement of the gland. (H&E stain)

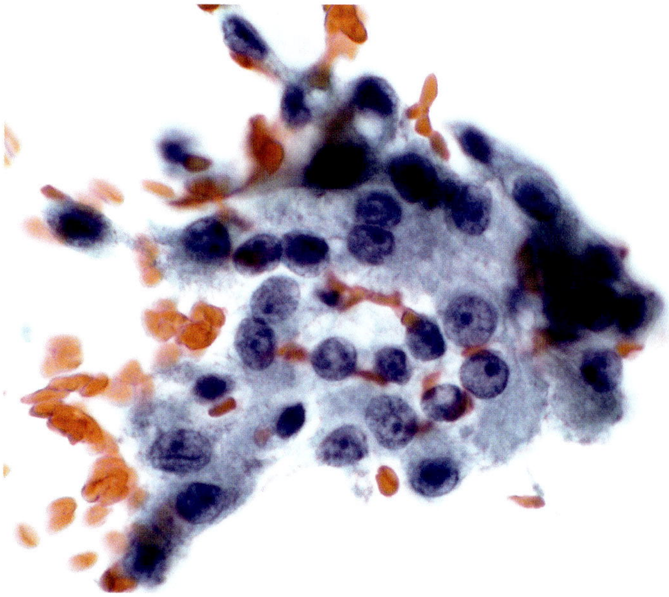

Figure 13.13 — Metastatic Renal Cell Carcinoma, FNA. In this example, the prominent nucleolus typical in renal cell carcinoma is readily appreciated in several cells. A longitudinal nuclear groove is present in a cell in the lower left portion of the image. The nucleus is hyperchromatic with coarse chromatin avoiding confusion with papillary carcinoma. The cytoplasm is more vacuolated and granular than in the prior images shown. (Papanicolaou stain)

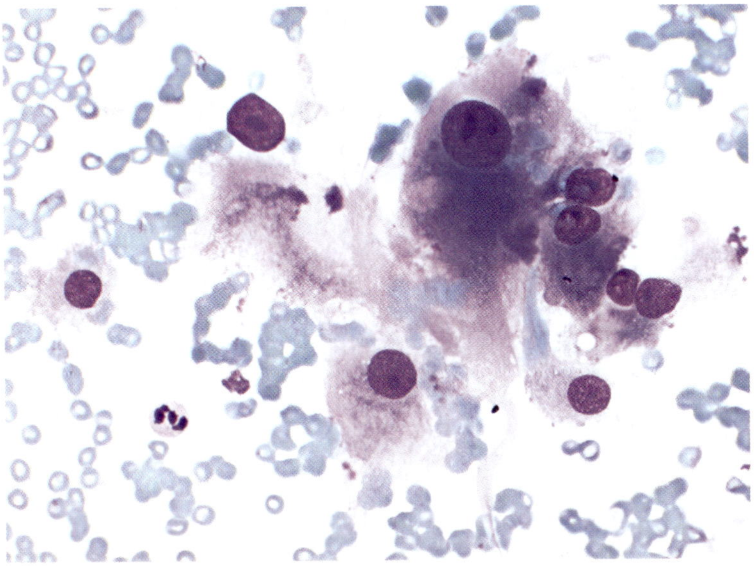

Figure 13.14 — Metastatic Renal Cell Carcinoma, FNA. Voluminous finely vacuolated cytoplasm is present in these cells. Marked nuclear size variation with prominent nucleoli is also seen. A single bare nucleus is present. Cell fragility often results in bare nuclei in the smear background. Metastasis from a renal primary can occur as long as twenty years following resection of the primary neoplasm. These tumors display moderately to highly cellular smears, often bloody, with cells appearing singly and in cohesive clusters, fragmented papillae, and small flat sheets. The neoplastic cells typically have abundant pale and finely vacuolated cytoplasm. (Diff Quik stain)

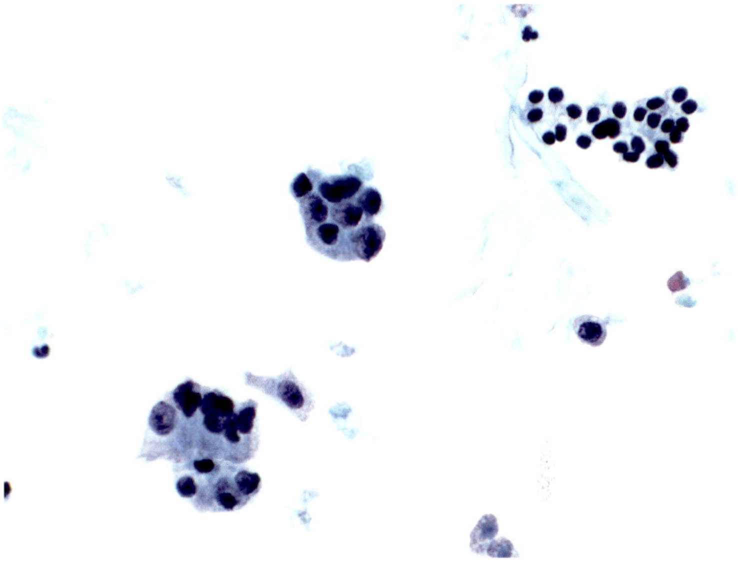

Figure 13.15a — Metastatic Lung Adenocarcinoma, FNA. Several clusters and individual malignant cells with enlarged hyperchromatic nuclei are present. Note the contrast with the group of benign follicular cells in the upper right of the image. The follicular cells are evenly spaced with small uniform nuclei with condensed chromatin. (Liquid based preparation, Papanicolaou stain)

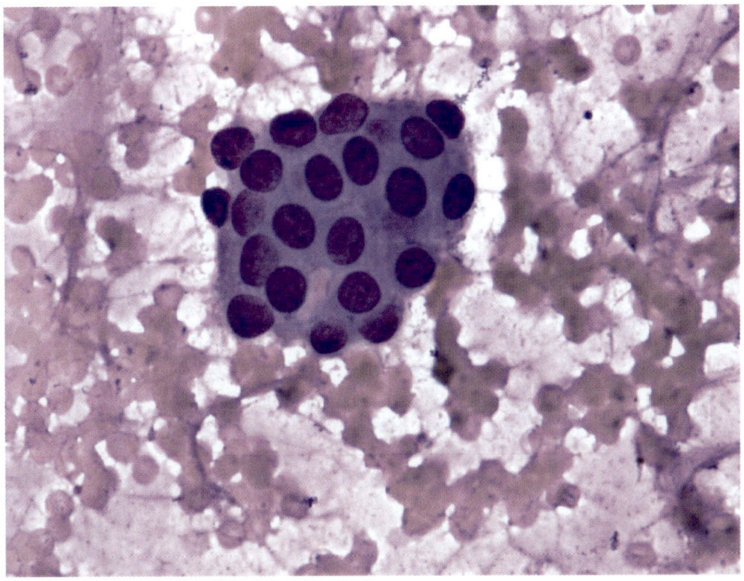

Figure 13.15b — Metastatic Lung Adenocarcinoma, FNA. This direct smear preparation displays a small three-dimensional gland-like fragment. N/C ratios are not high and cells do not show prominent nucleoli. If several of these small tissue fragments are present, a distinction has to be made with a primary follicular neoplasm. TTF-1 immunostain alone may not help and addition of thyroglobulin and Napsin-A in the immune panel is important for an accurate distinction. Lung adenocarcinomas are characteristically of higher nuclear grade than most thyroid follicular neoplasms. (Diff Quik stain)

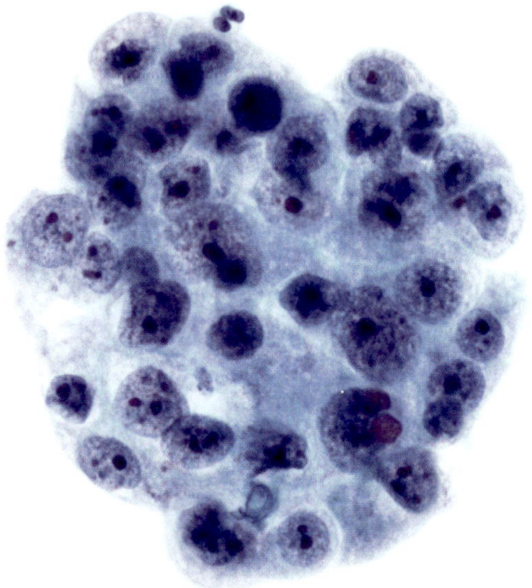

Figure 13.16a — Metastatic Lung Adenocarcinoma, FNA. Marked nuclear pleomorphism with a high nuclear:cytoplasmic ratio is seen. This poorly differentiated metastasis does not show clear evidence of glandular differentiation. The thyroid malignancy which might resemble this tumor would be undifferentiated (anaplastic) carcinoma. Undifferentiated thyroid carcinoma rarely expresses TTF-1. TTF-1 immunoreactivity in this case along with the clinical history supports a lung primary. (Liquid based preparation, Papanicolaou stain)

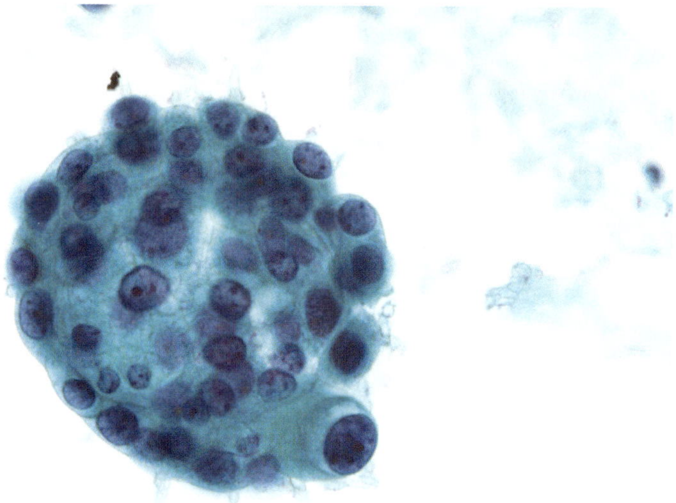

Figure 13.16b — Metastatic Lung Adenocarcinoma, FNA. Direct smear preparation of another case shows similar features. This patient had a known bronchioloalveolar carcinoma. Note the well-formed glandular morphology, vesicular nuclei, and macronucleoli. Lung adenocarcinomas are composed of medium to large cells displaying sheets and/or three-dimensional cell balls. The individual neoplastic cells often show columnar morphology with round to oval eccentric nuclei and prominent nucleoli. (Papanicolaou stain)

Figure 13.17 — Metastatic Breast Carcinoma, FNA. Few groups of malignant cells with enlarged hyperchromatic nuclei with irregular contours were present in this cytologic preparation from a patient with a known history of breast carcinoma. Metastases from a breast primary are one of the most common of the metastatic lesions to the thyroid. The majority of these are infiltrating ductal carcinomas. Although primary thyroid follicular neoplasms are in the differential, metastatic breast carcinoma cells (both ductal and lobular) have cells that are larger than most follicular neoplasms and may show distinct purple cytoplasmic inclusions on Diff Quik staining. (Liquid based preparation, Papanicolaou stain)

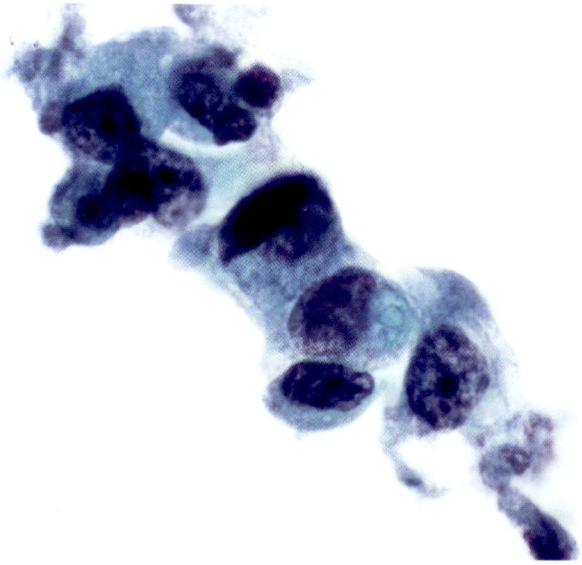

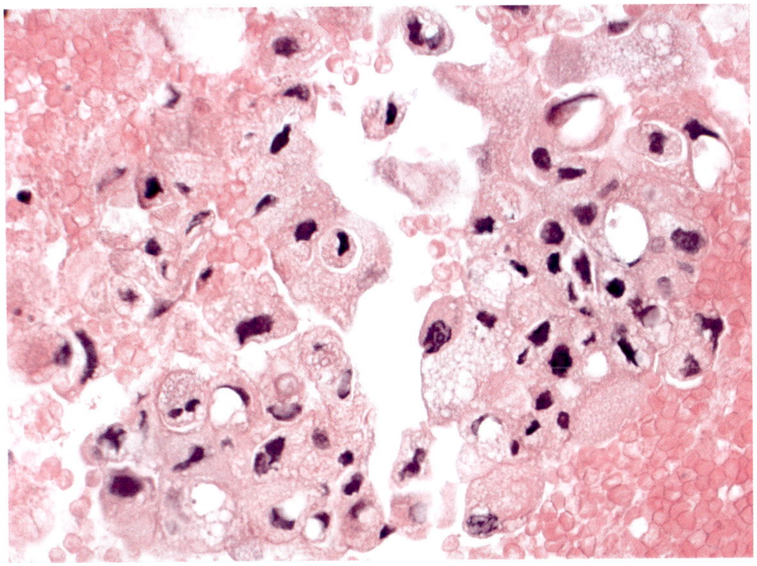

Figure 13.18 — Metastatic Breast Carcinoma, FNA. The cell block shows a large cluster of cells with abundant eosinophilic and vacuolated cytoplasm. Marked nuclear contour irregularities and hyperchromasia are present. Metastatic carcinomas are known to involve the thyroid in several distinct patterns; they may form multiple small discrete nodules (typically less than 2 mm in size) or a single large discrete mass or less likely, a diffuse involvement of the gland. (Cell block section, H&E stain).

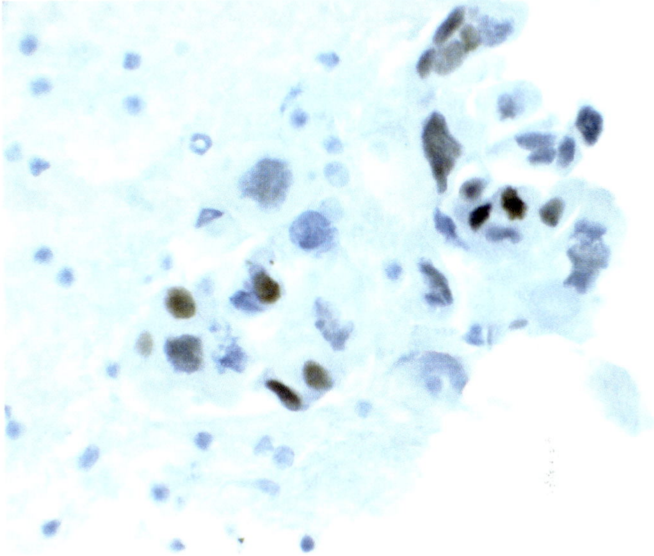

Figure 13.19 — Metastatic Breast Carcinoma, FNA. Immunostain for estrogen receptor (ER) is positive in some tumor cells supporting the diagnosis of metastatic breast carcinoma. Thyroid markers (TTF-1 and thyroglobulin) were negative. (ER immunolabeling, cell block section)

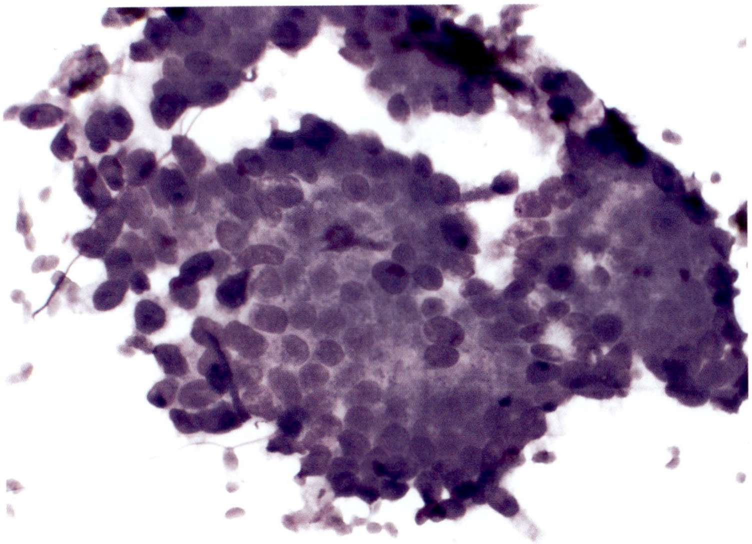

Figure 13.20a — Metastatic Colonic Adenocarcinoma, FNA. Although there is nuclear crowding and size variation, the overall appearance of this group resembles a macrofollicle. The initial impression of this aspirate was that it might represent a follicular neoplasm. A single cell at the lower right edge of the group has a more columnar configuration than can be appreciated in the rest of the image. (Diff Quik stain)

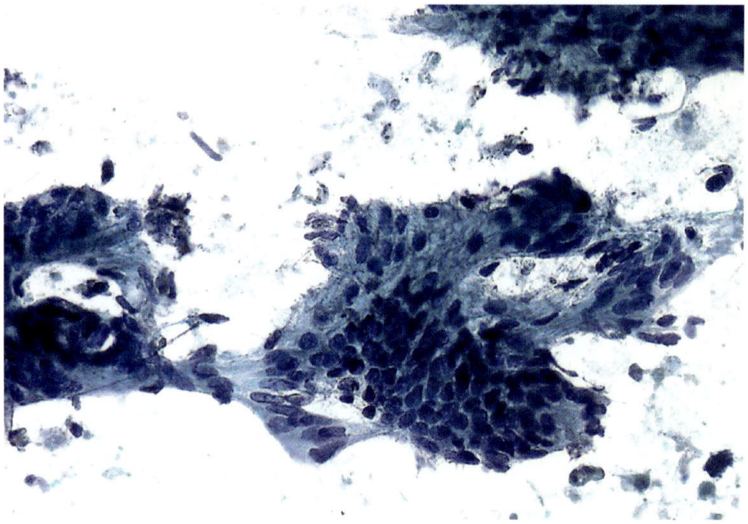

Figure 13.20b — Metastatic Colonic Adenocarcinoma, FNA. This case shows the characteristic elongated "cigar shaped" nuclei with focal palisading. Additionally, there is evidence of background necrosis so commonly seen in metastasis of colonic adenocarcinomas. Papillary thyroid carcinoma, tall cell variant has to be considered in the differential diagnosis if the history of a colonic primary is not available. (Papanicolaou stain)

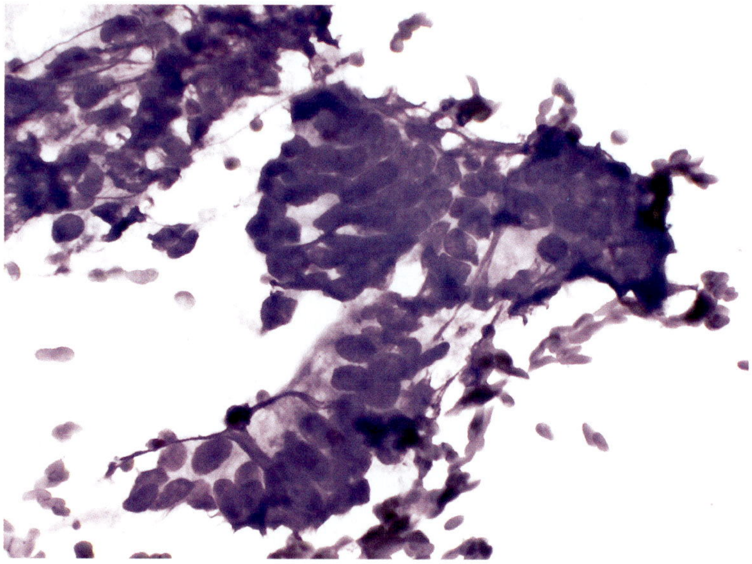

Figure 13.21 — Metastatic Colonic Adenocarcinoma, FNA. In this image, the group at the bottom shows columnar cells with nuclear crowding and stratification. The nuclei are hyperchromatic with round to oval shapes. These features are more typical of colonic adenocarcinoma, but a columnar variant of papillary carcinoma is in the differential diagnosis. (Diff Quik stain)

Figure 13.22 — Metastatic Colonic Adenocarcinoma, FNA. A columnar gland with hyperchromatic crowded nuclei is present. Immunostains supported a colonic origin (cytokeratin 20 and CDX-2 positive; cytokeratin 7, TTF-1, thyroglobulin negative). (Cell block section, H&E stain)

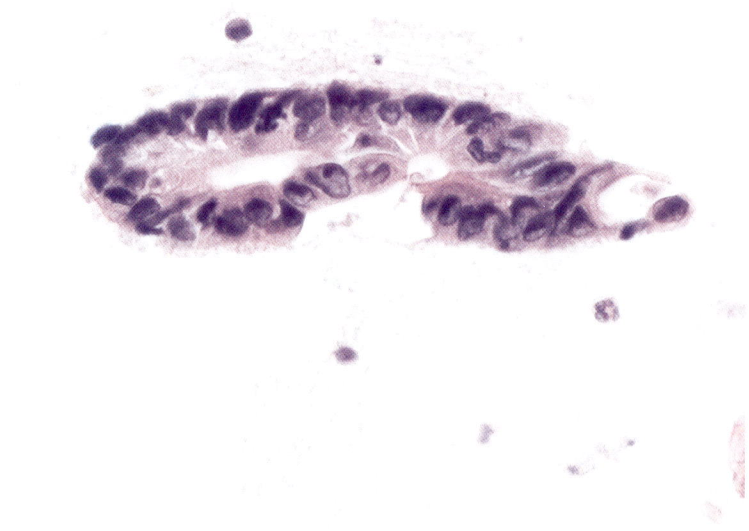

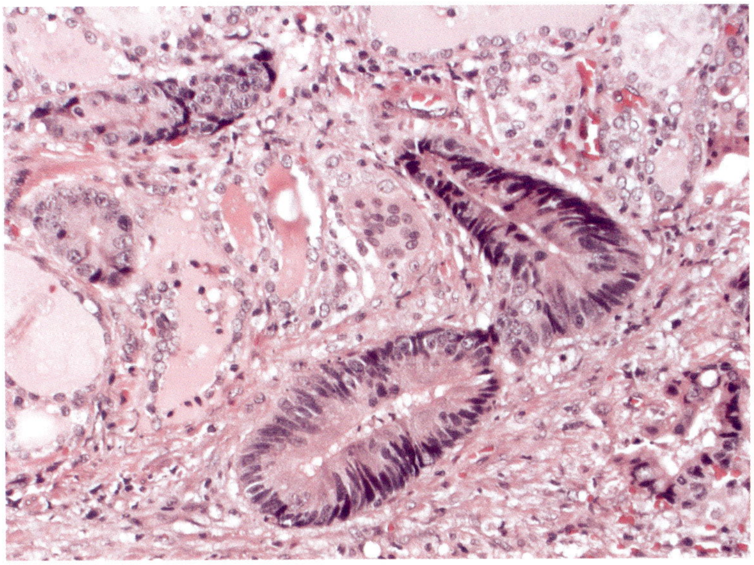

Figure 13.23 — Metastatic Colonic Adenocarcinoma, Histologic Section. The metastasis in the previous images was resected. The classic morphology of colonic adenocarcinoma with tall columnar glands with hyperchromatic nuclei can be seen interspersed with benign thyroid follicles. Both the cytology and histology of this tumor lacked the "dirty" necrosis characteristic of colonic adenocarcinoma. (H&E stain)

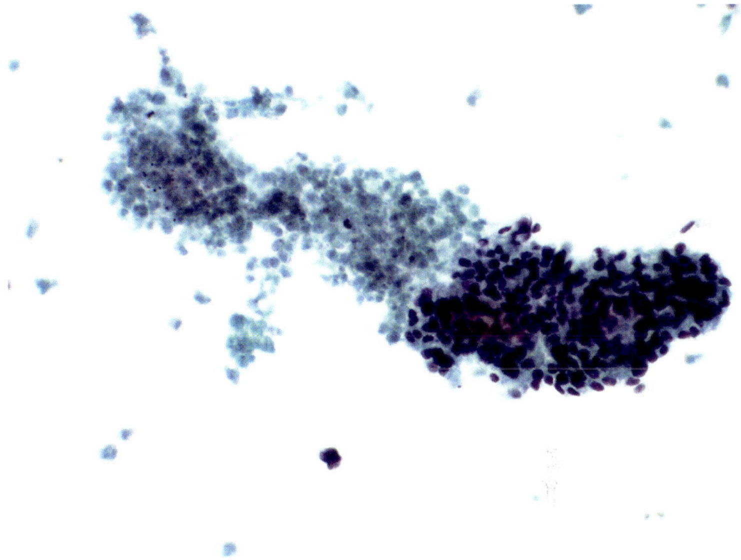

Figure 13.24 — Metastatic Esophageal Adenocarcinoma, FNA. A crowded three-dimensional group of fairly uniform cells with hyperchromatic nuclei is seen. Abundant necrosis is present adjacent to the viable cluster of malignant cells. In addition to metastasis, poorly differentiated thyroid carcinoma as well as undifferentiated (anaplastic) carcinoma would be diagnostic considerations. (Liquid based preparation, Papanicolaou stain)

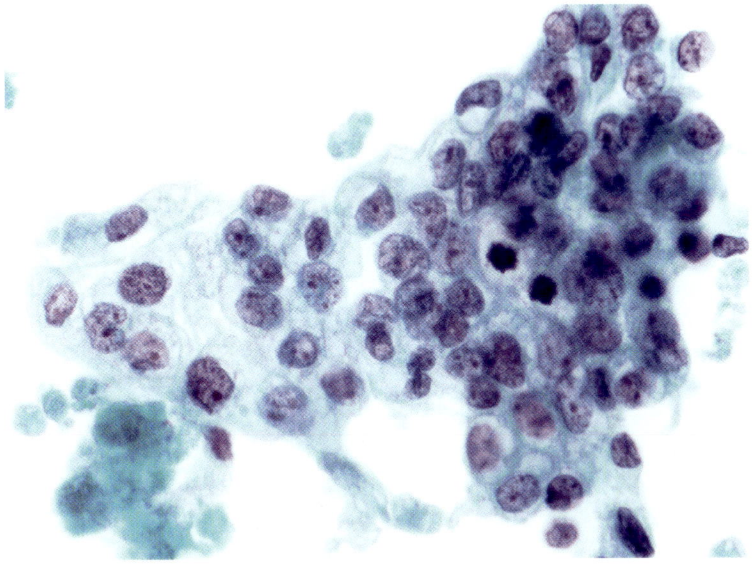

Figure 13.25 — Metastatic Esophageal Adenocarcinoma, FNA. The honeycombed configuration of this group with vacuolated cytoplasm and focally distinct cell membranes suggests the presence of glandular differentiation. The irregular spacing of the nuclei, marked anisonucleosis, chromatin abnormalities, and mitotic figures support the diagnosis of adenocarcinoma. Also note the necrotic cellular debris in the lower left corner. (Liquid based preparation, Papanicolaou stain)

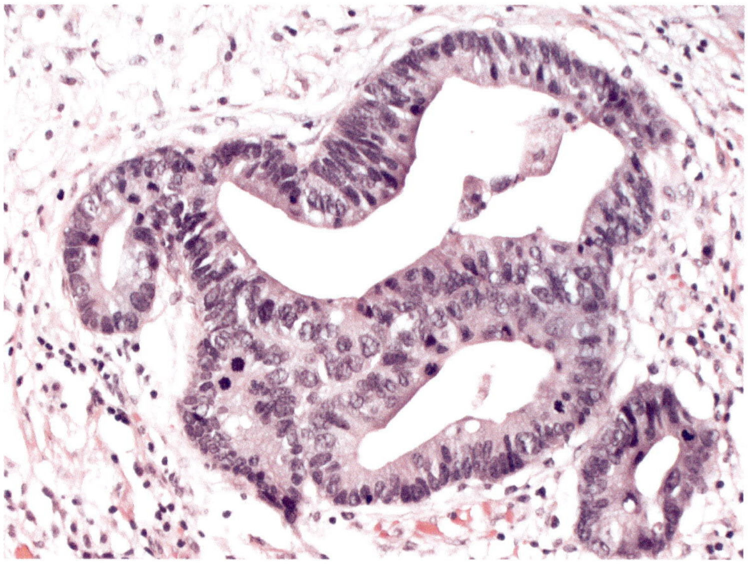

Figure 13.26 — Metastatic Esophageal Adenocarcinoma, Histologic Section. The esophageal primary shows columnar glands closely resembling the cells in the metastasis in the prior figure. (H&E stain)

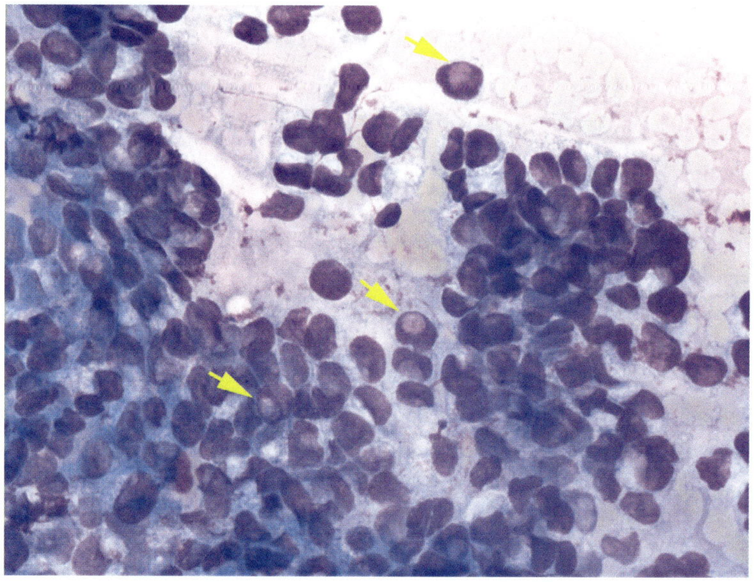

Figure 13.27 — Metastatic Gastric Adenocarcinoma, FNA. Loosely cohesive fragments of malignant cells appearing mostly as naked nuclei are shown. Cells are crowded, disorganized and have a three dimensional appearance. Notice glandular differentiation at 3 o'clock. Mucin vacuoles (arrows) overlap the nuclei and appear as "intranuclear inclusions" creating diagnostic confusion with a primary papillary carcinoma. The patient had a known gastric signet-ring cell adenocarcinoma. (Diff Quik stain)

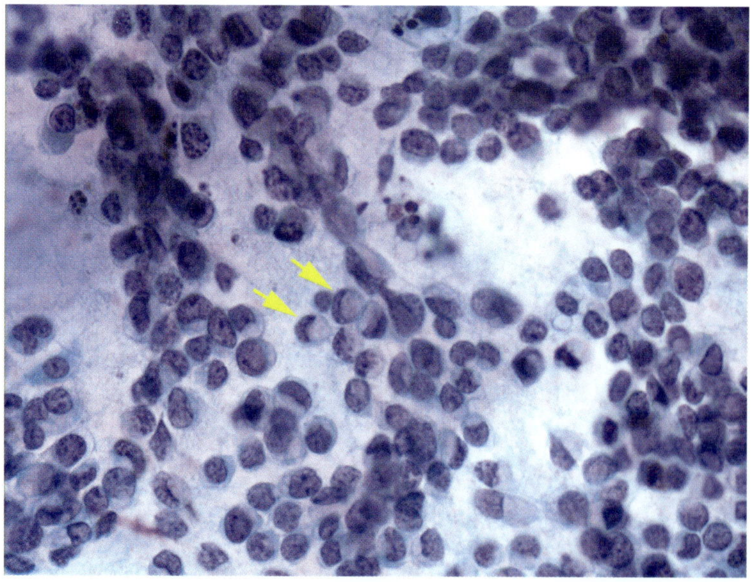

Figure 13.28 — Metastatic Gastric Adenocarcinoma, FNA. Similar features as the previous image are seen on Papanicolaou stain. Malignant cells are mostly singly dispersed and display classic signet-ring morphology (arrows). Free background mucin is noted as well. (Papanicolaou stain)

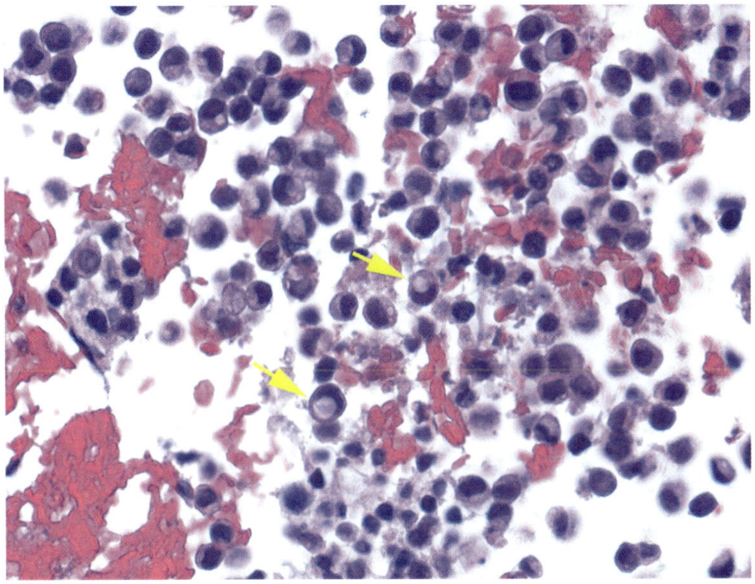

Figure 13.29 — Metastatic Gastric Adenocarcinoma, FNA. Cell block sections usually add limited information to most thyroid aspirates. However, in cases where the differential involves medullary thyroid carcinoma, lymphoma, or metastasis to the thyroid, cell block sections contain valuable material for confirmatory additional stains. A simple mucicarmine stain in this case would confirm the diagnosis by illustrating intracytoplasmic mucin vacuoles (arrows). (H&E stain, cell block section)

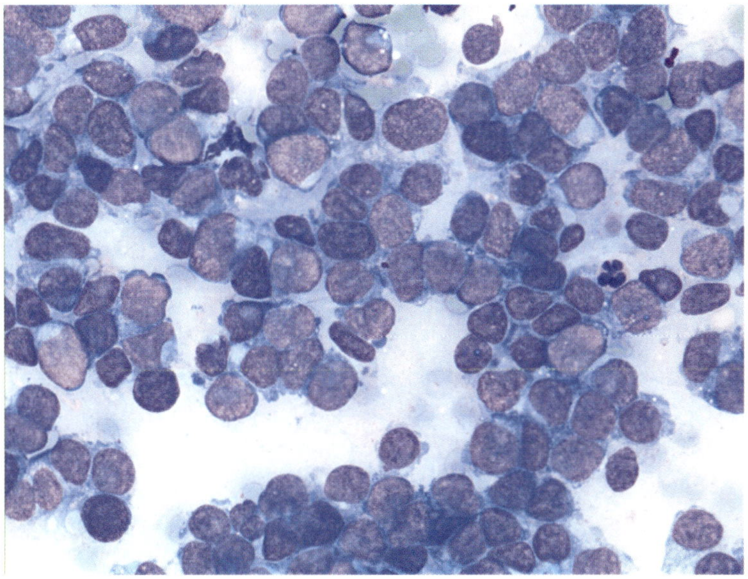

Figure 13.30 — Metastatic Merkel Cell Carcinoma, FNA. This patient did not disclose the previous resection of a skin/soft tissue tumor from his elbow performed a year before the thyroid nodule was aspirated. Based on the on-site evaluation the sample was sent for flow cytometry to rule out non-Hodgkin lymphoma. However, a negative flow and additional immune markers supported the diagnosis of a metastatic Merkel cell carcinoma, an extremely rare occurrence. Differential diagnosis would also include (along with malignant lymphoma), a primary medullary thyroid carcinoma and metastatic small cell carcinoma from lung and other primary sites. (Diff Quik stain)

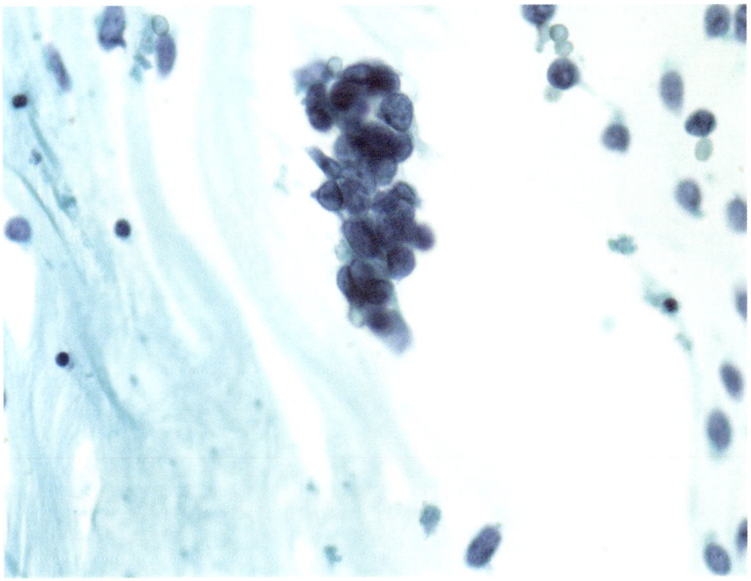

Figure 13.31 — Metastatic Merkel Cell Carcinoma, FNA. Classic features of a high-grade neuroendocrine carcinoma are seen, that is, small cells, high N/C ratios, nuclear hyperchromasia with fine dusty chromatin and nuclear molding. A cytologic distinction between small cell lung carcinoma, Merkel cell carcinoma and small cell carcinoma from other primary sites is not possible on morphology alone. A strong CK20 immunolabeling with the characteristic dot-shaped staining pattern would favor a metastatic Merkel cell carcinoma in this case. (Papanicolaou stain)

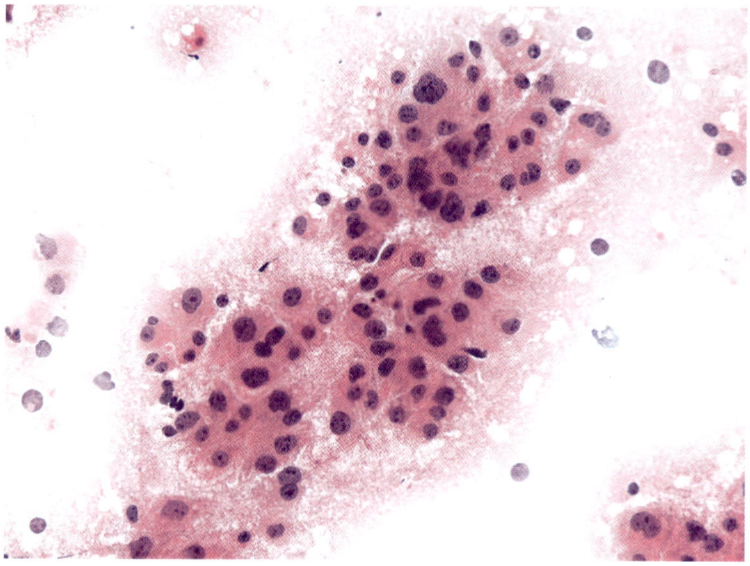

Figure 13.32 — Metastatic Hepatocellular Carcinoma, FNA. This unusual metastasis displays large polygonal cells with granular eosinophilic cytoplasm, large centrally placed nucleus with prominent nucleolus. Focal anisonucleosis is evident. A morphologic kinship to hepatocytes is clearly evident. However, without a known history of hepatocellular carcinoma, a Hürthle cell neoplasm would be on top of the list of differential diagnosis. (H&E stain) (Case courtesy of Dr. Pen Wang, Beijing Ditan Hospital, Beijing, China.)

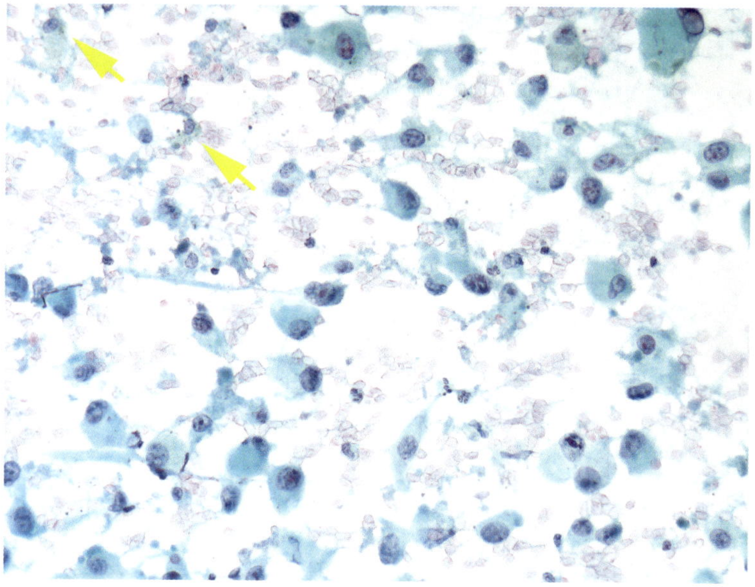

Figure 13.33 — Metastatic Malignant Melanoma, FNA. A dispersed population of epithelioid cells with eccentric nuclei, cytoplasmic tails, and macronucleoli is observed. There is focal evidence of pigment-laden cells (arrows). In older patients, a cytopathologic distinction from a primary anaplastic carcinoma can be difficult (especially when the later tumor shows a single cell "plasmacytoid" morphology). In such cases, immunostains are extremely helpful, as melanoma is positive for S-100 protein, HMB45, and melanA and anaplastic carcinoma typically shows (at least focally), cytokeratin, thyroglobulin, and PAX8 reactivity. (Papanicolaou stain)

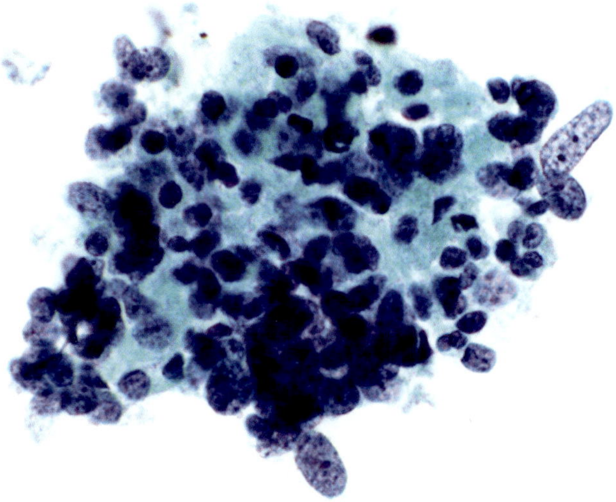

Figure 13.34 — Metastatic Ewing Sarcoma, FNA. A syncytial group of cells is present with round to elongate nuclei. Chromatin is uniformly granular with scattered indistinct nucleoli. The chromatin might suggest the possibility of a high-grade neuroendocrine carcinoma, but the cell configuration is not typical of a carcinoma. Undifferentiated (anaplastic) carcinoma is also in the differential diagnosis as are other sarcomas. The patient had a known history of Ewing sarcoma in the thigh as well as prior metastatic disease to the lung. (Liquid based preparation, Papanicolaou stain)

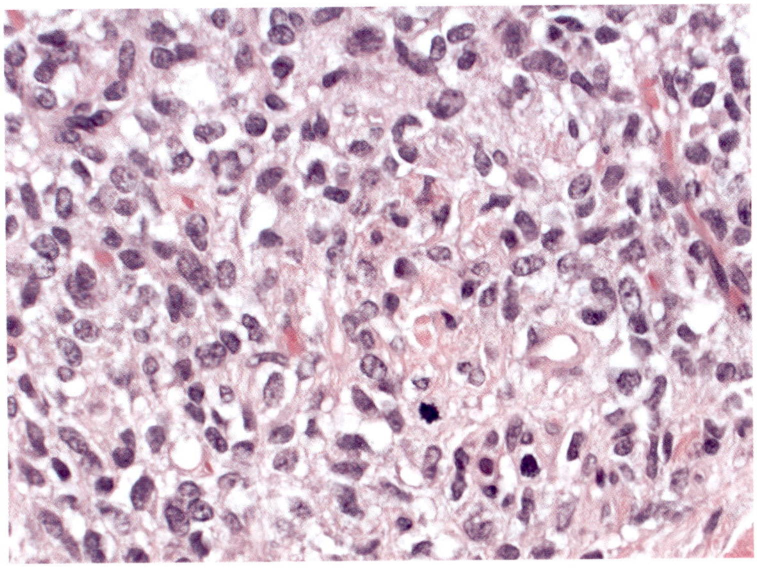

Figure 13.35 — Metastatic Ewing Sarcoma, Histologic Section. In the primary tumor, the histologic appearance is similar to the cytology in the prior figure. The cells exhibit indistinct cell borders with round to oval and elongate nuclei. (H&E stain)

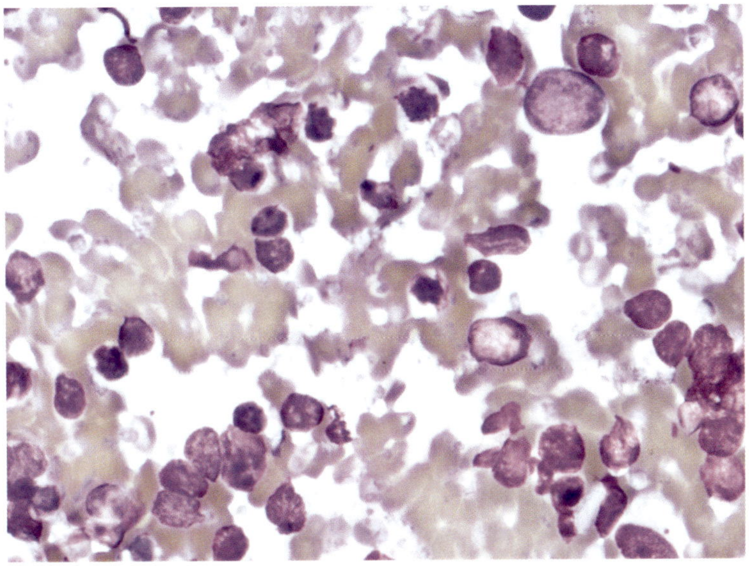

Figure 13.36 — Large Cell Lymphoma, FNA. A dispersed population of cells with scant cytoplasm is seen. Many of the cells are degenerating with few large preserved cells having clumped chromatin and a prominent nucleolus. Note the presence of cytoplasmic fragments ("lymphoglandular bodies") in the background supporting a lymphoid origin of the cells. (Diff Quik stain)

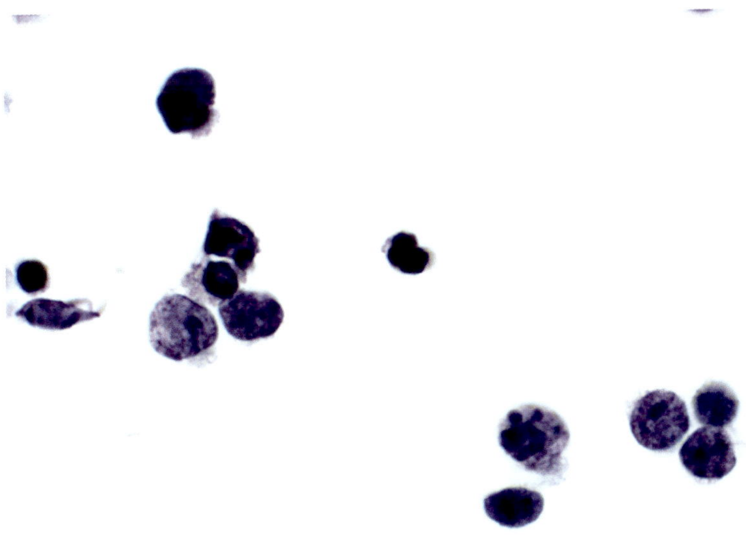

Figure 13.37 — Large Cell Lymphoma, FNA. The alcohol fixed counterpart to the prior image shows a similar population of large lymphoid cells with apoptotic cells present as well. Marker studies demonstrated that the malignant cells were CD20 positive B cells negative for CD10 and surface light chain immunoglobulins supporting the diagnosis. (Papanicolaou stain)

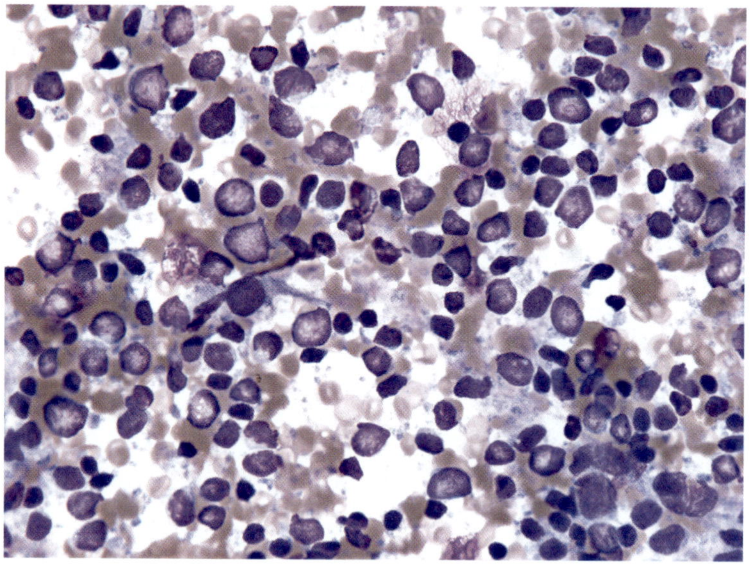

Figure 13.38 — MALT Lymphoma, FNA. Most primary lymphomas arising in the thyroid are non-Hodgkin B-cell type with over two-thirds arising in patients with previous history of Hashimoto thyroiditis. Both diffuse large B-cell lymphomas and extranodal marginal zone B-cell lymphomas of mucosa-associated lymphoid tissue (MALT) have been reported to arise in the thyroid. Based on cytomorphology and immunophenotyping by flow cytometry, this particular case was diagnosed as MALT lymphoma. An FNA distinction of thyroid MALT lymphoma from Hashimoto thyroiditis may be difficult on morphology alone. (Diff Quik stain)

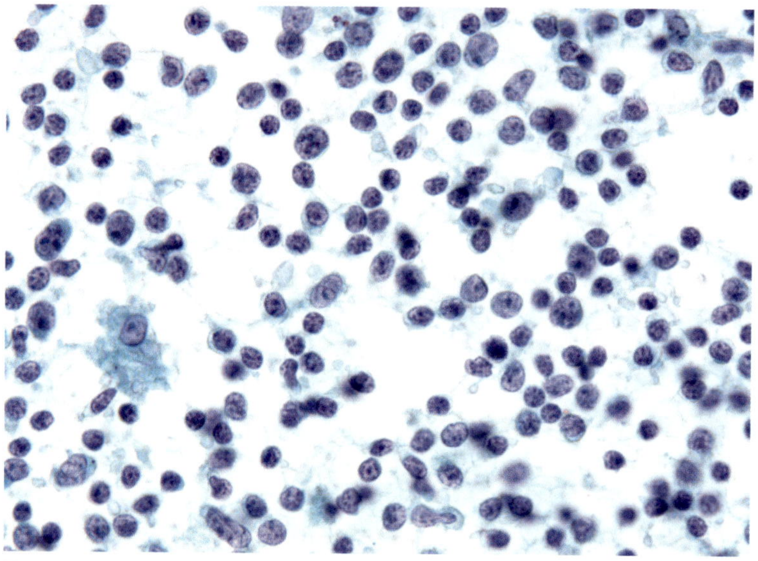

Figure 13.39 — MALT Lymphoma, FNA. The malignant cells in this case are twice the size of a small mature lymphocyte, display open chromatin and small nucleoli. A morphologic distinction with Hashimoto thyroiditis can be extremely difficult in a limited specimen and in the absence of flow cytometry analysis these cases are best diagnosed as atypia of undetermined significance (AUS). It's worthwhile to remember that small clonal B-cell populations have been reported in cases of Hashimoto thyroiditis on flow cytometry. Therefore, one needs to be careful when interpreting limited thyroid samples as malignant lymphoma in patients with an established diagnosis of Hashimoto thyroiditis. (Papanicolaou stain)

Index